Psychiatry of Intellectual Disability Across Cultures

Psychiatry of Intellectual Disability Across Cultures

Edited by

Regi T. Alexander,
Samuel J. Tromans, ˙
Satheesh Kumar Gangadharan,
Chaya Kapugama,
and Sabyasachi Bhaumik

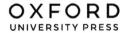

OXFORD
UNIVERSITY PRESS

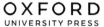

OXFORD
UNIVERSITY PRESS

Great Clarendon Street, Oxford, OX2 6DP,
United Kingdom

Oxford University Press is a department of the University of Oxford.
It furthers the University's objective of excellence in research, scholarship,
and education by publishing worldwide. Oxford is a registered trade mark of
Oxford University Press in the UK and in certain other countries

© Oxford University Press 2024

Published in the United States of America by Oxford University Press
198 Madison Avenue, New York, NY 10016, United States of America

British Library Cataloguing in Publication Data
Data available

Library of Congress Control Number: 2023940364

ISBN 978–0–19–885760–0

DOI: 10.1093/med/9780198857600.001.0001

Printed and bound by
CPI Group (UK) Ltd, Croydon, CR0 4YY

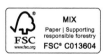

This book is dedicated to the fond memory of the late Professor Sabyasachi Bhaumik, an extraordinary psychiatrist, trainer, and leader who did much of the pioneering work focusing on the cultural aspects of health and social care for people with intellectual and other developmental disabilities.

Foreword

The global prevalence of intellectual disability (ID) is estimated to be around 1%—this equates to about 80 million people. It is highly unlikely that any clinician would not have come across ID in their clinical practice, irrespective of the field they practise in. Impacting cognitive skills and adaptive functioning, it is unsurprising that ID both in terms of their clinical presentation and adaptation are significantly influenced by cultural factors. It is this interaction of diversities—the diversity that resides within the umbrella term of ID multiplied by the cultural diversities in recognizing, accepting, and treating intellectual disability across communities and nations—that provides the main raison d-être for this book.

A compendium of literature on ID across cultures is needed for at least three reasons.

Firstly, *patient-related factors*. Disorders with the same taxonomy can present very differently in a different cultural setting. When I migrated from Mumbai, India, to Birmingham, UK, the subtle but significant differences in clinical features even in patients of Indian origin became readily apparent to me. Ensuring the delivery of safe and effective care across cultures requires an academic evidence-based assessment of the literature which this comprehensive resource provides.

Secondly, *clinician factors*. Clinicians across the world have variable training and local treatment protocols and pathways vary significantly depending on local cultures and customs. Add in the impact of a globally mobile workforce and then need for a primer on clinical practice across cultures becomes self-manifest.

Finally, and quite crucially, *systemic factors*. The doctor–patient interaction does not take place in a vacuum. Clinical system design, workplace cultures, funding and governance of systems of care, and geopolitical factors—all can play a role in influencing the clinical outcomes of an individual patient. Navigating this systems complexity requires a critical shift from seeing ID in isolation to viewing it as a condition that can be shaped and moulded by a range of systemic factors, the understanding of which in turn provides clinicians with an opportunity to shape the outcomes of the disability.

As Dean of the Royal College of Psychiatrists, I have tried to bring about a more explicit and direct link between our educational and training resources and patient outcomes. The twin lenses of *personalized or person-centred care* and *public mental health* (including wider sociocultural determinants of health) offer an opportunity to clinicians to make a difference to the care outcomes of not only their individual patients but also to the outcomes of the wider communities they care for.

A handbook of this nature needs delicate but elegant equipoise, ensuring academic rigour is matched by clinical usability. The editors and authors deserve praise for striking this balance consistently and accurately.

This essential compendium will certainly be of interest to every student and practitioner of ID psychiatry but will also be relevant to those who want to develop a culturally sensitive and culturally empowered practice for their patients with ID.

Professor Subodh Dave, FRCPsych, MMed (Clinical Education)
Dean of the Royal College of Psychiatrists, UK

Preface

Intellectual disability (ID) is a lifelong condition affecting both intellectual and adaptive functioning, with onset during the developmental period (i.e. from birth to 18 years of age). Individuals with ID experience significant mental and physical health problems relative to their peers, and often require a greater degree of professional and carer support. Additionally, their lives can be greatly influenced both positively and negatively by the cultures they exist within, including societal attitudes, belief systems, and norms.

This book, which is part of the Cultural Psychiatry series published by Oxford University Press, explores mental and physical health issues, support structures, and societal attitudes towards people with ID. It emphasizes the importance of cultural awareness and competency as essential requirements for good clinical practice, service provision, and managing population health.

The book is divided into four sections.

The first introduces the scientific and sociocultural concept of ID and focuses on the physical and mental health needs of this population. Exploring the epidemiological similarities and differences in different parts of the world, the chapters in this section explore how health needs of people with ID vary across different cultural groups, including the presentation of culturally bound syndromes.

The second section focuses on certain wider issues pertaining to people with ID, including anthropology, perceptions across cultures, human rights, abuse, sexuality, marriage and parenthood, spirituality, and social inclusion.

The third section explores how support for people with ID varies across cultures. Its chapters focus on models of healthcare provision, cultural variations in models of therapy, support from family networks, and spirituality and religious beliefs. Service delivery models across different cultures are explored along with informal support with an emphasis on the differences in practice across cultures and the underlying reasons for such variation.

The final section describes service models of psychiatric care provision in different geographical regions. With a fair representation from the East and West, it provides a brief oversight of services in countries across the world, for this the most vulnerable of populations.

As editors, we are very grateful to all our chapter authors. They are professionals who are at the forefront of practice in their respective areas. For sharing their expertise and finding the time to contribute, we are indebted to them. We hope that this book will be valuable in helping you explore models and practices from different cultures which you can share or adapt.

Professor Regi T. Alexander
Associate Professor Samuel J. Tromans
Professor Satheesh Kumar Gangadharan
Dr Chaya Kapugama

Contents

Abbreviations

AAIDD	American Association on Intellectual and Developmental Disabilities
AAMR	American Association on Mental Retardation
ADHD	attention deficit hyperactive disorder
ASD	autism spectrum disorder
BA	behaviour analyst
CJS	criminal justice system
CRPD	Convention on the Rights of Persons with Disabilities
DC-LD	Diagnostic Criteria for Psychiatric Disorders for Use with Adults with Learning Disabilities
DID	disorders of intellectual development
DSM	*Diagnostic and Statistical Manual of Mental Disorders*
ECHO	Extension for Community Healthcare Outcomes
FAS	fetal alcohol syndrome
FASD	fetal alcohol spectrum disorder
GLADS	Glasgow Level of Ability and Development Scale
HASI	Hayes Ability Screening Index
H-CARDD	Health Care Access Research and Developmental Disabilities
ICD	International Classification of Diseases
ICF	International Classification of Functioning
ID	intellectual disability
IDD	intellectual and developmental disabilities
IQ	intellectual quotient
ISRP	Integrated Service Response Programme (Australia)
LAMI	low- and middle-income
LeDeR	Learning Disabilities Mortality Review
LGBT	lesbian, gay, bisexual, and transgender
LMIC	low- and middle-income countries
MCCSS	Ministry of Children, Community and Social Services (Canada)
MMW	Mashkikiiwininiwag Mazinaatesijigan Wichiiwewin (Canada)
MRO	Means, Reasons, and Opportunities
NCD	non-communicable disease
NDD	neurodevelopmental disorder
NDIA	National Disability Insurance Agency (Australia)
NDIS	National Disability Insurance Scheme (Australia)
NGO	non-governmental organization
NHS	National Health Service (UK)
NIEPID	National Institute for the Empowerment of Persons with Intellectual Disabilities
OT	occupational therapist
RPWD	Rights of Persons with Disabilities
SD	standard deviation
SLT	speech and language therapist
SWID	Society for the Welfare of the Intellectually Disabled (Bangladesh)
SWO	State Welfare Organization (Iran)
UN	United Nations
VDDS	Victorian Dual Disability Services (Australia)
WHO	World Health Organization

Contributors

Javad Alaghband-Rad
Professor of Psychiatry & Child and
Adolescent Psychiatrist, Psychiatry
Department, Tehran University of
Medical Sciences, Iran

Regi T. Alexander
Consultant Psychiatrist,
Hertfordshire Partnership
NHS Foundation Trust, Little
Plumstead Hospital, Norwich, UK;
Visiting Professor, University of
Hertfordshire, Hatfield, UK

Mohammed Al-Uzri
Consultant Psychiatrist and
Honorary Professor, Health Sciences
Department, University of Leicester,
Leicester, UK

Ayomipo J. Amiola
Specialty Doctor, Little Plumstead
Hospital, Hertfordshire Partnership
University NHS, Norwich, UK

Rajnish Attavar
Hertfordshire Partnership NHS
Foundation Trust, Hatfield, UK

Aisha M. Bakhiet
Head of Department, Department
of Psychiatry, Faculty of Medicine,
University of Khartoum, Sudan

Mary Barrett
Consultant Psychiatrist in Intellectual
Disability, Agnes Unit, Leicestershire
Partnership NHS Trust, Leicester, UK

Marco O. Bertelli
Scientific Director, CREA (Research
and Clinical Centre), Fondazione San
Sebastiano, Misericordia di Firenze,
Florence, Italy

Asit Biswas
Consultant Psychiatrist,
Leicestershire Partnership NHS
Trust, Leicester; Honorary Professor,
University of Leicester, Leicester, UK

Harm Boer
Consultant Forensic Psychiatrist,
Coventry and Warwickshire
Partnership NHS Trust;
Honorary Professor,
University of Warwick, UK

Rosie Bunn
Rector, Church of England, Belton &
Burgh Castle, Norfolk, UK

Louis Busch
Community Support Specialist,
Behaviour Analyst, Centre for
Addiction & Mental Health,
Toronto, Canada

João Mauricio Castaldelli-Maia
Department of Neuroscience,
Fundação do ABC, Santo André;
Department of Psychiatry, University
of São Paulo, São Paulo, Brazil

Santosh K. Chaturvedi
Consultant Psychiatrist, Former
Dean and Senior Professor of
Psychiatry, National Institute of
Mental Health and Neurosciences
(NIMHANS), Bangalore, India

Ruth Chau
Memorial University of
Newfoundland, St. John's,
Newfoundland, Canada

Umesh Chauhan
Professor of Primary Care, School
of Medicine University of Central
Lancashire, Preston, UK

Verity Chester
Research Associate, Hertfordshire
Partnership University NHS Trust,
Hatfield, UK

Elen Cook
Head of International, Devolved
Nations and Divisions, Royal College
of Psychiatrists, London, UK

Ken Courtenay
Barnet, Enfield and Haringey Mental
Health NHS Trust, London, UK

Jessica Cremasco
Occupational Therapist, Surrey Place,
Toronto, Canada

Manji Daffi
Specialty Doctor, Little Plumstead
Hospital, Hertfordshire Partnership
University NHS, Norwich, UK

Romanie Dekker-Couchman
The Priory Group, Mildmay Oaks
Hospital, Winchfield, Hook, UK

Katerina Denediou Derrer
Higher Trainee in General Adult
Psychiatry, Hertfordshire Partnership
Foundation Trust, Hatfield, UK

Alison Drewett
Senior Lecturer in Speech and
Language Therapy, De Montfort
University, Leicester, UK

Soman Elangovan
Belmont Private Hospital, Carina,
Queensland; University of Southern
Queensland (USQ), Toowoomba,
Queensland, Australia

Mohamed O. El Tahir
Senior Consultant Psychiatrist,
Hamad Medical Corporation,
Doha, Qatar

Mo Eyeoyibo
Clinical Director and Consultant in
Psychiatry of Intellectual Disability,
Kent and Medway NHS and Social
Partnership Trust, Dartford, UK

Satheesh Kumar Gangadharan
Consultant Psychiatrist,
Leicestershire Partnership
NHS Trust, Leicester, UK;
Honorary Professor, University
of Leicester; Visiting Professor of
Neurodevelopmental Psychiatry,
Loughborough University, UK

Shweta Gangavati
Consultant Psychiatrist,
Leicestershire Partnership NHS
Trust, Leicester, UK

Rohit Gumber
Consultant Psychiatrist and Associate
Medical Director, Leicestershire
Partnership NHS Trust, Leicester, UK

Angela Hassiotis
UCL Division of Psychiatry,
London, UK

Chandanie G. Hewage
Department of Psychiatry, Faculty
of Medicine, University of Ruhuna
Galle, Sri Lanka

Avinash Hiremath
Consultant Psychiatrist and Medical
Director, Leicestershire Partnership
NHS Trust, Leicester, UK

Sheila Hollins, Baroness Hollins
Emeritus Professor of Psychiatry of
Intellectual Disability at St George's,
University of London, London,
UK; Member of the House of
Lords of UK.

Prabhleen Jaggi
Speciality Trainee in Psychiatry of
Intellectual Disability, Leicestershire
Partnership NHS Trust, Leicester,
UK; previously Fellow, US Fogarty
Training in Non-Communicable
Diseases & Diseases Across Lifespan

Amala Jesu
Consultant Psychiatrist and Clinical
Director, Leicestershire Partnership
NHS Trust, Leicester, UK

Muhammad Irfan Jiwa
Resident, Department of Family
Medicine, McMaster University,
Hamilton, Ontario, Canada

Keir Jones
Conbsultant Psychiatrist, Midlands
Partnership NHS Trust, UK

Chaya Kapugama
Consultant Psychiatrist, Sussex
Partnership NHS Foundation
Trust, UK

Nusra Khodabux
Specialist Registrar in Psychiatry of
Intellectual Disability, Agnes Unit,
Leicestershire Partnership NHS
Trust, Leicester, UK

Reza Kiani
Consultant Neuropsychiatrist,
Leicestershire Partnership NHS
Trust, Leicester; Honorary Senior
Lecturer, University of Leicester,
Leicester, UK

John Vijay Sagar Kommu
Professor and Head, Department of
Child and Adolescent Psychiatry,
National Institute of Mental Health
and Neurosciences (NIMHANS),
Bangalore, India

K.A.L.A. Kuruppuarachchi
Senior Professor of Psychiatry and
Cadre, Chair/Psychiatry, University
of Kelaniya, Faculty of Medicine,
Ragama, Sri Lanka

Thomas John Kuttichirayil
Consultant Psychiatrist, Ernakulam,
Kerala, India

Peter E. Langdon
Professor and Consultant Clinical
and Forensic Psychologist, Centre
for Educational Development,
Appraisal, and Research (CEDAR),
University of Warwick, Warwick;
Brooklands Hospital, Coventry and
Warwickshire Partnership NHS
Trust, Birmingham; Herefordshire
and Worcestershire Health and Care
NHS Trust, Worcester, UK

Yona Lunsky
Azrieli Adult Neurodevelopmental
Centre, Centre for Addiction and
Mental Health, Toronto and Temerty
Faculty of Medicine, University of
Toronto, Ontario, Canada

Chikkanna Manju
Consultant Psychiatrist, Sirona Care
& Health, South Gloucestershire, UK

Jane McCarthy
Honorary Associate Professor in
Psychological Medicine, University
of Auckland, New Zealand; Visiting
Senior Lecturer, Department of
Forensic & Neurodevelopmental
Sciences, King's College London,
London, UK

Patrick McKearney
Assistant Professor, University
of Amsterdam, Amsterdam, The
Netherlands

Michael McPartland
Academic Clinical Fellow, University
Hospitals of Leicester, Leicester, UK

Jayan Mendis
Senior Lecturer in Psychiatry;
Department of Psychiatry; Faculty
of Medicine, Kotalawala Defence
University, Ratmalana, Sri Lanka, &
Founder Director, National Institute
of Mental Health, Angoda, Sri Lanka
(2001–2015)

Dasari Michael
Consultant Psychiatrist, Humber
Teaching NHS Foundation Trust,
East Riding of Yorkshire, UK

Mahtab Motamed
Assistant Professor of Psychiatry
& General Adult Psychiatrist,
Psychiatry Department, Tehran
University of Medical Sciences, Iran

Kamalika Mukherji
Consultant Psychiatrist & Clinical
Director, Hertfordshire Partnership
University NHS Foundation Trust,
Hatfield, Herts UK

Kerim Munir
Associate Professor of Psychiatry and
Pediatrics, Harvard Medical School,
USA; Attending Clinical Psychiatrist,
Division of Developmental Medicine,
Boston Children's Hospital, USA

Arjun Nayar
Foundation year doctor, Royal
Devon and Exetor NHS Foundation
Trust, UK

Pauline Ndigirwa
Speech and Language Therapist,
Leicestershire Partnership NHS
Trust, UK

Marcelo O'Higgins
Department of Psychiatry, School of Medical Sciences, National University of Asunción, San Lorenzo, Paraguay

Mohammad Farhad Peerally
Associate Professor in Health Sciences, University of Leicester, Leicester, UK

Dhara N. Perera
Peninsula Mental Health Services, Mornington Adult Community Mental Health Programme, Victoria; Vita Healthcare, Mount Eliza, Victoria, Australia

Varghese Punnoose
Professor and Head of the Department of Psychiatry, Kottayam Medical College, Kerala, India

Raghu Raghavan
Professor of Mental Health, Director, Lifelong Health and Wellbeing Research; Director, Mary Seacole Research Centre; Co-Director, Leicester Centre for Mental Health Research (LCMHR), Faculty of Health and Life Sciences, De Montfort University, Leicester, UK

Ashok Roy
Consultant Psychiatrist and Associate Medical Director, Coventry and Warwickshire Partnership NHS Trust, Coventry; National Learning Disability & Autism Programme Clinical Lead, Health Education England; Co-Chair, Learning Disability Professional Senate; Chair, Birmingham Autism and ADHD Partnership Board, Birmingham, UK

Meera Roy
Consultant Psychiatrist, retired

Rachel Royston
Research Programme Manager, UCL Division of Psychiatry, London, UK

Sreeja Sahadevan
Specialty Registrar, Hertfordshire Partnership University NHS Foundation Trust, Little Plumstead Hospital, Norwich, UK

Rohit Shankar
Professor in Neuropsychiatry, Chy Govenck, Threemilestone Industrial Estate, Truro, UK

Sowmya Srikumar
MPhil in Psychiatric Social Work (NIMHANS), Dip. In Special Education Freelance consultant, Special Educator and Counsellor, Bengaluru
Director, Academic Programme, LeapYears Centre for special needs by Adiksha Foundation, Bengaluru Consultant (Faculty Counsellor), Christ University, Bengaluru

Inyang Takon
Consultant Community Paediatrician, East & North Hertfordshire NHS Trust, UK

Phil Temple
Locum Consultant Psychiatrist & Specialty Doctor, Hertfordshire Partnership University NHS Foundation Trust, Little Plumstead Hospital, Norwich, UK

Anupam Thakur
Azrieli Adult Neurodevelopmental
Centre, Centre for Addiction and
Mental Health, Toronto and Temerty
Faculty of Medicine, University of
Toronto, Ontario, Canada

Priyanka Tharian
Consultant General Adult
Psychiatrist, East London Foundation
Trust, London, UK

Lucretia Thomas
Medical Student, Medical School,
University of Birmingham,
Birmingham, UK

Julio Torales
Department of Medical Psychology
and Department of Psychiatry,
School of Medical Sciences, National
University of Asunción, San Lorenzo,
Paraguay

Samuel J. Tromans
Associate Professor of Psychiatry and
Honorary Consultant in Psychiatry
of Intellectual Disability, University
of Leicester, Leicester, UK

Ratnaraj Vaidya
Medical Student, Faculty of Medical
Sciences, Newcastle University,
Newcastle, UK

Natalie Yiu
Occupational Therapist, The Centre
for Addiction and Mental Health
(CAMH), Canada

Asif Zia
Consultant Psychiatrist & Executive
Medical Director, Hertfordshire
Partnership University NHS
Foundation Trust, Hatfield, Herts UK

Tyler Zoanni
Research Fellow, Max Planck
Institute of Social Anthropology,
Halle, Germany

Part 1

Introduction and epidemiology

Chapter 1

Concepts and prevalence of intellectual disability across cultures

Marco O. Bertelli, Elen Cook,
and Dasari Michael

Introduction

Culture and context are intertwined key concepts for understanding intellectual disability/disorders of intellectual development (ID/DID) and other neurodevelopmental disorders (NDDs), as well as providing and planning effective mental healthcare. There are additional implications for evaluating individual functioning impairments, support needs, and quality of life. In terms of identification, diagnosis, measurement of prevalence, and provision of support services, culture has been highlighted as a key factor. However, different definitions of culture have been employed, and it has often been discussed but not taken into consideration in analysis, evaluation, or planning. Definitions of disability, culture, and context are useful frameworks for thinking about and understanding ID/DID and overall human functioning. They can also be used to assess and improve support systems, other services, and care for people with ID/DID and/or other NDDs.

ID/DID concept and nomenclature across time and cultures

Various definitions of ID/DID have been offered throughout history in line with various conceptualizations, but with the emergence of worldwide classificatory systems for mental disorders and illnesses, a scientific dispute on description and nomenclature began. Until the mid-twentieth century, words like stupid, imbecile, cretin, moron, defective, and feebleminded or phrases like mental sub-normality and mental deficiency were used in these systems of classification and categorization (1–6). The two primary groups of idiots and imbeciles were defined in the first textbook on ID/DID, published in 1904 under the title *Mental Defectives*, with the former being ascribed a considerably more severe level of impairment and imbeciles being considered to be capable of learning some fundamental abilities with adequate training (4).

In the first edition of the *Diagnostic and Statistical Manual of Mental Disorders* of the American Psychiatric Association (DSM-I) (7), ID/DID was classified as 'chronic brain syndrome with mental deficiency' and 'mental deficiency', while the term 'mental retardation' was introduced by the American Association on Mental Deficiency in 1961 to replace the previous terms, which had become gravely stigmatized. This corresponded with the development of the first widely accepted definition and diagnostic criteria, which referred to 'sub-average general intellectual functioning which originates in the developmental period and is associated with impairment in adaptive behaviour' (8). In the mid-1970s, the terms 'sub-average' and 'impairment in adaptive functioning' were changed to 'significantly sub-average' and 'concurrent with deficits in adaptive behaviour', respectively, to correspond with the requirement to expand the intellectual quotient (IQ) standard deviation and to include adaptive behaviour among diagnostic criteria.

A paradigm change that characterized the DSM definitions until the fourth edition occurred in 1992, when the American Association on Mental Retardation (AAMR), formerly the American Association on Mental Deficiency, shifted the focus of the definition from a disorder (neither mental nor medical) to a disability: 'mental retardation refers to a particular state [not a trait] of functioning that begins in childhood in which limitations in intelligence coexist with related limitations in adaptive skills' (9). The individual condition is manifested through an interaction between the affected person and the environment.

The term 'intellectual disability' was proposed as a replacement for 'mental retardation' in the second part of the twentieth century, and it quickly became the most frequent term. In 2002, the AAMR aligned its definition with the World Health Organization's (WHO's) International Classification of Functioning (ICF) (10), emphasizing that mental retardation entails significant limitations in intellectual functioning and adaptive behaviour, with the two areas being treated equally and the latter being divided into conceptual, social, and practical domains. The AAMR, which changed its name to the American Association on Intellectual and Developmental Disabilities (AAIDD) in 2007, emphasized the primacy of the concept of disability in the 2010 edition of its manual, as well as the main causative role of the social–ecological context in the difficulty of the person with developmental impairment to achieve good adaptation to the environment (11,12).

The grading of ID/DID severity in this paradigm is indicated by 'patterns and intensity of supports needed', which differs significantly from the DSM severity codes.

To align with the first proposal of the WHO working group for the 11th revision of the (ICD-11), the American Psychiatric Association replaced 'mental retardation' with 'intellectual disability' and the parenthetical name 'intellectual developmental disorder' in the DSM-5 (13). This was done to emphasize that diagnosed deficits in cognitive and adaptive skills begin during the developmental period. The term 'disorders of intellectual development (DID)' has been approved by the ICD-11 (14).

In the previous decade, difficulties in defining and placing ID/DID have sparked a more intense scientific debate than ever before, which includes two main approaches: the first, promoted by the AAIDD and aligned with the ICF (11), focuses on disability as characterized by significant impairment of intellectual functioning and adaptive behaviour; the second, supported mainly by the Section of Psychiatry of Intellectual Disability of the World Psychiatric Association (WPA-SPID), is instead a polynomial-polysemic, multidimensional approach and interprets ID/DID as a condition to be defined differently in accordance with the specific context. With specific reference to the classificatory systems, it should be defined as a meta-syndromic group of 'intellectual development disorders' in the ICD, and as a condition of complex 'intellectual disability' in the ICF.

Extreme viewpoints in this discussion might have disastrous consequences. If ID/DID is defined just as a 'disability', it will be excluded from the ICD, resulting in a significant loss in eligibility for specific health services, especially mental health services, as well as educational and social services (15). In fact, it is the ICD and not the ICF that is used by the 194 WHO member countries to define the responsibilities of governments to provide healthcare and other services to their citizens. In contrast, treating ID/DID exclusively as a health issue would have negative repercussions for social and educational services, as well as public perception, policy development, and future legislation.

In most countries, for people with ID/DID, diagnostic categorization substantially influences service eligibility and treatment selection, and an accurate, valid, and practical diagnostic system appears to ensure improved healthcare. In low- and middle-income nations, however, mental health specialists of any sort may be scarce, and people with ID/DID may not even have access to basic health services. As a result, the ICD-11 and future worldwide mental health policies prioritize finding and delivering tools that enable broad, efficient, and accurate diagnosis and care for people with ID/DID. Furthermore, it is critical to emphasize the prevalence of ID/DID and its functional repercussions, because many people go years without being identified, particularly in low- and middle-income countries. Therefore, when developing healthcare programmes, one needs to consider the resources available for diagnosis rather than those just for therapy. However, it is worth noting that significant modifications to international categorization systems may take years to be implemented in clinical practice in many countries; hence, it is desirable to make evaluation as user-friendly as feasible to encourage its usage.

A public health approach to mental health for ID/DID is often inadequate in many middle- and lower-income countries, particularly in terms of preventive intervention. The number of psychiatrists in relation to the population is often insufficient, and an understanding of the mental health needs of individuals with ID/DID is not routinely included in the training of psychiatrists and other mental health professionals. These and other sociocultural and contextual variables contribute to challenges and delays in identifying people with ID/DID and implementing appropriate management. Diagnostic tests of ID/DID are not always available due to these being expensive. Diagnostic and treatment recommendations are frequently ineffective and incomplete. Most individuals with ID/DID in low- and middle-income countries are cared for by family members. Poverty and long hours of caregiving appear to have the greatest influence on carers' vulnerability to unsatisfactory well-being. Personal resources, such as religion or spirituality, and a positive perspective, become increasingly crucial in the absence of programmes and services to help carers and the people they care for.

Some caregiver support techniques, such as family-centred approaches or home-based community support, appear to be appreciated across cultures and contexts. In Africa, the lack of protective legislation and social policies exposes people with ID/DID to human rights violations and results in denial of basic services such as medical treatment and education. A significant percentage of the population in African nations attributes the aetiology or genesis of ID/DID and other NDDs to spiritual factors, which has an impact on perceived or felt stigma and help-seeking behaviour. Other variables, such as a lack of healthcare facilities and skilled staff for treatments, economic barriers, and stigma, are to blame for African and Asian children with ID/DID presenting late and receiving a delayed diagnosis. In Latin American countries, economic hardship, sociocultural issues, and political difficulties are the three main categories of causative reasons of social exclusion of people with ID/DID.

In Mexico, public policies, as well as an institutional model emphasizing self-sufficiency, social inclusion, and employment, are absent. In Argentina most health service providers are still understaffed and undertrained, despite the fact that the right of individuals with ID/DID to particular healthcare has been enshrined in domestic law for over 50 years. In Chile, although the existence of a national strategy for community inclusion of individuals with disabilities, the education sector is the only area where significant levels of integration have been achieved. In Asia, the prevalence of ID/DID appears to be comparable to that in other countries. As in other cultural, social, and economic contexts, discrimination and stigma can cause social exclusion of people with ID/DID as well their families and especially their caregivers. Cultural concerns that contribute to stigma and prejudice have been proven in Asian nations such as Vietnam where study has been conducted. One such issue is the perception that community harmony is upset when members with ID/DID are unemployed and unmarried (and with no evident prospects or opportunities for becoming employed or having social relationships). This is regarded as a danger to the individual's and family's standing. These cultural beliefs contribute to real stigmatization and discrimination, which can result in social isolation for both carers and their ID/DID family members (16).

People with ID/DID have not traditionally been institutionalized in many Asian nations; instead, they have lived with their family, albeit this does not always imply social inclusion. Discrimination and stigma in Asia can lead to social isolation for people with disabilities, as well as their family and carers (17). Despite the fact that many Asian nations do not have legislation that expressly attempt to segregate and institutionalize people with ID/DID, the relative lack of a culture of respect for human rights, inclusiveness, and non-discrimination in some, can lead to social exclusion.

Disability-rights activism, academic research interest, and public policies in Taiwan are greater than in other Asian nations, as is life expectancy for people with ID/DID; however, healthcare inequities persist, particularly in rural regions.

The context in India is influenced by the diversity of cultures, languages, customs, and beliefs. The recognition and prevalence of ID/DID is vastly influenced by these factors with estimates ranging from 0.07 to 40 per 1000 people. Over the past several decades India has seen a significant change in the provision for people with ID/DID through legislation and the involvement of the independent sector and government agencies. The National Institute for the Mentally Handicapped was established with a primary objective of empowering people with ID/DID. The projects delivered by the government and the independent sector are all aimed at raising awareness, prevention, early identification, intervention, special education, training professionals, and rehabilitation (18).

Organizational culture can influence the implementation of the model of care and quality of services. When staff acknowledge and accept the utility of a model of care's methods and goals (understood to be part of the overarching organization's formal culture) and attempt to execute them, presuming that the model of care is evidence based and successful, service and programme quality improves. Analysing the issue through the lens of culture can offer the possibility to assess the efficacy of the model of care as well as how it is being applied within the support networks of people with ID/DID. Contextual variables must be considered in policy formulation at all levels that impact human functioning outcomes, including the individual (microsystem), family (mesosystem), and society (macrosystem).

Prevalence of ID/DID across cultures

Over the centuries, people's perceptions of ID/DID and its definition have shifted (19,20). The community's treatment of people with ID/DID has also been tainted, with several reports of abuse and neglect (21). Even now, people with ID/DID continue to be stigmatized and abused in many regions, and their families are subjected to stigma and prejudice. Despite this, there have been positive developments over the decades that have improved the lives of people with ID/DID. Firstly, modern screening technologies have enabled not just early diagnosis of genetic problems but also remedial action in some cases. Secondly, a variety of evidence-based mental health services and supportive care facilities, as well as academic and vocational skills training, have been established to meet the needs of people with ID/DID. Thirdly, both national and international policies and conventions have been produced to protect the rights of people with disabilities across the world.

As more was learned about the aetiology of ID/DID and the capacity of people with ID/DID to adapt to their handicap and operate within society, the concept of ID/DID expanded as well. Currently, ID/DID is defined as a condition 'characterised by significantly below average intellectual functioning and adaptive behaviour that are approximately two or more standard deviations below the mean (approximately less than the 2.3rd percentile), based on appropriately normed, individually administered standardized tests' (14). ID/DID usually appears in early life and is caused by a combination of genetic and environmental factors. The behaviours of people with ID/DID change as they get older to meet their requirements. This is dependent on the severity of their condition and the accessible supportive services. People with ID/DID are able to contribute successfully to society at many levels of participation in the community, including ordinary activities, professional or academic activities. In addition to an IQ, the current standard for measuring ID/DID takes this into consideration and includes a comprehensive examination of adaptive behaviour. Adaptive behaviour includes three components: conceptual skills, practical skills, and social skills. Conceptual skills include those relating to language, literacy, money, time, number concepts, and self-direction. Social skills include interpersonal skills, social responsibility, self-esteem, gullibility, naïvety and wariness, social problem-solving, and the ability to follow rules/obey laws and avoid being victimized. Practical skills include activities of daily living. personal care, occupational skills, healthcare, travel/transportation, schedules/routines, safety, use of money, use of the telephone, and so on (22).

The incidence of ID/DID is reported to be approximately 1.8%, while the prevalence is considered to be between 1% and 3% (20,23). The prevalence of ID/DID is now less than 1% in developed countries such as Finland and the Netherlands, but it can grow to 4–5% in less developed areas of the world and up to 6% in some Eastern European countries (24). Eighty-five per cent have mild ID/DID, 10% have moderate ID/DID, 4% have severe ID/DID, and 2% have profound ID/DID, according to the four severity levels (19). It is because most of those with ID/DID fall in the mild category that the condition often goes undiagnosed in early childhood until they reach school age and begin having difficulty learning new skills (25). Borderline intellectual functioning is estimated to affect 12.3% of the population, Hassiotis et al. reported that one-eighth of 8450 individuals residing in a household in the UK had borderline intellectual functioning (26). In both adults and children/adolescents, males have a greater prevalence of ID/DID than females.

It is crucial to know not just the prevalence and aetiology of ID/DID, but also what kinds of health services are available to people with ID/DID. Better understanding of ID/DID epidemiology and existing services will aid in improving services, conducting research to fill information gaps, and informing policy-makers as they develop policies to enhance the lives of people with ID/DID.

The National Health Interview Survey shows changes in the frequency of ID/DID among 3–17-year-olds in the US from 1996 to 2008. While reporting on the trends, Boyle and colleagues (27) discovered that it has remained reasonably steady at around 0.7% of children, with the most recent batch of data from 2006 to 2008 providing an estimate of 0.67% of children. During the same time period, however, the incidence of learning disorders grew by 5.5% while the prevalence of ID/DID decreased significantly, which might be due to administrative data classifying more instances as learning disorders than ID/DID in order to lessen the stigma associated with ID/DID. According to a meta-analysis of 52 community-based research studies, the global prevalence of ID/DID is 1.04%. Low-income countries had the highest prevalence, with 1.64%, followed by middle-income countries (1.6%), and high-income countries (0.92%) (28). Children/adolescents, individuals from rural or urban slum communities, and females had the highest rates. McKenzie and colleagues (29) found a prevalence range of 0.05–1.55% in a systematic review of the prevalence and incidence of ID/DID between 2010 and 2015. According to King and colleagues (19), mild, moderate, severe, and profound ID/DID are recorded in 85%, 10%, 4%, and 2% of the population, respectively. Table 1.1 provides a review of more recent research on the prevalence of ID/DID.

Incidence is a more effective indicator of ID/DID significance than prevalence. However, there have been very few incidence investigations. In Sweden, a longitudinal study of children with a median age of 14 years found a cumulative incidence of 0.62% (46), whereas another study of adults aged 50 found a cumulative incidence of 1.58% for men and 0.96% for females (40). The cumulative incidence of ID/DID was reported to be 12.6/1000 in two cohort studies done in Finland in 1985–1986 ($n = 9432$) and 1966 ($n = 11,965$) (47). However, Heikura and colleagues (47) observed no change in the frequency of the severe category between the 1966 and 1986 cohorts, but a modest shift rate from severe to moderate to mild ID/DID. Mild ID/DID was shown to have a cumulative incidence of 7.5/1000, compared to 5/1000 in the younger group. In the US, Katusic and colleagues (48) found variations in the incidence of ID/DID based on sex and level of ID/DID. In a cohort of 5919 infants born between 1976 and 1980, the cumulative incidence of severe ID/DID was shown to be more than twice as high in females as it was in males, while the cumulative incidence of moderate ID/DID was found to be twice as high in males as females. The cumulative incidence of ID/DID in males was found to be 8.3/1000 population, while females had a rate of 10/1000 population. Males, on the other hand, had a cumulative incidence that was 1.7 times higher than females (48). The frequency of ID/DID was determined to be 0.87% in a Japanese epidemiological study of 5070 infants born between 1978 and 1987. The incidence of ID/DID was found to be 0.51% in the mild category and 0.36% in the severe category (49).

Prevalence of co-occurring autism spectrum disorder

Around 34% of people with ID/DID show widespread autistic characteristics (50–52), whereas up to 60% of those with autism have ID/DID (53–59). In people with ID/DID and a dual diagnosis (i.e. ID/DID plus another NDD or a psychopathological disorder), the risk of underestimating autism spectrum disorder (ASD) increases (60–62). When autism is present, over 40% of the items included in diagnostic tests for people with ID/DID and used to screen for psychosis obtain a high score (63). Another factor contributing to the growth of ASD incidence is incorrect diagnosis and a growing understanding that autistic disorders might be related to other conditions (64,65). Increases in prevalence were linked to decreases in other diagnostic categories in the US, showing that

Table 1.1 Prevalence of ID/DID in different countries

Country	Authors, year (reference)	Sample and methods features	Prevalence (%)
Australia	Australian Institute of Health and Welfare, 2004 (30)	503,000 people screened; any age	1.1
	Leonard et al., 2011 (31)	Children/adolescents and adult population survey	1.3
	Haider et al., 2013 (32)	Adult population survey	0.1
China	Zheng et al., 2011(33)	Nationally representative surveys conducted in 1987 and 2006; age-adjusted prevalence of ID estimated	1.3
India	Girimaji & Srinath, 2010 (34)	2064 children aged 0–16 years were screened for ID on ICD 10 criteria	3
	Lakhan et al., 2015 (35)	45,571 households in 4637 rural villages, and 24,731 households in 3354 urban blocks; children and adults	1.05–1.1
	Lakhan & Mawson, 2016 (36)	Community survey; a total of 8797 tribal population were screened for ID; prevalence of ID among children up to age 18 years was reported	0.6
Italy	ISTAT, 2018 (37) Salvini, 2018 (38)	Students with intellectual disability	1.9
UK	Emerson, 2012 (39)	Cross-sectional survey in a sample of 5.18 million children	1.5
Denmark	Pedersen et al., 2014 (40)	Data of residents who received health services between 2000 and 2012	0.1
South Africa	Christianson et al., 2002 (41)	6693 children screened	3.56
Canada	Lin et al., 2013 (42)	Administrative health data used to derive estimates of the prevalence of adult ID	0.1

(continued)

Table 1.1 Continued

Country	Authors, year (reference)	Sample and methods features	Prevalence (%)
US	Boyle et al., 2011 (27)	National Health Interview Survey datasets 1997–2008; data collected every 3 years from children aged 3–17 years	Rates at each time point 1997, 2000, 2003, 2006 were 0.68, 0.73, 0.75, and 0.67, respectively
	Van Naarden Braun et al. 2015 (43)	Population-based developmental disabilities surveillance programme data from 1991 to 2010 for 8-year-olds in metropolitan Atlanta	1.6
Mexico	Lazcano-Ponce et al., 2008 (44)	Estimate based on INDESOL (National Social Development Institute) data	2.54
Brazil	Malta et al., 2016 (45)	National Health Survey between August 2013 and February 2014; any age	0.8

diagnostic substitution had occurred (66). The need to clearly define the border between ASD and ID/DID is a key background issue in these discussions. ID/DID and ASD are both meta-syndromic groupings that include a wide range of clinical disorders (12). However, many people with ID/DID show autistic characteristics, and many individuals with ASD have worse cognitive performance than the general population (67,68).

Psychological and physical comorbid conditions

People with ID/DID have a greater incidence of physical and mental problems than the general population (69,70). According to Cooper and colleagues (69), specific physical and mental health issues were considerably greater in individuals with ID/DID, with epilepsy being the most prevalent. Hearing impairment is present in 10% of cases, while epilepsy is prevalent in 5–30% of cases, according to Harris (20). People with ID/DID are four to five times more likely to have mental health issues (71,72). According to Lundqvist (73), 62% of people with ID/DID had at least one self-injurious, stereotyped, or aggressive/destructive behaviour issue, with 18.6% having challenging behaviours.

Lakhan and Kishore (36) discovered a higher incidence of aggressive and destructive behaviours, as well as misbehaviour with others, in moderate and mild ID/DID, and self-injurious behaviour, temper tantrums, and stereotypical behaviours in profound and severe ID/DID. Physical health issues can contribute to behavioural issues in people with ID/DID (74). However, the aetiology and comorbid disorders may differ depending on the age group studied and the context in which the study is conducted.

Discussion on variations in prevalence across cultures

It is important to recognize the difficulty of comparing prevalence studies as they vastly differ in terms of the conceptualization of ID/DID, diagnostic criteria followed, and the methods adopted to identify ID/DID. King and colleagues (19) while discussing the various factors that tend to influence the prevalence of ID/DID globally observed that definitions used for ID/DID by different surveys determine how ID/DID is identified in the community. As discussed earlier, the definition of ID/DID has changed through time as standard diagnostic methods have been revised, resulting in changes to ID/DID diagnostic criteria. Researchers are currently debating whether to utilize adaptive behaviour capabilities in addition to IQ scores or to use each of them independently. The AAIDD defines ten areas of adapted behaviour and employs both IQ and adaptive behaviour to determine the severity of ID/DID (22).

Age of ascertainment also plays a crucial role because with age, adaptive behaviours modify the functional ability of people with ID/DID. Ten years is now the global mean age for identification. The mortality rates for people with ID/DID also vary by age. When a child begins school, he or she is more likely to be identified, and this is frequently the age at which point prevalence peaks. Prevalence is also determined by the survey tools used and the people polled, such as research conducted in the community, clinics, and special institutions. Because of conceptual and practical difficulties with the criteria used, data on the prevalence of ID/DID among ethnic groups and communities throughout the world may be skewed. In general, although epidemiological research in rich countries produce reasonably consistent rates, observed rates in low- and middle-income countries are higher and more varied, most likely due to methodological issues as well as variations in risk exposure.

Surveillance methods focused on impairments indicate lower rates of disability, whereas indicators based on limited activity provide the highest rates. Variations in disability classification among national surveillance systems have long been acknowledged by analysts as a key obstacle to our understanding of disability on a global scale. IQ tests can also affect rate differences, though to a lesser extent, since they present some level of cultural bias against minority populations. They gave numerous explanations for the differences. IQ tests do not dependably represent the general population's IQ levels, which rise at regular periods owing to environmental variables, a phenomenon known as the Flynn effect. To counteract the Flynn effect, IQ tests are re-standardized at regular intervals to make the test items more challenging. However, there is a disadvantage in that more people have IQs less than 70 (75,76). As a result, IQ levels alone are not enough to diagnose ID/DID.

As discussed before, ID/DID is strongly related with ASDs, and statistics suggest that in many countries the incidence of ASD is growing while the prevalence of ID/DID is decreasing due to administrative policies of providing resources that favour autism (77–79). It is estimated that 40–60% of people with ASDs have ID/DID (43,67). In high-income countries, medical terminations of pregnancies due to prenatal diagnosis of specific types of ID/DID, such as Down syndrome, Edwards syndrome, and Patau syndrome, are leading to a decline in ID/DID prevalence. Furthermore, increased public health and risk preventive efforts such as teaching about alcohol use during pregnancy and reducing lead contamination in drinking water may have reduced the risk of ID/DID in the community (80).

Variations in the frequency and incidence of ID/DID have also been linked to changes in demographic characteristics, average parental age, rising maternal age, and sex ratio (29,81), which show significant differences between different countries and cultural contexts.

Arguably, economic and social variables are the most important influencing elements determining prevalence. Harriss-White (82) describes a disability notion based on the absence of local economic skills in a field study of three communities in rural south India. At the end of the last century, when the US chose to broaden the diagnostic criteria for ID/DID to include anybody with an IQ of less than 75, the government's acceptance of that would have implications on the ability to afford support to a considerably greater number of people who would be eligible for services. In Italy, the diagnosis of ID/DID in adults has implications for access to mental health services, also on the basis of organizational and economic aspects (83). In the UK, ID/DID services have been in danger of being cut in order to manage scarce resources while believing that mainstream services would have covered the gap (84).

Regarding strict social factors, in many cultural contexts survey questions concerning disability are more likely to be linked with stigma and hence underreported, as are queries about terms that respondents do not understand or misinterpret (85).

Clearly, comparing prevalence rates across nations and cultural settings within the same country cannot give insight into cultural differences in ID/DID conceptualization and the dynamic of the disablement process. These figures, by contrast, may be utilized to improve policymaking and advocacy in different countries, as well as to raise awareness of the link between societies and its citizens with ID/DID. In the preface of its Atlas-ID project (86), the WHO hoped that the project (aimed to map resources and services for ID/DID across the world) could have been 'the first step towards global empowerment of people with intellectual disabilities and their families through awareness of the need to implement policies and programmes to fill the gap of services and resources across the globe'.

Gaps in knowledge and future research needs

There are significant gaps in the existing research on epidemiology of ID/DID in low- and middle-income countries. Although these countries have some research available, the quality of these studies is frequently restricted due to the fact that they are small clinic-based studies. There are no big cohorts that give as much data as other cohort studies in Europe, such as the Olmstead County study or other cohort studies (87). The difficulty in determining incidence rates, causative variables, trends in prevalence, risk factors susceptible to embedding intervention and outcomes, and mortality is hampered by the lack of such research. There is also a lack of clarity about how and to what extent mental disorders affect behavioural manifestations in people with ID/DID (88).

Research into the genetics of ID/DID is another area that is advancing but still has a long way to go (89). While new exome and genome sequencing tools have enhanced our understanding of the genetic sequence in many situations, others remain unclear. There are few treatments based on genetic research, and more study is needed to determine how treatment based on genetic modification may be administered in a cost-effective way at the population level.

According to the US Centres for Disease Control and Prevention estimates, in 2003 the lifetime cost of ID/DID in the Atlanta metropolitan area was around USD 1.01 million per person (54), and data from Australia suggest that the cost of managing care for people with ID/DID is about AUD 14.7 billion per year, with 85% of the cost being opportunity cost owing to missed time (90). Low- and middle-income countries, in contrast, have done very little related research. One of the primary reasons for the WHO and the World Bank Burden of Disease study's exclusion was a lack of appropriate and reliable epidemiological data. Other implications include insufficient consideration of global health concerns and a growing gap between available health services and clients' needs (86).

References

1. **Esquirol É.** Mental Maladies; A Treatise on Insanity. Translated from the French by Ebenezer Kingsbury Hunt. Philadelphia, PA: Lea and Blanchard; 1845 [1838 (original French edition)].
2. **Down JLH.** Observation on an ethnic classification of idiots. Journal of Mental Science 1867;**13**(61):121–3.
3. **Griesinger W.** Die Pathologie und Therapie der psychischen Krankheiten, 4th edition. Braunschweig: Wreden; 1876.
4. **Barr MW.** Sketch of the history of the treatment of mental defect. Charities 1904;879–83.
5. **Scheerenberger RC.** A History of Mental Retardation. Baltimore, MD: Paul H. Brookes; 1983.
6. **Goodey CF.** A History of Intelligence and 'Intellectual Disability': The Shaping of Psychology in Early Modern Europe. Farnham: Ashgate; 2011.
7. **American Psychiatric Association**. Diagnostic and Statistical Manual of Mental Disorders. Washington, DC: American Psychiatric Association; 1952.
8. **Heber R.** Modifications in the manual on terminology and classification in mental retardation. American Journal of Mental Deficiency 1961;**65**:499–500.
9. **Luckasson R, Coulter DL, Polloway EA, Reese S, Schalock RL, Snell ME**, et al. Mental Retardation: Definition, Classification, and Systems of Supports, 9th edition. Washington, DC: American Association on Mental Retardation; 1992.
10. **World Health Organization**. ICF: International Classification of Functioning, Disability and Health. Geneva: WHO Press; 2001.
11. **Schalock RL, Luckasson RA, Shogren KA, Borthwick-Duffy S, Bradley V, Buntinx WH**, et al. The renaming of mental retardation: understanding the change to the term intellectual disability. Intellectual and Developmental Disabilities. 2007;**45**(2):116–24.
12. **Salvador-Carulla L, Bertelli M.** 'Mental retardation' or 'intellectual disability': time for a conceptual change. Psychopathology 2008;**41**(1):10–16.
13. **American Psychiatric Association.** Diagnostic and Statistical Manual of Mental Disorders, 5th edition (DSM-5). Washington, DC: American Psychiatric Association; 2013.
14. **World Health Organization**. 6A00 Disorders of intellectual development. In: International classification of diseases for mortality and morbidity statistics (11th revision). 2018. Available from: https://icd.who.int/browse11/l-m/en#/ http%3a%2f%2fid.who.int%2ficd%2fentity%2f605267007
15. **Bertelli MO, Munir K, Harris J, Salvador-Carulla L.** 'Intellectual developmental disorders': reflections on the international consensus document for redefining 'mental retardation-intellectual disability' in ICD-11. Advances in Mental Health and Intellectual Disabilities 2016;**10**(1):36–58.
16. **Ngo H, Shin JY, Nhan NV, Yang LH.** Stigma and restriction on the social life of families of children with intellectual disabilities in Vietnam. Singapore Medical Journal 2012;**53**(7):451–7.
17. **Jansen-van Vuuren J, Aldersey HM.** Stigma, acceptance and belonging for people with IDD across cultures. Current Developmental Disorders Reports 2020;**7**(3):163–72.

18. Girimaji SC, Kommu JVS. Intellectual disability in India: Recent trends in care and services. In: Rubin IL, Merrick J, Greydanus DE, Patel DR, editors. Health Care for People with Intellectual and Developmental Disabilities across the Lifespan. Springer, Cham; 2016.

19. King BH, Toth KE, Hodapp RM, Dykens EM. Intellectual disability. In: Sadock BJ, Sadock VA, Ruiz P, editors. Comprehensive Textbook of Psychiatry, 9th edition. Philadelphia, PA: Lippincott Williams & Wilkins; 2009: 3444–74.

20. Harris JC. The classification of intellectual disability. In: Intellectual Disability: Understanding its Development, Causes, Classification, Evaluation, and Treatment. New York: Oxford University Press; 2006: 42–98.

21. Maulik PK, Harbour CK, McCarthy J. History and epidemiology of intellectual disorders. In: Tsakanikos E, McCarthy J, editors. Handbook of Psychopathology in Intellectual Disability: Research, Practice and Policy. New York: Springer; 2013: 9–21.

22. American Association on Intellectual and Developmental Disabilities. Definition of intellectual disability. 2021. Available from: https://www.aaidd.org/intellectual-disability/definition

23. Heikura U, Taanila A, Olsen P, Hartikainen AL, von Wendt L, Jarvelin MR. Temporal changes in incidence and prevalence of intellectual disability between two birth cohorts in Northern Finland. American Journal of Mental Retardation: AJMR 2003;108(1):19–31.

24. Durkin M. The epidemiology of developmental disabilities in low-income countries. Mental Retardation and Developmental Disabilities Research Reviews 2002;8(3):206–11.

25. Schalock RL, Reeve A, Shogren KA, Snell ME, Spreat S, Tasse MJ, et al. Intellectual Disability: Definition, Classification, and Systems of Supports, 11th edition. Washington, DC: American Association on Intellectual and Developmental Disabilities. 2010.

26. Hassiotis A, Strydom A, Hall I, Ali A, Lawrence-Smith G, Meltzer H, et al. Psychiatric morbidity and social functioning among adults with borderline intelligence living in private households. Journal of Intellectual Disability Research 2008;52(2):95–106.

27. Boyle CA, Boulet S, Schieve LA, Cohen RA, Blumberg SJ, Yeargin-Allsopp M, et al. Trends in the prevalence of developmental disabilities in US children, 1997–2008. Paediatrics 2011;127(6):1034–42.

28. Maulik PK, Mascarenhas MN, Mathers CD, Dua T, Saxena S. Prevalence of intellectual disability: a meta-analysis of population-based studies. Research in Developmental Disabilities 2011;32(2):419–36.

29. McKenzie K, Milton M, Smith G, Ouellette-Kuntz H. Systematic review of the prevalence and incidence of intellectual disabilities: current trends and issues. Current Developmental Disorders Reports 2016;3(2):104–15.

30. Australian Institute of Health and Welfare (AIHW). Estimates of prevalence of intellectual disability in Australia. Journal of Intellectual and Developmental Disability 2004;29(3):284–9.

31. Leonard H, Glasson E, Nassar N, Whitehouse A, Bebbington A, Bourke J, et al. Autism and intellectual disability are differentially related to sociodemographic background at birth. PLoS One 2011;6(3):e17875.

32. **Haider SI, Ansari Z, Vaughan L, Matters H, Emerson E.** Health and wellbeing of Victorian adults with intellectual disability compared to the general Victorian population. Research in Developmental Disabilities 2013;**34**(11):4034–42.

33. **Zheng X, Chen G, Song X, Liu J, Yan L, Du W**, et al. Twenty-year trends in the prevalence of disability in China. Bulletin of the World Health Organization 2011;**89**(11):788–97.

34. **Girimaji SC, Srinath S.** Perspectives of intellectual disability in India: epidemiology, policy, services for children and adults. Current Opinion in Psychiatry 2010;**23**(5):441–6.

35. **Lakhan R, Ekúndayò OT, Shahbazi M.** An estimation of the prevalence of intellectual disabilities and its association with age in rural and urban populations in India. Journal of Neurosciences in Rural Practice 2015;**6**(4)523–8.

36. **Lakhan R, Kishore MT.** Mortality in people with intellectual disability in India: correlates of age and settings. Life Span and Disability 2016;**19**:45–56.

37. **ISTAT —Istituto nazionale di statistica.** L'integrazione degli alunni con disabilità nelle scuole primarie e secondarie di primo grado, anno scolastico 2016/2017. Statistiche Report. 2018. Available from: https://www.istat.it/it/files//2018/03/alunni-con-disabi lit%C3%A0-as2016-2017.pdf

38. **Salvini F.** I principali dati relativi agli alunni con disabilità per l'a.s. 2016/2017. Ufficio Statistica e Studi. 2018. Available from: https://www.miur.gov.it/documents/20182/0/ FOCUS_I+principali+dati+relativi+agli+alunni+con+disabilit%C3%A0_a.s.2016_2 017_def.pdf/1f6eeb44-07f2-43a1-8793-99f0c982e422

39. **Emerson E.** Deprivation, ethnicity and the prevalence of intellectual and developmental disabilities. Journal of Epidemiology and Community Health 2012;**66**(3):218–24.

40. **Pedersen CB, Mors O, Bertelsen A, Waltoft BL, Agerbo E, McGrath JJ**, et al. A comprehensive nationwide study of the incidence rate and lifetime risk for treated mental disorders. JAMA Psychiatry. 2014;**71**(5):573–81.

41. **Christianson AL, Zwane ME, Manga P, Rosen E, Venter A, Downs D, Kromberg JG.** Children with intellectual disability in rural South Africa: prevalence and associated disability. Journal of Intellectual Disability Research 2002;**46**(Pt 2):179–86.

42. **Lin E, Balogh R, Cobigo V, Ouellette-Kuntz H, Wilton AS, Lunsky Y.** Using administrative health data to identify individuals with intellectual and developmental disabilities: a comparison of algorithms. Journal of Intellectual Disability Research 2013;**57**(5):462–77.

43. **Van Naarden Braun K, Christensen D, Doernberg N, Schieve L, Rice C, Wiggins L**, et al. Trends in the prevalence of autism spectrum disorder, cerebral palsy, hearing loss, intellectual disability, and vision impairment, metropolitan Atlanta, 1991–2010. PLoS One 2015;**10**(4):e0124120.

44. **Lazcano-Ponce E, Rangel-Eudave G, Katz G.** Intellectual disability and its effects on society. Salud Pública de México 2008;**50**(Suppl 2):S119–20.

45. **Malta DC, Stopa SR, Canuto R, Gomes NL, Mendes VL, Goulart BN, Moura L.** Self-reported prevalence of disability in Brazil, according to the National Health Survey, 2013. Ciência and Saúde Coletiva 2016;**21**(10):3253–64.

46. **Sandin S, Nygren KG, Iliadou A, Hultman CM, Reichenberg A.** Autism and mental retardation among offspring born after in vitro fertilization. JAMA 2013;**310**(1):75–84.

47. **Heikura U, Taanila A, Olsen P, Hartikainen AL, von Wendt L, Jarvelin MR.** Temporal changes in incidence and prevalence of intellectual disability between two birth cohorts in Northern Finland. American Journal of Mental Retardation: AJMR 2003;**108**(1):19–31.

48. **Katusic SK, Colligan RC, Beard CM, O'Fallon WM, Bergstralh EJ, Jacobsen SJ, et al.** Mental retardation in a birth cohort, 1976–1980, Rochester, Minnesota. American Journal of Mental Retardation: AJMR 1996;**100**(4):335–44.

49. **Yamada K.** Incidence rates of cerebral palsy, mental retardation and Down syndrome in Sodegaura City, Chiba Prefecture. No to hattatsu. Brain and Development 1994;**26**:411–17.

50. **Morgan CN, Roy M, Nasr A, Chance P, Hand M, Mlele T, Roy A.** A community study establishing the prevalence rate of autistic disorder in adults with learning disability. Psychiatric Bulletin 2002;**26**(4):127–9.

51. **La Malfa G, Lassi G, Bertelli M, Salvini R, Placidi GF.** Autism and intellectual disability: a study of prevalence on a sample of the Italian population. Journal of Intellectual Disability Research 2004;**48**(3):262–7.

52. **Cooper SA, Smiley E, Morrison J, Williamson A, Alla L.** Mental ill-health in adults with intellectual disabilities: prevalence and associated factors. British Journal of Psychiatry 2007;**190**:27–35.

53. **Hoekstra R, Happé F, Baron-Cohen S, Ronald A.** Association between extreme autistic traits and intellectual disability: insights from a general population twin study. British Journal of Psychiatry 2009;**195**(6):531–6.

54. **Centres for Disease Control and Prevention.** Intellectual disability among children. 2006. Available from: https://www.cdc.gov/ncbddd/developmentaldisabilities/docume nts/intellectualdisabilities.pdf

55. **Edelson MG.** Are the majority of children with autism mentally retarded? A systematic evaluation of the data? Focus on Autism and Other Developmental Disabilities 2006;**21**(2):66–83.

56. **Matson JL, Shoemaker M.** Intellectual disability and its relationship to autism spectrum disorders. Research in Developmental Disabilities 2009;**30**(6):1107–14.

57. **Baird G, Simonoff E, Pickles A, Chandler S, Loucas T, Meldrum D, Charman T.** Prevalence of disorders of the autism spectrum in a population cohort of children in South Thames: the Special Needs and Autism Project (SNAP). Lancet 2006;**368**(9531):210–15.

58. **Noterdaeme MA, Wriedt E.** Comorbidity in autism spectrum disorders—I. Mental retardation and psychiatric comorbidity. Zeitschrift fur Kinder und Jugendpsychiatrie und Psychotherapie 2010;**38**(4):257–66.

59. **Bryson SE, Smith IM.** Epidemiology of autism: prevalence, associated characteristics, and implications for research and service delivery. Mental Retardation and Developmental Disabilities Research Reviews 1998;**4**(2):97–103.

60. **Palucka AM, Lunsky Y, Gofine T, White SE, Reid M.** Brief report: comparison of referrals of individuals with and without a diagnosis of psychotic disorder to a specialized dual diagnosis program. Journal on Developmental Disabilities 2009;**15**(2):103–9.

61. **Savage M, Benia F, Balanquit M., Palucka AM.** Unrecognized medical concern as cause of 'psychiatric' disorder and challenging behaviour in developmental disability: a case study. Journal on Developmental Disabilities 2007;**13**(3):205–10.

62. **Bradley E, Lunsky Y, Palucka A, Homitidis S.** Recognition of intellectual disabilities and autism in psychiatric inpatients diagnosed with schizophrenia and other psychotic disorders. Advances in Mental Health and Intellectual Disabilities 2011;**5**(6):4–18.

63. **Helverschou SB, Bakken TL, Martinsen H.** Identifying symptoms of psychiatric disorders in people with autism and intellectual disability: an empirical conceptual analysis. Advances in Mental Health and Intellectual Disabilities 2008;**11**(4):105–15.

64. **Wing L, Potter D.** The epidemiology of autistic spectrum disorders: is the prevalence rising? Mental Retardation and Developmental Disabilities Research Reviews 2002;**8**(3):151–61.

65. **Matson JL, Kozlowski AM.** The increasing prevalence of autism spectrum disorders. Research in Autism Spectrum Disorders 2011;**5**(1):418–25.

66. **Shattuck PT.** The contribution of diagnostic substitution to the growing administrative prevalence of autism in US special education. Pediatrics. 2006;**117**(4):1028–37.

67. **Fombonne E.** Epidemiological surveys of autism and other pervasive developmental disorders: an update. Journal of Autism and Developmental Disorders 2003;**33**(4):365–82.

68. **Ghaziuddin M.** Mental Health Aspects of Autism and Asperger Syndrome. London: Jessica Kingsley Publishers; 2005.

69. **Cooper SA, McLean G, Guthrie B, McConnachie A, Mercer S, Sullivan F,** et al. Multiple physical and mental health comorbidity in adults with intellectual disabilities: population-based cross-sectional analysis. BMC Family Practice 2015;**16**:1.

70. **Kwok H, Cheung PW.** Co-morbidity of psychiatric disorder and medical illness in people with intellectual disabilities. Current Opinion in Psychiatry 2007;**20**(5):443–9.

71. **Rojahn J, Meier L.** Epidemiology of mental illness and maladaptive behavior in intellectual disabilities. In: **Hodapp R,** editor. International Review of Research in Mental Retardation, Volume 38. London: Academic Press; 2009; 239–87.

72. **Yoo JH, Valdovinos MG, Schroeder SR.** The epidemiology of psychopathology in people with intellectual disability. International Review of Research in Developmental Disabilities 2012;**42**(4):31–56.

73. **Lundqvist LO.** Prevalence and risk markers of behavior problems among adults with intellectual disabilities: a total population study in Örebro County, Sweden. Research in Developmental Disabilities 2013;**34**(2):1346–56.

74. **May ME, Kennedy CH.** Health and problem behavior among people with intellectual disabilities. Behavior Analysis in Practice 2010;**3**(3):4–12.

75. **Flynn JR.** Wechsler intelligence tests: do we really have a criterion of mental retardation? American Journal of Mental Deficiency 1985;**90**(6):236–44.

76. **Kanaya T, Ceci SJ, Scullin MH.** The rise and fall of IQ in special education: historical trends and their implications. Journal of School Psychology 2003;**41**(6):453–65.

77. **Croen LA, Grether JK, Hoogstrate J, Selvin S.** The changing prevalence of autism in California. Journal of Autism and Developmental Disorders 2002;**32**(3):207–15.

78. **Coo H, Ouellette-Kuntz H, Lloyd JE, Kasmara L, Holden JJ, Lewis MS.** Trends in autism prevalence: diagnostic substitution revisited. Journal of Autism and Developmental Disorders 2008;**38**(6):1036–46.

79. **National Academies of Sciences, Engineering, and Medicine.** Mental Disorders and Disabilities Among Low-Income Children. Washington, DC: The National Academies Press; 2015.

80. **Hanna-Attisha M, LaChance J, Sadler RC, Champney Schnepp A.** Elevated blood lead levels in children associated with the Flint drinking water crisis: a spatial analysis of risk and public health response. American Journal of Public Health 2016;**106**(2):283–90.

81. **Lakhan R, Mawson AR.** Identifying children with intellectual disabilities in the Tribal Population of Barwani District in State of Madhya Pradesh, India. Journal of Applied Research in Intellectual Disabilities 2016;**29**(3):211–19.

82. **Harriss-White B.** Staying Poor: Chronic Poverty and Development Policy. Oxford: Oxford University Press; 2003.

83. **Bertelli MO, Bianco A, Forte L.** Psicopatologia e disabilità dello sviluppo: Servizi e Formazione in Italia. Il Sirente: Fagnano Alto; 2021.

84. **O'Hara J, Bouras N.** Intellectual disabilities across cultures. In: **Bhugra D, Bhui K,** editors. Textbook of Cultural Psychiatry. Cambridge: Cambridge University Press; 2007; 493–502.

85. **Fujiura GT, Park HJ, Rutkowski-Kmitta V.** Disability statistics in the developing world: a reflection on the meanings in our numbers. Journal of Applied Research in Intellectual Disabilities 2005;**18**(4):295–304.

86. **World Health Organization.** Atlas: Global Resources for Persons with Intellectual Disabilities. Geneva: World Health Organization; 2007.

87. **Katusic SK, Colligan RC, Myers SM, Voigt RG, Yoshimasu K, Stoeckel RE,** et al. What can large population-based birth cohort study ask about past, present and future of children with disorders of development, learning and behaviour? Journal of Epidemiology and Community Health 2017;**71**(4):410–16.

88. **Allen D, Davies D.** Challenging behaviour and psychiatric disorder in intellectual disability. Current Opinion in Psychiatry 2007;**20**(5):450–5.

89. **Vissers LE, Gilissen C, Veltman JA.** Genetic studies in intellectual disability and related disorders. Nature Reviews Genetics 2016;**17**(1):9–18.

90. **Doran CM, Einfeld SL, Madden RH, Otim M, Horstead SK, Ellis LA, Emerson E.** How much does intellectual disability really cost? First estimates for Australia. Journal of Intellectual and Developmental Disability 2012;**37**(1):42–9.

Chapter 2

Physical health of people with intellectual disability across cultures

Katerina Denediou Derrer, Rachel Royston, Reza Kiani, Umesh Chauhan, and Angela Hassiotis

Impact of the disability models on health-seeking behaviour

In the last 100 years, the biomedical, or individual model has been influential in conceptualizing intellectual disability (1). It is characterized by the belief that disability is the result of a deficit located within the individual. This model acknowledges the disability before the person and places a duty on society to work towards preventing conditions causing the disability (e.g. by genetic screening), rehabilitating individuals (to reduce the effect of their deficits), and providing social care (to support the individual). Families of higher socioeconomic position tend to adopt this model of cultural understanding.

An alternative explanatory model is the social model, characterized by the belief that disability is a social construct, not inherent in the individual, but the result of inequitable practices and a general lack of understanding of people with intellectual disability (2,3). This differs from other models including the biomedical, charitable (disability is something that should be pitied), and religious (disability is related to supernatural beliefs) models (4). The social model distinguishes between impairment (an injury, illness, or condition that is associated with long-term differences and/or limitations in potential functioning) and disability (the economic, social, physical, and cultural barriers that exclude people with impairments from fully participating in society as equal citizens) (5,6).

The biopsychosocial model combines elements of both models to provide a more comprehensive and dynamic approach to explain intellectual disability

(1,7). It recognizes the complex interactions between biological factors, emotions, behaviour, social factors, and the environment. The environment is recognized as being particularly crucial in influencing the person's level of functioning and social participation. For instance, when people are confronted with social conditions or environmental barriers that prevent them from participating in society, this is likely to exacerbate their disability.

Morbidity and mortality from non-communicable diseases in people with intellectual disabilities

Non-communicable diseases (NCDs) are those that are not directly transmissible between people. According to the World Health Organization (WHO), NCDs kill 41 million people each year, equivalent to 71% of all deaths globally (8). Many are chronic diseases such as cardiovascular disease, most cancers, chronic lung diseases, diabetes, epilepsy, kidney disease, osteoarthritis, dementias, and Parkinson's diseases. The first four groups of NCDs also account for over 80% of all premature deaths. Poorer people are disproportionally affected by NCDs and mental health conditions (9). Moreover, NCDs tend to co-occur and this poses significant challenges for individuals, their families, and health providers (10). Multimorbidity can lead to polypharmacy and is compounded by limited access to health promotion, disease self-management strategies, and screening programmes (11).

Epidemiological studies indicate that people with intellectual disability have higher rates of physical disabilities (30%), mental health problems (30%), communication difficulties (30%), visual impairments (20%), and hearing impairments (10%) compared to peers without intellectual disability (3). People with intellectual disabilities are also more likely to suffer from multiple NCDs, in part due to underlying factors such as genetic and biological associations with certain causes of intellectual disability (e.g. autism, intellectual disability, and epilepsy; Down syndrome with dementia and cardiovascular disease) (12,13), but also greater exposure to environmental and social risk factors such as obesity, unhealthy diets, and substance use (8,14).

A recent review of 54 studies by Tyrer et al., published between 2010 and 2019 (15), found a continuing trend in mortality disparities in people with intellectual disability, consistent across countries and publication years and with no evidence of a decrease over time. The review revealed that people with intellectual disability can still expect to live 12–23 years less than the general population. This is despite the development of many national and international health and social care policy initiatives over the past few decades.

Impact of the disability models on health-seeking behaviour in ethnically diverse populations

Treatment approaches for intellectual disabilities vary widely from culture to culture, due to differences in the public health systems and the impact of prevailing intellectual disability models on available healthcare and health-seeking behaviour. Families who value a biomedical explanatory model of intellectual disability may be more likely to access formal healthcare and be more accepting of available therapies to improve health and well-being.

Families who view intellectual disability through the sociocultural model lens may not seek treatment or support from those they see as 'outsiders' (16,17). This has been reported in some Southeast Asian cultures and the Sami people in Northern Scandinavia, who are culturally less inclined to discuss their difficulties or seek help outside the family (17). Some communities discourage seeking formal healthcare, saying 'this is the way the person is', and hope the condition will improve with time or with marriage. For example, in a study in Ghana on the perceived causes of cerebral palsy, over half (54%) of respondents were unaware of any risk factors for the disorder and 40% thought it was caused by witchcraft and were thus more likely to seek treatment from traditional healers (18). In Somalia, there are at least three established healing systems, and such beliefs persist even when Somalis emigrate, with people continuing to seek traditional approaches in their new country (19,20). In some Southeast Asian cultures, such as in Laos, a shaman—a healthcare and spiritual provider—is called on to perform healing, preventive, and diagnostic rituals. Social relationships are often important in influencing the interpretation of illness, treatment, and healing. Indian families may combine yoga, Ayurveda, and homeopathy with conventional medicine (21).

Morbidity and mortality from non-communicable diseases in people from ethnically diverse groups with intellectual disabilities

The Confidential Inquiry into Premature Death of people with Learning Disability (CIPOLD) (22,23) reviewed 247 deaths between 2010 and 2012 across five primary care trusts in the UK. It was found that death certification data only mentioned intellectual disability in 23% of cases, with a lower number of deaths referred to the coroner for people with intellectual disabilities compared to the general population (38% vs 46%, respectively) (22,24). Tyrer et al. (25) explored differential cause-specific mortality and trends in mortality over time in England using the Clinical Practice Research Datalink and the Office for National Statistics mortality data from 2000 to 2019. Among 1.4 million patients studied (n = 33,855 with intellectual disability), mortality rates were consistently higher in people with intellectual disabilities compared with the general population.

Due to a significant under-representation of non-White UK individuals in both the CIPOLD report and the study by Tyrer et al., analyses were unable to explore ethnicity and this has been a common theme in morbidity and mortality intellectual disability research (22,25,26). However, in recent years there has been emerging global evidence of an association between ethnicity and mortality in people with intellectual disability, with ethnic minority status being predictive of higher mortality (27). For instance, Santoro et al. found that for children with Down syndrome, being from a Black African/Caribbean background significantly increased the risk of mortality compared to White counterparts (28).

In 2017, NHS England established the Learning Disability Observatory (Learning Disabilities Mortality Review (LeDeR) programme) to improve care, reduce health inequalities, and reduce premature mortality in people with an intellectual disability. LeDeR produces annual reports on mortality in people with intellectual disabilities and estimates it is notified of 65% of deaths (27,29). The 2020 LeDeR report found a higher risk of mortality in people of Asian/ Asian British ethnicity (9.2 times greater than a White British person), mixed/ multiple ethnicities (3.9 times greater than a White British person), and Black/ African/Caribbean/ Black British ethnicity (3.6 times greater than a White British person) (27,29).

A recent systematic review into early mortality identified specific NCDs, namely respiratory and circulatory diseases, as the main causes of death for people with intellectual disability, although rates of cancer deaths were reportedly lower than those found in the general population (30). Disparities in morbidity by ethnicity within people with intellectual disability have scarcely been explored. However, the 2019 LeDeR report found some health conditions were more common among people from certain ethnic groups. For example, they reported South Asians to be at higher risk of acute glaucoma, chronic kidney disease, coronary heart disease, and diabetes. Further studies have started to explore ethnic differences in NCDs within the intellectual disability community, finding higher rates of some diseases (e.g. diabetes and heart disease) in South Asian and Black communities (31,32). It has also been found that people from ethnic minority backgrounds are more likely to have profound and multiple intellectual disabilities (26,33).

Studies in the US found that Latinos and Black people with intellectual disability are significantly more likely than White counterparts and people without intellectual disability to describe their physical and mental health as fair or poor (34). They are also more likely to be obese than White adults with intellectual disability, with around 40% of Black and Latino adults having a BMI greater than 30 kg/m^2, compared with 33% of White adults (34–36).

Prevention of non-communicable diseases

Prevention of physical illness in people from ethnically diverse groups can be achieved through reducing risk factors, adapting lifestyles, and increasing awareness of screening programmes (35). The take-up of physical activity in people with intellectual disability tends to be low (36). This may be due to negative health perceptions (e.g. exercise is inappropriate or unnecessary) and personal barriers (e.g. time constraints, distance to sports facilities). For people from ethnically diverse backgrounds, an additional constraint may also relate to cultural expectations relating to sex and religion (e.g. certain religious clothes may make exercise difficult) (35–38).

Important public health measures, including immunizations and screening programmes, can reduce/prevent infectious diseases and lifestyle interventions (e.g. increasing physical activity, changes to diet) can be implemented to improve general wellness. However, intervention programmes need to be tailored specifically to the needs of ethnically diverse groups to address underlying barriers to behaviour change that are often seen in multicomponent interventions (38,39).

Access to healthcare for ethnic minority groups with intellectual disability: barriers and facilitators

Healthcare access is a sociological concept of how easily an individual can obtain needed medical services. It implies that the individual can recognize his or her need and that services are readily accessible in terms of their physical location, affordability, and cultural acceptability. The notion of candidacy was constructed by Mary Dixon-Woods and colleagues to describe the ways in which people's eligibility for medical attention and intervention is jointly negotiated between individuals and healthcare services (40–42). Vulnerable groups, such as immigrants, refugees, people with intellectual disability, and people from ethnic minority groups are often under-represented in health services. This may be explained by a reduced awareness of available services and being unable to negotiate or meet service eligibility criteria. Although the need is present, family carers may provide care for many years and services may only be accessed when a crisis occurs due to parental ill-health or the onset of mental ill-health in the person with intellectual disability (26,43,44). Unfortunately, very few studies worldwide examine how people with intellectual disability experience health and social care services, with even fewer in those from Black and other ethnic minority populations, despite these people facing a double disadvantage when seeking to access healthcare. People with intellectual disability are known to have low health literacy and have a low tendency to access primary care and secondary specialist services (45). However, a study by Ali et al. in 2016 (46) indicated they may attend such services in cases where they suffer psychological distress due to stigmatization.

Some patients or carers from ethnic minority backgrounds cannot read or speak the majority language, and there are often limited numbers of available professionals who can speak the required languages. Patients and carers report this as a significant barrier to accessing help (47). Health services therefore often rely on interpreters, although this introduces a 'third person' in the therapeutic relationship and is not considered universally satisfactory (48). For example, less than 30% of paediatricians in California offered autism screening in Spanish to children of Latino families and only 10% offered both general developmental and autism spectrum disorder screening in Spanish, even though both are available as per the American Academy of Paediatrics guidelines (49). A UK study by Ali and colleagues (2013) found that carers are often not provided with an interpreter and struggle to complete benefit forms, feel ignored at consultations, and are not kept up to date (47). It was also reported that carers found the health service complex and often suffered from stress and poor emotional well-being, sometimes leading to certain health needs of the person with intellectual disability remaining unmet, and carers not having the confidence to complain (47). It has been indicated that services can be improved and are preferred by people from ethnic minorities when members of staff are from the same culture as them (26,50).

People with intellectual disability also often experience barriers due to healthcare professionals' misconceptions about them and diagnostic overshadowing, whereby health problems are misattributed to the person's disability. This has been shown as a problem for people with intellectual disability accessing sexual and reproductive health services, with a lack of proactive support from professionals, despite many people being victims of sexual abuse (51). Access to such services is likely to be even more challenging for those from some religious groups or cultural backgrounds. Healthcare professionals need to be adequately trained to ensure cultural sensitivity and how to best treat and support people with intellectual disability.

Further adjustments also need to be made to encourage and promote access to services. In terms of physical accessibility, services need to account for motor impairments and musculoskeletal problems that prohibit the person from using standard equipment (52). Communication supports and intellectual disability-friendly environments are also essential (47). This should include the use of communication passports, such as the 'Grab and Go Guide', a short hospital passport designed specifically for COVID-19 (53). It is also important to educate healthcare professionals to recognize early signs of physical health problems, take observations, respond, and escalate concerns about patients (54,55). For people from ethnically diverse communities, interpreters and information printed in various languages should be available to promote effective communication and to ensure needs are met (56).

A summary of healthcare barriers and facilitators can be found in Box 2.1.

Initiatives and interventions

One of the possible reasons for the slow pace in the development of culturally sensitive care and responsiveness to cultural diversity initiatives is institutional racism (57). This refers to the systematic, yet often hard to detect, discrimination and suboptimal care for people because of their culture, ethnicity, or colour (58). Such racism has recently been further exposed through records of mortality rates during the COVID-19 pandemic, with people from Black and Asian ethnic groups being three to four times more likely to die from the virus (59). In order to address institutional racism, the Cultural Formulation Interview (60,61) has embedded the relevance of culture within the patient–clinician encounter around five dimensions, which are integrated with clinical opinion to formulate a diagnosis. The dimensions are (i) the cultural identity of the individual, (ii) the cultural explanations of the individual's illness, (iii) the cultural factors related to psychosocial environment and levels of functioning, (iv) cultural elements of the relationship between the individual and the clinicians, and (v) the overall cultural assessment for diagnosis and care. Although it is fairly long, the Cultural Formulation Interview has been called the most important contribution of anthropology to psychiatry (2,60,61).

In the UK, the '#MyGPandMe' (26,62,63) campaign focuses on informing people of reasonable adjustments that can be made to make a service accessible for someone with a disability inclusive of intellectual disability; however, the effectiveness of the initiative to improve care for ethnically marginalized groups is unclear. Other research has indicated that four factors influence culturally sensitive care: patient factors, parent factors, professional factors, and institutional resources (40,64,65). Adjustments that can assist healthcare delivery to people with intellectual disabilities and their families from ethnically diverse

Box 2.1 Barriers and facilitators to access healthcare by patients with intellectual disability from diverse backgrounds

Barriers

- Comprehension of the majority language.
- Unvalidated diagnostic tools across languages and across degrees of intellectual disability.
- Insufficient time.
- Conflict between staff and families/service users in relation to decision-making.
- Diagnostic overshadowing.
- Healthcare professionals inadequately trained in transcultural healthcare.
- Culture not supportive of supported decision-making or positive behaviour support.

Facilitators

- Reasonable adjustments.
- 'Grab and Go guide'—a COVID-19-specific short hospital passport (53).
- Educating healthcare professionals working in care/nursing homes on recognizing early soft signs, responding, and escalating concerns (54,55).
- Educating healthcare professionals on diagnostic overshadowing.
- Employing healthcare professionals from diverse cultural backgrounds.
- Employing interpreters and advocates.
- Employing an accessible information officer to create easy-read literature.
- Communication supports such as objects of reference, picture association cards, modified sign language, and Makaton.
- Intellectual disability-friendly environment, such as low sensory stimulation, being ramp accessible, and a clock with large font numbers.
- Diagnostic tools validated in people with varying degrees of intellectual disability.

groups need to take into account the communication barriers and adopt pro-grammes that increase professional awareness of the disease patterns in people with intellectual disabilities.

There are also further UK policy initiatives that aim to improve access to healthcare for people with intellectual disability. These include the policy re-sponses to the LeDeR programme which have recommended mandatory intellectual disability awareness training, greater health and social care coord-ination, improving uptake of vaccinations, and a focus on care pathways sup-ported by the NHS Rightcare programme on the prevention and treatment of sepsis, pneumonia, and aspiration pneumonia in patients who have dysphagia (66–72).

The Annual Health Check that is known to reduce morbidity in people with intellectual disability is another nationwide intervention in England that fa-cilitates early identification and treatment of unmet health needs (15,25,26). Similarly, the ongoing national project 'Stopping over medication of people with a learning disability, autism or both' (STOMP) could reduce cardiovas-cular mortality due to inappropriate prescription of antipsychotic medication (73,74).

Fundamental constituents to achieving cultural competency are education of healthcare professionals, non-judgemental environments, effective com-munication, and advocacy. Of these four, communication is often substandard as many people with intellectual disability may need additional support to get their views across. The ACCESS model (57,75) has been deemed an effective framework to implement transcultural healthcare in the UK. The acronym ACCESS stands for:

(A)ssessment.

(C)ommunication.

(C)ultural negotiation and compromise.

(E)stablishing respect and rapport.

(S)ensitivity.

(S)afety.

This model embodies delivery of culturally specific care by assessing cultural aspects of the individual's life, beliefs, and practices, encouraging his/her ex-pression, within a non-judgemental environment, understanding others' point of view, and creating a mutually respectful relationship (2). This model could also be utilized in people from ethnic minorities with intellectual disability to ensure culturally competent services that promote physical and mental well-being in this population.

Discussion

There is a wealth of literature highlighting the physical health inequalities for people with intellectual disabilities, and emerging evidence to suggest even further disparities in morbidity and mortality for people with intellectual disability from ethnic minorities (26,76). However, focus in this area is only just emerging and further research is warranted to investigate the extent of health problems, risk factors, and service use in ethnically diverse communities. Access to healthcare may be inhibited by beliefs and perceptions of health, discrimination, lack of cultural or religious sensitivity within services, and community stigma (56,77,78).

Comorbidity of multiple long-term conditions and their impact on mortality are commonly reported in people with intellectual disability; however, little is known about multimorbidity in relation to ethnic background (11,25). Hence, the needs and comorbidities associated with people with intellectual disabilities from ethnically diverse backgrounds should be addressed as a priority.

NCDs can be prevented through the adoption of targeted and specific lifestyle interventions and the current barriers that exist which prevent people with intellectual disability from accessing healthcare can be overcome through more sensitive and transcultural healthcare. Several initiatives are already in place to address these concerns; however, more time is required to determine their effectiveness. More ambitious population-level approaches (e.g. specially tailored health promotion strategies, prevention programmes, or training to improve quality of care for people with intellectual disabilities across health and social care settings) should be considered regardless of their costs and challenges (40,42).

Future research directions

There are a number of ideas which could be explored in future research if services are to address health inequalities and mortality disparities in people with intellectual disability. Some of these potential projects have been briefly discussed below (see also Box 2.2).

People with intellectual disabilities, and particularly those from ethnic minority groups, are more likely to live in deprived areas and have limited opportunities for paid employment (79). Deprivation, as a social determinant of health, may disadvantage people with intellectual disabilities and is already known to be a key risk factor for premature mortality in the general population (80,81). A study by Tyrer et al. (25) was unable to identify an association between deprivation and higher mortality in people with intellectual disabilities. However, this finding may be explained by the study's small sample size and/

Box 2.2 Future research directions

- ◆ International multicentre studies to capture potential differences in health inequalities and mortality to tackle causes and predictors across various cultural and ethnic backgrounds.

- ◆ Research on the impact of COVID-19 on exacerbating the mortality disparities to develop preventative strategies on a global scale for similar events in future.

- ◆ Studies on potential benefits of artificial intelligence and digital technologies in reducing the rate of multiple long-term conditions and premature mortality.

- ◆ More research on the impact of socioeconomic disadvantages and deprivation on the premature mortality of people with intellectual disability.

or the use of a deprivation measure designed for the general population that may not be robust enough to capture deprivation in people with intellectual disabilities. The correlation between deprivation and health outcome may also be lower for people living in care homes or those who travel to access healthcare services in more affluent rural areas (82). Hence, area-based socioeconomic indicators might not be appropriate predictors of comorbidities in people with intellectual disabilities. This highlights an area requiring further research as findings related to socioeconomic factors such as deprivation will have significant implications for the development of targeted interventions to reduce health inequalities and mortality in the most vulnerable postcode areas (83,84).

Data shows that COVID-19 has had a devastating impact on people with intellectual disabilities with an increased risk of premature mortality compared to the general population (85). This is likely due to an increased risk of transmission, increased rate of known risk factors, and lack of enough testing and vaccination opportunities (86–88). Public Health England have also reported a disproportionately higher death rate in people with intellectual disabilities from ethnic minority backgrounds in the UK (85). It is essential that further national and international research is conducted using routine data and patient-reported outcomes. Adapted interventions will also be needed to ensure inequalities that have always existed but have been further exposed by the COVID-19 pandemic are finally addressed.

Though still in its infancy, another emerging research direction is the use of artificial intelligence to analyse big-scale data collated by digital and mobile sensors. This will no doubt have a significant impact on prevention and reduction of multiple long-term conditions and, as a result, help to combat premature mortality in people with intellectual disability. Health promotion strategies, especially those utilizing digital technologies and online and educational programmes, must be adjusted for people with intellectual disability and backed up by evidence-based interventions that are easily accessible and appropriate (89,90).

All major studies published on mortality in people with intellectual disability originate from high-income countries (15). An internationally coordinated effort is required to support a culture of research collaboration between high-income countries and low- and middle-income countries to identify and tackle the causes and predictors of mortality globally and across different ethnic and cultural backgrounds.

Conclusion

It is evident there are many remaining gaps in our understanding of the health and care needs of people with intellectual disability, and even more so for those from Black, Asian, and minority ethnic backgrounds. People with intellectual disability and their families experience challenges navigating health and social care services to seek support, and it is likely that cultural misconceptions and institutionalized racism further hinder appropriate diagnosis and treatment of physical and mental health problems. Furthermore, there is limited available information on the health patterns relating to particular ethnic minority populations and the extent that service users are able to access screening, treatment, or other preventative measures. In order to make service access truly equitable, further research is needed to examine how physically, culturally, and financially accessible services currently are for people with intellectual disability, with a specific focus on those from ethnic minorities. Finally, given the mortality gap does not appear to be decreasing, a more collective response may be needed to implement both population and individual-level prevention approaches to tackle the continuing health inequalities and mortality disparities in people with intellectual disability.

References

1. **Emerson E, Hatton C.** The health of people with intellectual disabilities. In: Health Inequalities and People with Intellectual Disabilities. Cambridge: Cambridge University Press; 2013: 1–10.
2. **Crotty G, Doody O.** Transcultural care and individuals with an intellectual disability. Journal of Intellectual Disabilities 2016;20(4):386–96.

3. **Ouellette-Kuntz H, Minnes P, Garcin N, Martin C, Lewis MES, Holden JJA.** Addressing health disparities through promoting equity for individuals with intellectual disability. Canadian Journal of Public Health 2005;**96**(Suppl 2):S8–22.

4. **Haihambo C, Lightfoot E.** Cultural beliefs regarding people with disabilities in Namibia: implications for the inclusion of people with disabilities. International Journal of Special Education 2010;**25**(3):76–87.

5. **Mostert M.** Stigma as barrier to the implementation of the convention on the rights of persons with disabilities in Africa. African Disability Rights Yearbook 2016;**4**:3–24.

6. **Rohwerder B.** Disability stigma in developing countries. Institute of Development Studies; 2018. Available from: https://assets.publishing.service.gov.uk/media/5b18fe324 0f0b634aec30791/Disability_stigma_in_developing_countries.pdf

7. **McKenzie JA.** Models of intellectual disability: towards a perspective of (poss)ability. Journal of Intellectual Disability Research 2013;**57**(4):370–9.

8. **World Health Organization.** Noncommunicable diseases. 2021. Available from: https://www.who.int/news-room/fact-sheets/detail/noncommunicable-diseases

9. **World Health Organization.** Noncommunicable diseases (NCDs) and mental health: challenges and solutions. 2021. Available from: https://www.who.int/nmh/publi cations/ncd-infographic-2014.pdf?ua=1

10. **Eyowas FA, Schneider M, Yirdaw BA, Getahun FA.** Multimorbidity of chronic non-communicable diseases and its models of care in low- and middle-income countries: a scoping review protocol. BMJ Open 2019;**9**(10):e033320.

11. **Hanlon P, MacDonald S, Wood K, Allan L, Cooper S-A.** Long-term condition management in adults with intellectual disability in primary care: a systematic review. BJGP Open 2018;**2**(1):bjgpopen18X101445.

12. **Hithersay R, Startin CM, Hamburg S, Mok KY, Hardy J, Fisher EMC, et al.** Association of dementia with mortality among adults with Down syndrome older than 35 years. JAMA Neurology 2019;**76**(2):152–60.

13. **Amiet C, Gourfinkel-An I, Bouzamondo A, Tordjman S, Baulac M, Lechat P, et al.** Epilepsy in autism is associated with intellectual disability and gender: evidence from a meta-analysis. Biological Psychiatry 2008;**64**(7):577–82.

14. **Heslop P, LeDeR Team.** Learning Disability Mortality Review (LeDeR): Action from Learning 2020–21. University of Bristol; 2021. Available from: https://www.england.nhs.uk/wp-content/uploads/2021/06/LeDeR-Action-from-learning-report-202021.pdf

15. **Tyrer F, Kiani R, Rutherford MJ.** Mortality, predictors and causes among people with intellectual disabilities: a systematic narrative review supplemented by machine learning. Journal of Intellectual & Developmental Disability 2021;**46**(2):102–14.

16. **Linehan C.** Epidemiology of intellectual disability. In: **Scheepers M, Kerr M**, editors. Seminars in the Psychiatry of Intellectual Disability. Cambridge: Cambridge University Press; 2019: 1–11.

17. **Gjertsen H.** Mental health among Sami people with intellectual disabilities. International Journal of Circumpolar Health 2019;**78**(1):1565860.

18. **Kyei EA, Dogbe J.** Perceptions of primary caregivers about causes and risk factors of cerebral palsy in Ashanti Region, Ghana. Disability, CBR & Inclusive Development 2019;**30**(2):37.

19. **Rivelli F.** A situational analysis of mental health in Somalia. 2010. Available from: https://applications.emro.who.int/dsaf/EMROPUB_2010_EN_736.pdf

20. **Samatar A.** Somali parents and their perceptions of the autism spectrum disorder diagnosis. 2016. Available from: https://sophia.stkate.edu/msw_papers/668

21. **Baxter C, Mahoney W.** Developmental disability across cultures. 2018. Available from: https://www.kidsnewtocanada.ca/mental-health/developmental-disability

22. **Heslop P, Blair P, Fleming P, Hoghton M, Marriott A, Russ L.** Confidential Inquiry into Premature Deaths of People with Learning Disabilities (CIPOLD): Final Report. CIPOLD; 2013. Available from: https://www.bristol.ac.uk/media-library/sites/cipold/migrated/documents/fullfinalreport.pdf

23. **Heslop P, Blair PS, Fleming P, Hoghton M, Marriott A, Russ L.** The Confidential Inquiry into premature deaths of people with intellectual disabilities in the UK: a population-based study. Lancet 2014;**383**(9920):889–95.

24. **Heslop P, Lauer E, Hoghton M.** Mortality in people with intellectual disabilities. Journal of Applied Research in Intellectual Disabilities 2015;**28**(5):367–72.

25. **Tyrer F, Morriss R, Kiani R, Gangadharan SK, Rutherford MJ.** Mortality disparities and deprivation among people with intellectual disabilities in England: 2000–2019. Journal of Epidemiology and Community Health 2022;**76**(2):168–74.

26. **Robertson J, Raghavan R, Emerson E, Baines S, Hatton C.** What do we know about the health and health care of people with intellectual disabilities from minority ethnic groups in the United Kingdom? A systematic review. Journal of Applied Research in Intellectual Disabilities 2019;**32**(6):1310–34.

27. **Heslop P, Byrne V, Calkin R, Pollard J, Sullivan B, Daly P,** et al. The Learning Disabilities Mortality Review (LeDeR) programme annual report 2020. University of Bristol; 2021 Available from: https://leder.nhs.uk/images/annual_reports/LeDeR-bristol-annual-report-2020.pdf

28. **Santoro SL, Esbensen AJ, Hopkin RJ, Hendershot L, Hickey F, Patterson B.** Contributions to racial disparity in mortality among children with Down syndrome. Journal of Pediatrics 2016;**174**:240–6.e1.

29. **Learning Disabilities Mortality Review.** About LeDeR. n.d. Available from: https://leder.nhs.uk/about

30. **O'Leary L, Cooper S, Hughes-McCormack L.** Early death and causes of death of people with intellectual disabilities: a systematic review. Journal of Applied Research in Intellectual Disabilities 2018;**31**(3):325–42.

31. **Tyrer F, Ling S, Bhaumik S, Gangadharan SK, Khunti K, Gray LJ,** et al. Diabetes in adults with intellectual disability: prevalence and associated demographic, lifestyle, independence and health factors. Journal of Intellectual Disability Research 2020;**64**(4):287–95.

32. **Landes SD, Turk MA, Bisesti E.** Uncertainty and the reporting of intellectual disability on death certificates: a cross-sectional study of US mortality data from 2005 to 2017. BMJ Open 2021;**11**(1):e045360.

33. **NHS England and NHS Improvement.** Learning Disability Mortality Review (LeDeR) Programme: action from learning. 2019. Available from: https://www.england.nhs.uk/wp-content/uploads/2019/05/action-from-learning.pdf

34. **Magaña S, Parish S, Morales MA, Li H, Fujiura G.** Racial and ethnic health disparities among people with intellectual and developmental disabilities. Intellectual and Developmental Disabilities 2016;**54**(3):161–72.

35. **Koshoedo SA, Paul-Ebhohimhen VA, Jepson RG, Watson MC.** Understanding the complex interplay of barriers to physical activity amongst black and minority ethnic groups in the United Kingdom: a qualitative synthesis using meta-ethnography. BMC Public Health 2015;**15**(1):643.

36. **Temple VA.** Barriers, enjoyment, and preference for physical activity among adults with intellectual disability. International Journal of Rehabilitation Research 2007;**30**(4):281–7.

37. **Smith B, Kirby N, Skinner B, Wightman L, Lucas R, Foster C.** Physical activity for general health benefits in disabled adults: summary of a rapid evidence review for the UK Chief Medical Officers' update of the physical activity guidelines. Public Health England; 2018. Available from: https://assets.publishing.service.gov.uk/government/uploads/system/uploads/attachment_data/file/748126/Physical_activity_for_general_health_benefits_in_disabled_adults.pdf

38. **Taggart L, Doherty AJ, Chauhan U, Hassiotis A.** An exploration of lifestyle/obesity programmes for adults with intellectual disabilities through a realist lens: impact of a 'context, mechanism and outcome' evaluation. Journal of Applied Research in Intellectual Disabilities 2021;**34**(2):578–93.

39. **Bergström H, Hagströmer M, Hagberg J, Elinder LS.** A multi-component universal intervention to improve diet and physical activity among adults with intellectual disabilities in community residences: a cluster randomised controlled trial. Research in Developmental Disabilities 2013;**34**(11):3847–57.

40. **Dixon Woods M, Kirk D, Agarwal S, Annandale E, Arthur T, Harvey J,** et al. Vulnerable groups and access to health care: a critical interpretive review. Report for the National Coordinating Centre for NHS Service Delivery and Organisation R&D (NCCSDO). NCCSDO; 2005. Available from: https://njl-admin.nihr.ac.uk/document/download/2027192

41. **Gulliford MC, Khoshaba B, McDermott L, Cornelius V, Ashworth M, Fuller F,** et al. Cardiovascular risk at health checks performed opportunistically or following an invitation letter. Cohort study. Journal of Public Health (Oxford, England) 2018;**40**(2):e151–6.

42. **Potter J.** Qualitative Health Research Network seminar on candidacy. University College London; 2020. Available from: https://www.ucl.ac.uk/qualitative-health-research-network/dr-jessica-potter

43. **Durà-Vilà G, Hodes M.** Ethnic factors in mental health service utilisation among people with intellectual disability in high-income countries: systematic review. Journal of Intellectual Disability Research 2012;**56**(9):827–42.

44. **Parker R, Balaratnasingam S, Roy M, Huntley J, Mageean A.** Intellectual disability in Aboriginal and Torres Strait Islander people. In: **Dudgeon P, Milroy H, Walker R,** editors. Working Together: Aboriginal and Torres Strait Islander Mental Health and Wellbeing Principles and Practices. Canberra: Commonwealth of Australia. 2014: 307–34. Available from: https://www.telethonkids.org.au/globalassets/media/documents/aboriginal-health/working-together-second-edition/working-together-aboriginal-and-wellbeing-2014.pdf

45. **Scott HM, Havercamp SM.** Race and health disparities in adults with intellectual and developmental disabilities living in the United States. Intellectual and Developmental Disabilities 2014;**52**(6):409–18.

46. **Ali A, King M, Strydom A, Hassiotis A.** Self-reported stigma and its association with socio-demographic factors and physical disability in people with intellectual disabilities: results from a cross-sectional study in England. Social Psychiatry and Psychiatric Epidemiology 2016;**51**(3):465–74.

47. **Ali A, Scior K, Ratti V, Strydom A, King M, Hassiotis A.** Discrimination and other barriers to accessing health care: perspectives of patients with mild and moderate intellectual disability and their carers. PLoS One 2013;**8**(8):e70855.

48. **Albores-Gallo L, Roldán-Ceballos O, Villarreal-Valdes G, Betanzos-Cruz BX, Santos-Sánchez C, Martínez-Jaime MM,** et al. M-CHAT Mexican version validity and reliability and some cultural considerations. ISRN Neurology 2012;**2012**:1–7.

49. **Zuckerman KE, Sinche B, Mejia A, Cobian M, Becker T, Nicolaidis C.** Latino parents' perspectives on barriers to autism diagnosis. Academic Pediatrics 2014;**14**(3):301–8.

50. **Bonell S, Ali A, Hall I, Chinn D, Patkas I.** People with intellectual disabilities in out-of-area specialist hospitals: what do families think? Journal of Applied Research in Intellectual Disabilities 2011;**24**(5):389–97.

51. **Garbutt R.** Sex and relationships for people with learning disabilities: a challenge for parents and professionals. Mental Health and Learning Disabilities Research and Practice 2008;**5**(2):266–77.

52. **Yalon-Chamovitz S.** Invisible access needs of people with intellectual disabilities: a conceptual model of practice. Intellectual and Developmental Disabilities 2009;**47**(5):395–400.

53. **National Health Service.** COVID-19 Grab and Go guide. I have a learning disability or I am autistic. To be read in conjunction with my hospital passport. 2020. Available from: https://www.england.nhs.uk/coronavirus/wp-content/uploads/sites/52/2020/03/C0381-nhs-covid-19-grab-and-go-lda-form.pdf

54. **National Health Service.** Clinical guide for front line staff to support the management of patients with a learning disability, autism or both during the COVID-19 pandemic, relevant to all clinical specialties. 2021. Available from: https://www.nice.org.uk/media/default/about/covid-19/specialty-guides/management-patients-learning-disability-autism-during-pandemic.pdf

55. **Hampshire and Isle of Wight Integrated Care Board.** Recognising Early Soft signs, Take Observations, Respond, Escalate: RESTORE-2 adult physiological observation and escalation chart. 2021. Available from: https://www.hantsiowhealthandcare.org.uk/your-health/schemes-and-projects/restore2

56. **Raghavan R, Small N.** Cultural diversity and intellectual disability. Current Opinion in Psychiatry 2004;**17**(5):371–5.

57. **Narayanasamy A.** The ACCESS model: a transcultural nursing practice framework. British Journal of Nursing 2002;**11**(9):643–55.

58. **Elias A, Paradies Y.** The costs of institutional racism and its ethical implications for healthcare. Journal of Bioethical Inquiry 2021;**18**(1):45–58.

59. **Aldridge RW, Lewer D, Katikireddi SV, Mathur R, Pathak N, Burns R,** et al. Black, Asian and Minority Ethnic groups in England are at increased risk of death from COVID-19: indirect standardisation of NHS mortality data. Wellcome Open Research 2020;**5**:88.

60. **Aggarwal NK.** The psychiatric cultural formulation: translating medical anthropology into clinical practice. Journal of Psychiatric Practice 2012;**18**(2):73–85.

61. **Lewis-Fernández R, Krishan Aggarwal N.** Culture and psychiatric diagnosis. In: **Alarcon RD,** editor. Advances in Psychosomatic Medicine. Volume 38. Basel: Karger; 2013: 15–30.

62. **Chaplin R.** Mental health services for people with intellectual disabilities. Current Opinion in Psychiatry 2011;**24**(5):372–76.

63. **Dimensions.** #MyGPandMe. 2021. Available from: https://dimensions-uk.org/dimensi ons-campaigns/mygpandme-campaign-health-inequalities/

64. **van Herwaarden A, Rommes EWM, Peters-Scheffer NC.** Providers' perspectives on factors complicating the culturally sensitive care of individuals with intellectual disabilities. Research in Developmental Disabilities 2020;**96**:103543.

65. **Heer K, Rose J, Larkin M.** The challenges of providing culturally competent care within a disability focused team. Journal of Transcultural Nursing 2016;**27**(2):109–16.

66. **Department of Health and Social Care.** The Government response to the Learning Disabilities Mortality Review (LeDeR) programme second annual report. 2018. Available from: https://assets.publishing.service.gov.uk/government/uploads/system/ uploads/attachment_data/file/739560/government-response-to-leder-programme-2nd-annual-report.pdf

67. **Department of Health and Social Care.** The Government response to the third annual Learning Disabilities Mortality Review (LeDeR) Programme report. 2020. Available from: https://assets.publishing.service.gov.uk/government/uploads/system/uploads/atta chment_data/file/865288/government-response-to-leder-third-annual-report.pdf

68. **NHS England.** NHS RightCare pathways. 2020. Available from: https://www.england. nhs.uk/rightcare/products/pathways/

69. **Epilepsy Action, SUDEP Action, Young Epilepsy.** RightCare: epilepsy toolkit: optimising a system for people living with epilepsy. 2020. Available from: https://www.england.nhs.uk/rightcare/products/pathways/epilepsy-toolkit/

70. **Perez CM, Wagner AP, Ball SL, White SR, Clare ICH, Holland AJ,** et al. Prognostic models for identifying adults with intellectual disabilities and mealtime support needs who are at greatest risk of respiratory infection and emergency hospitalisation. Journal of Intellectual Disability Research 2017;**61**(8):737–54.

71. **Robertson J.** Health checks for people with learning disabilities: a systematic review of evidence. Improving Health and Lives: Learning Disabilities Observatory. 2010. Available from: http://www.improvinghealthandlives.org.uk/uploads/doc/vid_7646_I HAL2010-04HealthChecksSystemticReview.pdf

72. **Robertson J, Hatton C, Emerson E, Baines S.** The impact of health checks for people with intellectual disabilities: an updated systematic review of evidence. Research in Developmental Disabilities 2014;**35**(10):2450–62.

73. **NHS England.** Stopping over medication of people with a learning disability, autism or both (STOMP). 2016. Available from: https://www.england.nhs.uk/learning-disabilit ies/improving-health/stomp/

74. **Correll CU, Solmi M, Veronese N, Bortolato B, Rosson S, Santonastaso P,** et al. Prevalence, incidence and mortality from cardiovascular disease in patients with pooled and specific severe mental illness: a large-scale meta-analysis of 3,211,768 patients and 113,383,368 controls. World Psychiatry 2017;**16**(2):163–80.

75. **Heer K, Rose J, Larkin M, Singhal N.** The experiences of mothers caring for a child with developmental disabilities: a cross cultural perspective. International Journal of Human Rights in Healthcare 2015;**8**(4):218–32.

76. **Krahn GL, Hammond L TA.** A cascade of disparities: health and health care access for people with intellectual disabilities. Mental Retardation and Developmental Disabilities Research Reviews 2006;**12**(1):70–82.

77. **Raghavan R, Waseem F.** Services for young people with learning disabilities and mental health needs from South Asian communities. Advances in Mental Health and Learning Disabilities 2007;**1**(3):27–31.

78. **Roberts T, Miguel Esponda G, Krupchanka D, Shidhaye R, Patel V, Rathod S.** Factors associated with health service utilisation for common mental disorders: a systematic review. BMC Psychiatry 2018;**18**(1):1–19.

79. **Public Health England.** People with learning disabilities in England 2015: main report. 2016. Available from: https://assets.publishing.service.gov.uk/government/uploads/system/uploads/attachment_data/file/613182/PWLDIE_2015_main_report_NB090517.pdf

80. **Office for National Statistics, John S.** Changing trends in mortality by national indices of deprivation, England and Wales: 2001 to 2018. Analysis of the recent changes in the trends of mortality rates in England and Wales, by deprivation (Experimental Statistics). 2020. Available from: https://www.ons.gov.uk/peoplepopulationandcommunity/birthsdeathsandmarriages/deaths/articles/changingtrendsinmortalitybynationalindicesofdeprivationenglandandwales/2001to2018

81. **Marmot M, Allen J, Boyce T, Goldblatt P, Morrison J.** Health equity in England: the Marmot Review 10 years on. Institute of Health Equity; 2020. Available from: http://www.instituteofhealthequity.org/resources-reports/marmot-review-10-years-on

82. **Local Government Association and Public Health England.** Health and wellbeing in rural areas. 2017. Available from: https://www.local.gov.uk/publications/health-and-wellbeing-rural-areas

83. **Tyrer F, Dunkley AJ, Singh J, Kristunas C, Khunti K, Bhaumik S,** et al. Multimorbidity and lifestyle factors among adults with intellectual disabilities: a cross-sectional analysis of a UK cohort. Journal of Intellectual Disability Research 2019;**63**(3):255–65.

84. **Cooper SA, McLean G, Guthrie B, McConnachie A, Mercer S, Sullivan F,** et al. Multiple physical and mental health comorbidity in adults with intellectual disabilities: population-based cross-sectional analysis. BMC Family Practice 2015;**16**:110.

85. **Glover G, Public Health England.** Deaths of people identified as having learning disabilities with COVID-19 in England in the spring of 2020. 2020. Available from: https://www.gov.uk/government/publications/covid-19-deaths-of-people-with-learning-disabilities/covid-19-deaths-of-people-identified-as-having-learning-disabilities-summary

86. **Heslop P, Byrne V, Calkin R, Huxor A, Sadoo A, Sullivan B,** et al. Deaths of people with learning disabilities from COVID-19. University of Bristol; 2020. Available from: https://www.bristol.ac.uk/media-library/sites/sps/leder/Deaths%20of%20people%20with%20learning%20disabilities%20from%20COVID-19.pdf

87. **Public Health England.** COVID-19 deaths of people identified as having learning disabilities: report. 2020. Available from: https://www.gov.uk/government/publications/

covid-19-deaths-of-people-with-learning-disabilities/covid-19-deaths-of-people-ide
ntified-as-having-learning-disabilities-summary

88. **Tromans S, Kinney M, Chester V, Alexander R, Roy A, Sander JW**, et al. Priority
concerns for people with intellectual and developmental disabilities during the COVID-
19 pandemic. BJPsych Open 2020;**6**(6):e128.

89. **Department of Health and Social Care**. Advancing our health: prevention in the
2020s—consultation document. 2019. Available from: https://www.gov.uk/government/
consultations/advancing-our-health-prevention-in-the-2020s/advancing-our-health-
prevention-in-the-2020s-consultation-document

90. **Office of Communications (Ofcom)**. Disabled users access to and use of
communication devices and services. Research summary: learning disability. 2019.
Available from: https://www.ofcom.org.uk/__data/assets/pdf_file/0026/132965/Resea
rch-summary-learning-disability.pdf

Chapter 3

Neurodevelopmental disorders in people with intellectual disability across cultures

Rohit Shankar, Mary Barrett,
John Vijay Sagar Kommu, and Asit Biswas

Introduction

Culture is a constantly evolving shared pattern of customs, ideas, and behaviours by a particular society (1). Culture refers to the characteristics passed between generations which distinguish one society from another (2). It is a dynamic, active state of being and therefore subject to change and will evolve over time. Culture can have a significant influence on health and social outcomes particularly in approaches to disability (3,4). It can affect understanding of a disability, management options, and relationships with professional caregivers (4). Perspectives on disability can hinge on the differing cultural values of social interdependence and individual autonomy. Personal and environmental factors, including culture, share a complex relationship with functional capabilities and participation (5). Some cultures emphasize social relationships rather than a person's cognitive abilities thus providing fluctuation on societal expectations of an individual's overall competence (1,6). It is important for care providers for people with neurodevelopmental conditions to be intimately aware of cross-cultural challenges which influence care delivery (7–9). This chapter provides an oversight of how different cultures can influence care and management of people with neurodevelopmental conditions. To help provide a cohesive view, some large assumptions have been made, chief among which is division of cultural models where examples are given based on the World Bank economic model of high-income countries and low- and middle-income countries (LMICs) (10).

Definitions

The major conditions of intellectual disability (ID), autism spectrum disorder (ASD), and attention deficit hyperactive disorder (ADHD) will be discussed in detail as templars for neurodevelopmental disorders.

Intellectual disability

It has been argued that ID is a legitimate culture, often lost within other defined cultures. Communication, health inequity, and challenging behaviour are key elements of this culture (11). Descriptions of ID are found across all cultures and societies throughout history, although definition, diagnosis, and treatment have changed over time. Changes occurred in parallel with the philosophical, political, and economic trends of the period but remained distinct from mental illness (12,13). Terminology continues to change, with the World Health Organization International Classification of Diseases (ICD) Working Group on the Classification of Intellectual Disabilities recommending a move to intellectual developmental disorders (IDDs) and its incorporation into the parent category of neurodevelopmental disorders (14).

Autism spectrum disorder

ASD is characterized by deficits in social communication, social interaction, and restricted repertoire of behaviours and interests (15). Over the years there has been an increase in awareness and diagnosis of ASD across the world. However, there are wide cultural variations in clinical presentation, parental beliefs, explanatory models, help seeking, processes of evaluation and diagnosis, barriers for delivery of interventions, models of intervention, and sociolegal aspects.

Attention deficit hyperactive disorder

ADHD is characterized by symptoms of inattention and/or hyperactivity and impulsivity (15). Symptoms of ADHD are first evident during the developmental period, causing functional impairments in more than one domain in life and continue into adulthood. Wide variations in the diagnosis and management rates of ADHD across cultures question the validity of the ADHD construct and hence its universal acceptance. The making of a diagnosis of ADHD is a situated process, shaped by both global standards, and local, culturally specific norms of knowledge and experience.

Diagnostic thresholds

Intellectual disability

The World Health Organization Working Group has defined IDDs as 'a group of developmental conditions characterized by significant impairment of cognitive functions, which are associated with limitations of learning, adaptive behaviour and skills' (14).

Assessment of both intellectual functioning and adaptive behaviour may be influenced by a range of factors, including sociocultural background. Adaptive functioning includes social, conceptual, and practical domains, with 'deficits resulting in failure to meet developmental and sociocultural standards for personal independence and social responsibility' (16). Sociocultural experience can also impact adaptive functioning, along with educational opportunities, socialization, and support systems (16).

Evidence supports sociocultural factors as the key feature determining what is seen as 'competent behaviour'. Within Western high-income countries, the construct of ID has been defined to meet the needs of urban, industrialized societies, with the identification of large numbers of individuals with below-average intellectual functioning coinciding with the industrial revolution and the growth of schooling. In non-industrialized societies, competence may be demonstrated through collaborative, interpersonal problem-solving skills (17).

Different communities are noted to have different tolerance levels for departure from social norms (18). It has been argued that intellectual disability is a social concept which fluctuates with the thresholds of community tolerance and is thus arbitrary (19). Thus, as the concept of 'normalcy' gets redefined, the prevalence rate will change (12). The classification of borderline intellectual functioning is a good example of these issues, being subject to changing nomenclature and status in both the *Diagnostic and Statistical Manual of Mental Disorders* (DSM) and ICD systems over time. It is now excluded from the category of ID in both systems, resulting in a still vulnerable group being excluded from specialist services in most countries. Interestingly, in the Netherlands, individuals with borderline intellectual functioning and comorbid psychiatric disorders are eligible for the same specialized mental healthcare services as people with ID; however, this is the exception rather than the rule (20).

The recognition of ID in LMICs depends on local factors, which influence interpretation of measures of intellectual and adaptive functioning. Such factors include expectations arising from educational provision and adaptive capacity (21).

Autism spectrum disorder

ASD is a complex and heterogeneous disorder presenting with varying symptoms across the range of mild to severe intensity (22). The diagnostic criteria for ASD in DSM-5 compared to DSM-IV have increased specificity but reduced sensitivity especially for adolescents, those with ID, and those who had an earlier diagnosis of Asperger syndrome or pervasive developmental disorder—not otherwise specified (23,24). DSM-5 criteria have certain advantages, namely inclusion of sensory issues, change in age of onset criterion to early childhood, removing the requirement of language delay, and allowing comorbid diagnosis like ADHD. Parental recognition of symptoms usually happens before 30 months; however, there is often a delay in diagnosis, usually based on cultural and resource issues (25–29). Recognition of autism depends on sex, ethnicity, residing areas, previous contact with ASD, and educational level of the parents (30,31).

Studies from the US have reported a delay in diagnosis for children of African American and Latin American ethnicity and those from a lower socioeconomic status (32–35). There are also reports of an increased number of children from a Caucasian background diagnosed with mild ASD compared to children from other racial backgrounds (36,37).

The tools available for screening and diagnosis are mostly developed in the Western countries and many not have been adapted to the cultural context of other countries (38). Any adaptation is mostly limited to language translation (39). A few tools have recently been developed in the LMICs and are outlined in Table 3.1 (40).

Attention deficit hyperactive disorder

The principal criteria for diagnosis of ADHD (15) include (i) the presence of five or more symptoms (in adulthood) from the inattention and/or hyperactivity domains, (ii) the symptoms must be present before the age of 12 years, and (iii) functional impairments are present in two or more areas of life. ADHD can be further categorized into three types: combined, predominantly inattentive, or predominantly hyperactivity/impulsive type.

A 10-year literature review focusing on cultural influences in the diagnosis of adult ADHD and respective societal burden found few papers focused on cultural factors influencing diagnosis (41). The review further commented that the onset, course, and outcomes of ADHD are highly heterogeneous with a wide range of clinical presentations and impairments, and these can be modified by social, cultural, and environmental factors in addition to underlying genetic and non-familial environmental aetiologies, concluding that better

Table 3.1 Autism screening tools developed in low- and middle-income countries

Tool name/ description	Country	Reference
HIVA screening tool	Iran	Samadi SA, McConkey R. Screening for autism in Iranian preschoolers: contrasting M-CHAT and a scale developed in Iran. Journal of Autism and Developmental Disorders 2015;45(9):2908–16
INCLEN diagnostic tool	India	Juneja M, Mishra D, Russell PS, Gulati S, Deshmukh V, Tudu P, et al. INCLEN Study Group. INCLEN Diagnostic Tool for Autism Spectrum Disorder (INDT-ASD): development and validation. Indian Pediatrics 2014;51(5):359–65
23-item screener	Uganda	Kakooza-Mwesige A, Ssebyala K, Karamagi C, Kiguli S, Smith K, Anderson MC et al. Adaptation of the 'ten questions' to screen for autism and other neurodevelopmental disorders in Uganda. Autism 2014;18(4):447–57
Chandigarh Autism Screening Instrument (CASI)	India	Arun P, Chavan BS. Development of a screening instrument for autism spectrum disorder: Chandigarh Autism Screening Instrument. Indian Journal of Medical Research 2018;147(4):369–75
Indian Scale for Assessment of Autism (ISAA)	India	Mukherjee SB, Malhotra MK, Aneja S, Chakraborty S, Deshpande S. Diagnostic accuracy of Indian Scale for Assessment of Autism (ISAA) in children aged 2–9 years. Indian Pediatrics 2015;52(3):212–16
Three-Item Direct Observation Screen (TIDOS)	Turkey	Oner P, Oner O, Munir K. Three-item Direct Observation Screen (TIDOS) for autism spectrum disorder. Autism 2014;18(6):733–42
Pictorial Autism Assessment Schedule (PAAS)	Sri Lanka	Perera H, Jeewandara KC, Seneviratne S, Guruge C. Culturally adapted pictorial screening tool for autism spectrum disorder: a new approach. World Journal of Clinical Pediatrics 2017;6(1):45–51

understanding of the factors that contribute to accurate diagnosis is needed for improving the low recognition of ADHD in many world regions.

Prevalence

Intellectual disability

The World Health Organization estimates the prevalence of ID to be between 1% and 3% (42). Among those with ID, mild, moderate, severe, and profound mental retardation affects about 85%, 10%, 4%, and 2% of the population, respectively (43). Although the prevalence of mild ID has declined somewhat in recent years, the prevalence of severe ID has remained the same during that time at approximately 0.3–0.5% of the population. ID is consistently found to be more common in males, with a male-to-female ratio of 2:1 (16).

It has been acknowledged that prevalence of ID cross-culturally is more difficult to estimate. In addition to differences in definition, confounders such as the effect of education, especially in studies of children, and the cultural appropriateness of intellectual quotient tests need to be considered (44). A meta-analysis of population-based studies between 1980 and 2009 (45) found estimates of prevalence varied according to income group of the country of origin, being highest in LMICs; the age-group of the study population, being higher in studies based on children/adolescents than adults; and by study design, with studies using psychological assessments or scales showing higher prevalence than those using standard diagnostic systems and disability instruments. Some variation in ID rates between groups and over time can be expected, due to factors such as antenatal and neonatal care, screening for genetic abnormalities, and socioeconomic factors such as poverty and nutrition (45). It is notable that the prevalence rates of ID in LMICs were found to be almost twice that in high-income countries (45). Explanatory factors included socioeconomic disadvantage, for example, lack of adequate antenatal screening methods may lead to proportionately higher number of births with hereditary illnesses, iodine deficiency, birth-related infections and injuries due to poor healthcare facilities, and intrauterine growth retardation (45).

Autism spectrum disorder

Globally there has been an increase in the prevalence rates of ASD over the past few decades (46). A comprehensive review of studies done until 2012 reported a wide variation in the prevalence of 0.9–11.9 per 1000 (47). The wide variation in the prevalence rates is due to differences in awareness, sample sizes, study design, assessment tools, and case definition (48). It has been reported that approximately 30% who met DSM-IV criteria for autistic disorder and other categories under pervasive developmental disorder do not meet the criteria for ASD under DSM-5 (49). However, studies after 2014 still continue to report wide variation in prevalence rates (48). The prevalence in European studies ranges from 5.2 to 17.4 per 1000 (50–53). Studies from North America have reported prevalence rates ranging from 8.7 to 16.8 per 1000 (54–58). There is a wide variability in the prevalence rates of ASD in Asian countries as reported in a recent review (59).

Attention deficit hyperactive disorder

A systematic review of 102 population-based studies of ADHD showed significant differences in the reported worldwide prevalence of adult ADHD, with estimates between 2.3% and 4.5%. It found differences could be attributed to methodological differences, specifically in the way diagnostic criteria were used and the evaluation of what constitutes impairment, suggesting cultural context contributes to variability in the estimated prevalence rates (60). The systematic review commented further that geographic location plays a limited role in the reasons for the large variability of ADHD prevalence estimates worldwide, explaining the differences by the methodological characteristics of studies.

Variations in presentation

Intellectual disability

ID is universally recognized; however, its understanding, meaning, and subsequent treatment are culturally specific (61). Literature relating to variations in presentation of ID across cultures is limited. Significantly fewer behaviour problems in people with ID in the South Asian population compared to the White population in Leicester, UK, were identified (62). It was hypothesized that the South Asian culture may be more successful in limiting adaptive behaviour problems and/or more tolerant of such problems. This is in keeping with previous reports that individuals with ID were spoken of favourably in parts of Southeast Asia and may even be offered religious roles (61). Alternatively, it could be due to increased reluctance to identify this milder group to service providers (62).

Diagnosis of mental illness in people with ID remains challenging in part because of the lack of standardized instruments and this is a developing area (63).

Autism spectrum disorder

There is a normal variation in social behaviour of children across cultures. This usually manifests in eye contact, facial expressiveness and recognition, interpretations and usage of non-verbal cues and language, types of games and objects used during play, and expression of emotions (64–66). Parents in the Western countries are more likely to recognize and report developmental delay whereas those in Asian countries are likely to report social skill deficits (67).

The symptoms of ASD across different cultures may vary in qualitative and quantitative differences, the extent to which symptoms result in clinical impairment in day-to-day functioning, and how these symptoms cluster together in broad domains (68). Studies have also reported variations in symptoms like eye contact, stereotyped behaviours, and imaginative play (69–73). A greater degree of impairment in functioning has been reported in children with ASD from Taiwan compared to those from Australia (74). Few studies have reported an increased burden of non-verbal cases and comorbid ID (75).

Attention deficit hyperactive disorder

ADHD diagnosis and treatment rates vary across countries and within countries which have multi-ethnic populations. Ethnic minorities refer to people whose ethnic origins, religious beliefs, language or cultural identity, and self-identity differs from that of the majority population in a defined geographical area (76).

In the US, possible reasons for the disparities in the diagnosis and treatment of ADHD in the Hispanic population may be partly explained by language barriers that interfere with the ability to report ADHD symptoms to the physician, degree of acculturation (less acculturated mothers may not recognize symptoms of ADHD), different developmental expectations by Hispanic mothers, or physician bias that may cause dismissal of concerns regarding ADHD symptoms in the Hispanic population (77).

Medical and biological dysfunction

Intellectual disability

Underlying cause, risk factors, and likelihood of early detection varies with the level of ID. Mild ID is less likely to be recognized before the age of 6 years and less likely to have a specific aetiology identified. Environmental and psychosocial factors are the major risk factors for mild ID; however, malnutrition and inadequate access to healthcare both play a significant role. In severe ID, a specific underlying cause, such as a genetic disorder or inborn error of metabolism, can be identified in more than 75% of cases (16).

ID has been long associated with increased morbidity and early mortality compared to the general population, with high rates of individual disorders, for example, 40% for additional mental ill-health conditions, 30% for epilepsy, and 50% for gastro-oesophageal reflux. In addition, there is now evidence of a greater multimorbidity burden at an early age (78). Medical advances have enabled people with ID to live longer but also brought new challenges, for example, a higher incidence of dementia, which will have implications for services (79).

Autism spectrum disorder

Common medical comorbidities include epilepsy, gastrointestinal disorders, mitochondrial dysfunction, immune-mediated conditions, and sleep difficulties (80,81). Comorbid medical conditions influence the clinical presentation, developmental trajectory, treatment planning, and outcomes (82).

Attention deficit hyperactive disorder

A population-based prospective nationwide Danish cohort of children with and without ADHD during the first 12 years of life identified higher prevalence of recorded diagnoses across all included chapters of medical disorders in the ICD-10, except neoplasm, with the highest relative risks for diseases of the nervous system, with episodic and paroxysmal disorders (G40–G47) being the most frequently registered category (83). A systematic review synthesized evidence from 126 studies connecting adult ADHD with somatic disease (84). The review found obesity, sleep disorders, and asthma were all documented and there was tentative evidence for an association between adult ADHD and migraine and coeliac disease.

Legal structures

Intellectual disability

'It is a mark of civilised societies to grant meaningful rights to their citizens' (85). Internationally, the Universal Declaration of Human Rights and the Convention on the Rights of Persons with Disabilities provide a moral steer to countries; however, it is an individual country's legal framework that sets out the rights enforceable for its citizens, including those with ID (85–87). The United Nations Convention on Rights of Persons with Disabilities (UNCRPD) is an international treaty which identifies the rights of people with disabilities and aims to ensure that disabled people enjoy the same human rights as everyone else and that they can participate fully in society by receiving the same opportunities as others. UNCRPD has been ratified by 174 countries (87). It has been acknowledged that people with ID continue to experience social exclusion, stigma, discrimination, and human rights violations across a wide range of low-resource settings, in particular in LMICs (88).

In most countries, laws, acts, or regulations provide the framework for both the legal rights of people with ID as well as the services they receive. Funding for these services may be provided through governmental and/or non-governmental means. Such services include interventional, educational, vocational, and social services (16).

Few studies have compared the legal aspects of service provision for people with ID across countries. One study conducted across five European countries found that the principles of normalization were embodied across the legislative frameworks of all five countries and initiatives had focused on integration into community care. However, policy and legislation tended to separate the disability aspects of people with ID from their mental health needs and the specific needs of adults with ID and additional mental health problems had not been fully addressed (89).

Autism spectrum disorder

International legal frameworks applying to ID also apply to ASD (87). In the US, various pieces of legislation ensure early identification, early intervention, special education services, prevention of discrimination, and access to social security benefits (89). Several European countries, like France, the UK, Bulgaria, Hungary, and Denmark, and Australia have specific legislations and policies for autism (91–93). Among LMICs, few have legislation. Some exceptions are India, Philippines, Thailand, Malaysia, and Singapore which have enacted legislations related to disability. Lack of comprehensive legislation and poor implementation of the existing legislation are the major challenges in many LMICs (94).

Attention deficit hyperactive disorder

ADHD is over-represented in the criminal justice system. A meta-analysis of 42 studies indicated 25.5% of the prison population in the UK met the criteria for ADHD (95). The prevalence of ADHD is fivefold higher in youth prison populations (30.1%).

Models of care

Intellectual disability

Care systems for people with ID have varied over time and between cultures. Interestingly, the historical context dating as far back as ancient Greece and Rome still has parallels in certain tribal cultures today (96,97).

Family and community responsibility for care is a theme across cultures. Family caregiving is the prevailing norm in some countries and there are a growing number of older family members who continue to provide primary care for relatives with ID well into old age (98). The importance of informal social support systems for families, including intergenerational support, in caring for children with ID has been demonstrated across cultures (99,100). The negative impact of the decline of informal networks as societies shift from a collectivist to an industrialized, modernized model has also been recognized (101).

Whole community responsibility is found in a range of societies including certain East African cultures, the American Hutterite community, and Flanders in Belgium (61,102,103). As cultures shift from collectivist towards a more in-dustrialized model, changes in provision may occur in parallel, with social care structures assuming increasing responsibility, often underpinned by legisla-tion (21).

In other societies, most commonly Western countries, the prevailing norm for many decades has been care supervised by the state, through health and social care structures. De-institutionalization and community integration has been the focus of social care policy in Western countries for several decades; however, the rate of progress varies considerably (44). Changing attitudes, public opinion, and perception are key in achieving acceptance of people with ID into local communities and can remain a challenge even after physical inte-gration has taken place (89,104).

Policies and services for people with ID in Western countries are becoming increasingly organized in accordance with an ideology that emphasizes market efficiencies, privatization, outcome orientation, and consumer responsiveness, along with individual responsibility, personal choice, and self-determination (105). Most commonly, provision is through independent or supervised living in private or public accommodation with direct support needs organized by a service provider (106–108).

Autism spectrum disorder

Models of intervention for ASD are classified broadly into two groups, biologic-ally based and educational, as outlined in Box 3.1 (109).

Recently, 'naturalistic developmental behavioural interventions' are being used with increased frequency and have been found to be effective. These are implemented in natural settings, involve shared control between child and ther-apist, utilize natural contingencies, and use a variety of behavioural strategies to teach developmentally appropriate and prerequisite skills (110).

Parent-mediated intervention models and interventions delivered by trained primary healthcare workers have been found effective in LMICs (111–115).

Attention deficit hyperactive disorder

Models of care in low-resource settings, whether in low-, middle-, or high-income countries, include assessment and screening in non-specialist psychiatric and paediatric clinics for children and psychiatric clinics for adults. Interventions are focused on use of medication for ADHD and also psychoeducational and behavioural interventions. In higher-resource settings, routine screening with confirmation of diagnosis by a skilled specialist clinician with a structured plan of treatment and monitoring is seen in addition (116).

Box 3.1 Models of intervention for autism spectrum disorder

Each of these groups is subclassified as follows:

Biologically based interventions

◆ Medication.

◆ Complementary and alternative medicine.

Educational interventions

1. Behavioural interventions:
   - Early intensive behavioural intervention (EIBI).
   - Contemporary applied behaviour analysis:
     - Pivotal response training (PRT).
     - Natural Language Paradigm (NLP).
     - Incidental teaching.
2. Developmental interventions:
   - Floor time (Developmental, Individual-differences, & Relationship-based model (DIR)).
   - Responsive teaching (RT).
   - Relationship Development Intervention (RDI).
3. Therapy-based interventions:
   - Communication focused interventions:
     - Visual strategies and visually cued instruction.
     - Manual signing.
     - The Picture Exchange Communication System (PECS).
     - Social stories.
     - Speech-generating devices.
     - Facilitated communication (FC).
     - Functional communication training (FCT).
   - Sensory-motor interventions:
     - Auditory integration training (AIT).
     - Sensory integration.

Box 3.1 Continued

4. Combined interventions:
   - The SCERTS model.
   - Treatment and Education of Autistic and related Communication Handicapped Children (TEACCH).
   - Learning Experiences—An Alternative Program for Preschoolers and Parents (LEAP).
5. Family-based interventions:
   - Family-centred positive behaviour support (PBS) programmes.
   - The Hanen programme (More than Words).

Availability and access to resources

Intellectual disability

People with ID remain among the most vulnerable members of society and often face many barriers in healthcare (11). The current key challenges, particularly for LMICs, can occur across cultures irrespective of economic status (21). Access to care for physical and mental health-related comorbidities is a key issue, with up to 94% of people with ID in rural populations having one or more unmet health needs (21). The role of psychiatrists in the care of people with ID in LMICs includes prevention, early screening, and identification of developmental delay (21). There is a need for globally agreed effective models of prevention, care, and treatment (21). Support from high-income countries to LMICs is needed, but the individual country's health system, resources, skilled personnel, and psychiatric leadership are key in facilitating change.

Worldwide, few people with ID receive treatment for comorbid mental disorders despite experiencing disproportionately high rates of mental illness. The World Psychiatric Association Presidential Action Plan 2020–2023 aims to address this and has set priorities that will affect the mental healthcare of people with ID (21). As a general principle, the development of policy and models for mental health services for people with ID must be tailored to local cultures, particularly given the influence of a society on the lives of those with ID (117).

Autism spectrum disorder

Access to diagnostic and therapeutic resources is essential for improving outcomes among children with ASD. There are significant challenges to get access to these resources on time (118). The gap for availability and access to these resources exist even in the developed countries (119).

Ethnic and socioeconomic disparities seem to influence the access to re-sources in developed countries (120). Rural communities face significant chal-lenges regarding the adequate availability of services for children diagnosed with ASD. Geographical distance, cultural beliefs, and stigma limit the access to the meagre resources. Limited access to services adversely impacts the out-comes (121).

Attention deficit hyperactive disorder

Little is known of availability of resources for children and adults with ADHD globally. Global use of ADHD medications rose threefold from 1993 through to 2003. The reported per capita gross domestic product robustly predicted use of medications for ADHD across countries (122). The US, Canada, and Australia showed significantly higher than predicted use. An electronic review covering 46 countries in Latin America concluded that children and adolescents are undertreated in Latin America and the Caribbean (123).

Societal explanatory model

Intellectual disability

ID has been subject to a wide range of explanatory causes across different cul-tures as well as within the same culture at different times (124). Spiritual causes are found across cultures as far back as the ancient world, among primitive nomadic tribes as well as early Christianity and still feature today in certain African cultures (125–127).

Many Western societies have traditionally focused on biomedical explan-ations for ID, for example, the presence of an underlying genetic, biological, or neurological disorder (16). In contrast, others see ID as a social construct, sub-ject to change according to the prevailing culturally accepted 'norms' of social interaction and behaviour. In practice, many individuals and societies now use both sociocultural and biomedical models of ID and normative development to facilitate their understanding of ID (128). In line with this, ID nursing in the UK has shifted from an illness-based model of disability to a social model, where disability is seen as a problem that exists within the environment rather than the person (129).

Autism spectrum disorder

Common medical explanatory models attribute ASD to the influence of her-editary factors, complications during pregnancy/childbirth, infections, and malnutrition (130–133). Religious models are common across all the major religious denominations across cultures (132–135). Parents can have multiple explanatory models at a given point of time and these can vary before and after diagnostic evaluation (136–138). A questionnaire to elicit explanatory models has been proposed (139).

Attention deficit hyperactive disorder

Social representation of attention deficit, hyperactivity, or impulsivity symptoms is critical in the recognition of ADHD as a disorder that may be best perceived in some communities as extremes of the dimensions of normal behaviour. When defined as a categorical disorder (DSM-5) when symptoms are extreme and give rise to meaningful impairments, diagnosis of ADHD, and interventions, including psychosocial and pharmacological, in others.

Cultural and family attitudes

Intellectual disability

Attitudes are acquired by an individual from the societal culture in which they live (140). There is recognition that ID cannot be considered separately from societal attitudes towards it (126). The frequent changes in terminology of how people with ID are referred to are an example of the stigma that the diagnosis carries. Longitudinal work on attitudes to people with ID over time is limited, although there is some suggestion of a positive shift (141). A systematic review of cross-cultural comparisons in attitudes to people with ID between 1990 and 2011 showed ongoing evidence of stigma and of lay people wanting to maintain social distance from people with ID across a range of ethnic groups (142).

A summary of the key literature on attitudes to people with ID, noted it to be predominantly Western in origin (2). The study noted principal factors affecting attitudes as being sex, formal educational experience, and previous personal experience of people with ID. Family attitudes to ID are influenced by having a family member with ID but vary across different ethnic groups (Table 3.2) (143–147).

In contrast, there is growing evidence across cultures of the negative impact of caring responsibilities for a child with ID on maternal well-being compared to a child without ID (148). Higher levels of malaise, depression, and anxiety have been reported. A study across mothers of children with ID in Ireland, Taiwan, and Jordan found consistent themes of poor maternal mental health, increased levels of child-related stress, and poorer family functioning, suggesting a common impact of having a child with ID, irrespective of culture (148).

Paradoxically, in spite of positive perceptions in certain cultures such as the Latino group, self-sacrificial caregiving behaviours could lead to the mothers becoming overextended with household and caring responsibilities and increased carer strain from less use of out-of-home placements, with this in turn causing higher level of depression and lower morale (150).

Table 3.2 Societal explanatory models

Ethnic group	Attitudes and beliefs finding
African American mothers	Perceived less carer burden and more satisfaction than Caucasian counterparts possibly due to intergenerational family support and religious connectedness
Latino mothers	More positive attitude, attribution, and acceptance towards negative behaviours than Caucasian counterparts
South-Asian parents	Religious beliefs, God's will, and destiny seen as a major influencer leading to better and resilient coping strategies

Autism spectrum disorder

The conceptualization of ASD is variable across different cultures (151). The term 'autism' is considered a 'new word' in many languages and the disorder is perceived as a condition affecting mainly White populations (152). In certain communities, the hidden nature of autism and poor awareness gives raise to misconceptions such as being considered dangerous (153). Stigma towards the children with ASD and their parents is common. Parenting stress is influenced by social support, severity of autism symptoms, financial difficulty, parents' understanding and perception towards ASD, parents' anxiety and worries about their child's future, and religious beliefs (154).

The majority of parents who recognize their children's atypical development and behaviour are anxious, uncertain, and confused (155–157). Acceptance that the child's behaviour is related to a disorder is less likely in Asian and Pacific Islander families compared to European families. Experiences of social exclusion and negative judgement even from extended family members have been reported in a meta-synthesis of studies (158). In South Korea, parents prefer to call their child a 'border child'. This substitute explanation focuses primarily on the social domain rather than on more generalized developmental problem and frames the child's symptoms as temporary difficulties rather than a long-term condition (159). Similarly, parents in Vietnam often prefer to refer to ASD as a disease rather than disorder, viewing the condition as temporary and emphasizing the possibility of a cure (160).

Attention deficit hyperactive disorder

In cross-cultural studies, major and significant differences between raters from different cultures in the way they rated symptoms of ADHD are apparent (161). Regarding the recent rise of rates of diagnosis of ADHD, a cultural perspective is necessary. In modern Western culture many factors adversely affect the mental health of children and their families. These include loss of extended family support, mother blame, pressure on schools, a breakdown of the moral authority of adults, parents being put in a double bind on the question of discipline, family life being busy and 'hyperactive', and a market economy value system that emphasizes individuality, competitiveness, and independence (162).

References

1. **Oxford English Dictionary.**
2. **Benomir AM, Nicolson RI, Beail N.** Attitudes towards people with intellectual disability in the UK and Libya: a cross-cultural comparison. Research in Developmental Disabilities 2016;**51–52**:1–9.
3. **Matsumoto D,** editor. The Handbook of Culture and Psychology. Oxford: Oxford University Press; 2001.
4. **Ravindran N, Myers BJ.** Cultural influences on perception of health, illness, and disability: a review and focus on autism. Journal of Child and Family Studies 2012;**21**(2):311–19.
5. **World Health Organization.** International Classification of Functioning, Disability and Health (ICF). n.d. Available from: https://www.who.int/classifications/international-cla ssification-of-functioning-disability-and-health
6. **Odom SL, Horner RH, Snell ME, Blacher J,** editors. Handbook of Developmental Disabilities. New York: Guilford Press; 2007.
7. **McLean M, Wolery M, Bailey DB** Jr. Assessing Infants and Preschoolers With Special Needs, 3rd edition. Upper Saddle River, NJ: Pearson Education; 2004.
8. **Summers SJ, Jones J.** Cross-cultural working in community learning disabilities services: clinical issues, dilemmas and tensions. Journal of Intellectual Disability Research 2004;**48**(Pt 7):687–94.
9. **Bernier R, Mao A, Yen J.** Psychopathology, families, and culture: autism. Child and Adolescent Psychiatric Clinics of North America 2010;**19**(4):855–67.
10. **Serajuddin U, Hamadeh N.** New World Bank country classifications by income level: 2020–2021. World Bank Blogs; 1 July 2020. Available from: https://blogs.worldb ank.org/opendata/new-world-bank-country-classifications-income-level-2020-2021
11. **Crotty G, Doody O.** Transcultural care and individuals with an intellectual disability. Journal of Intellectual Disabilities 2016;**20**(4):386–96.
12. **Manion ML, Bersani HA.** Mental retardation as a western sociological construct: a cross-cultural analysis. Disability, Handicap & Society 1987;**2**(3):231–45.
13. **Littlewood R.** Mental health and intellectual disability: culture and diversity. Journal of Intellectual Disability Research 2006;**50**(Pt 8):555–60.
14. **Salvador-Carulla L, Reed GM, Vaez-Azizi LM, Cooper SA, Martinez-Leal R, Bertelli M,** et al. Intellectual developmental disorders: towards a new name, definition and framework for 'mental retardation/intellectual disability' in ICD-11. World Psychiatry 2011;**10**(3):175–80.
15. **American Psychiatric Association.** Diagnostic and Statistical Manual of Mental Disorders, 5th edition. Arlington, VA: American Psychiatric Association; 2013.

16. **Patel DR, Cabral MD, Ho A, Merrick J.** A clinical primer on intellectual disability. Translational Pediatrics 2020;**9**(Suppl 1):S23–35.

17. **Parmenter TR.** The present, past and future of the study of intellectual disability: challenges in developing countries. Salud Publica de Mexico 2008;**50**(Suppl 2):S124–31.

18. **McCullough TL.** Reformulation of the problem of mental deficiency. American Journal of Mental Deficiency 1947;**52**:130–6.

19. **Clarke AM, Clarke ADB.** Mental Deficiency: The Changing Outlook. Glencoe, IL: Free Press; 1958.

20. **Manion ML, Bersani HA.** Mental retardation as a western sociological construct: a cross-cultural analysis disability. Handicap & Society 1987;**2**(3):231–45.

21. **Roy A, Courtenay K, Odiyoor M, Walsh P, Keane S, Biswas A,** et al. Setting priorities for people with intellectual disability/intellectual developmental disorders across the lifespan: a call to action by the World Psychiatric Association. BJPsych International 2021;**18**(3):54–7.

22. **Lai MC, Lombardo MV, Baron-Cohen S.** Autism. Lancet 2014;**383**(9920):896–910.

23. **Lord C, Bishop SL.** Recent advances in autism research as reflected in DSM-5 criteria for autism spectrum disorder. Annual Review of Clinical Psychology 2015;**11**:53–70.

24. **Huerta M, Bishop SL, Duncan A, Hus V, Lord C.** Application of DSM-5 criteria for autism spectrum disorder to three samples of children with DSM-IV diagnoses of pervasive developmental disorders. American Journal of Psychiatry 2012;**169**(10):1056–64.

25. **Daley TC.** From symptom recognition to diagnosis: children with autism in urban India. Social Science & Medicine 2004;**58**(7):1323–35.

26. **Tait K, Fung F, Hu A, Sweller N, Wang W.** Understanding Hong Kong Chinese families' experiences of an autism/ASD diagnosis. Journal of Autism and Developmental Disorders 2016;**46**(4):1164–83.

27. **Kommu JVS, Gayathri KR, Srinath S, Girimaji SC, P Seshadri S, Gopalakrishna G,** et al. Profile of two hundred children with autism spectrum disorder from a tertiary child and adolescent psychiatry centre. Asian Journal of Psychiatry 2017;**28**:51–6.

28. **Kandasamy P, Srinath S, Seshadri S, Girimaji S, Kommu J.** Lost time—need for more awareness in early intervention of autism spectrum disorder. Asian Journal of Psychiatry 2017;**25**:13–15.

29. **Ribeiro SH, Paula CS, Bordini D, Mari JJ, Caetano SC.** Barriers to early identification of autism in Brazil. Brazilian Journal of Psychiatry 2017;**39**(4):352–4.

30. **Wang J, Zhou X, Xia W, Sun C, Wu L, Wang J.** Autism awareness and attitudes towards treatment in caregivers of children aged 3–6 years in Harbin, China. Social Psychiatry and Psychiatric Epidemiology 2012;**47**(8):1301–8.

31. **Donohue MR, Childs AW, Richards M, Robins DL.** Race influences parent report of concerns about symptoms of autism spectrum disorder. Autism 2019;**23**(1):100–11.

32. **Mandell DS, Listerud J, Levy SE, Pinto-Martin JA.** Race differences in the age at diagnosis among medicaid-eligible children with autism. Journal of the American Academy of Child and Adolescent Psychiatry 2002;**41**(12):1447–53.

33. **Liptak GS, Benzoni LB, Mruzek DW, Nolan KW, Thingvoll MA, Wade CM, Fryer GE.** Disparities in diagnosis and access to health services for children with autism: data from

the National Survey of Children's Health. Journal of Developmental and Behavioral Pediatrics 2008;**29**(3):152–60.

34. Mandell DS, Wiggins LD, Carpenter LA, Daniels J, DiGuiseppi C, Durkin MS, et al. Racial/ethnic disparities in the identification of children with autism spectrum disorders. American Journal of Public Health 2009;**99**(3):493–8.

35. Thomas P, Zahorodny W, Peng B, Kim S, Jani N, Halperin W, et al. The association of autism diagnosis with socioeconomic status. Autism 2012;**16**(2):201–13.

36. Jarquin VG, Wiggins LD, Schieve LA, Van Naarden-Braun K. Racial disparities in community identification of autism spectrum disorders over time; Metropolitan Atlanta, Georgia, 2000–2006. Journal of Developmental and Behavioral Pediatrics 2011;**32**(3):179–87.

37. Baio J, Wiggins L, Christensen DL, Maenner MJ, Daniels J, Warren Z, et al. Prevalence of autism spectrum disorder among children aged 8 years—Autism and Developmental Disabilities Monitoring Network, 11 Sites, United States, 2014. Morbidity and Mortality Weekly Report. Surveillance Summaries 2018;**67**(6):1–23.

38. Durkin MS, Elsabbagh M, Barbaro J, Gladstone M, Happe F, Hoekstra RA, et al. Autism screening and diagnosis in low resource settings: challenges and opportunities to enhance research and services worldwide. Autism Research 2015;**8**(5):473–6.

39. Al Maskari TS, Melville CA, Willis DS. Systematic review: cultural adaptation and feasibility of screening for autism in non-English speaking countries. International Journal of Mental Health Systems 2018;**8**(12):22.

40. Marlow M, Servili C, Tomlinson M. A review of screening tools for the identification of autism spectrum disorders and developmental delay in infants and young children: recommendations for use in low- and middle-income countries. Autism Research 2019;**12**(2):176–99.

41. Asherson P, Akehurst R, Sandra Kooij JJ, Huss M, Beusterien K, Sasane R, et al. Under diagnosis of adult ADHD: cultural influences and societal burden. Journal of Attention Disorders Supplement 2012;**16**(5):20S–38S.

42. Raghavan R, Small N. Cultural diversity and intellectual disability. Current Opinion in Psychiatry 2004;**17**(5):371–5.

43. King BH, Toth KE, Hodapp RM, Dykens EM. Intellectual disability. In: Sadock BJ, Sadock VA, Ruiz P, editors. Comprehensive Textbook of Psychiatry, 9th edition. Philadelphia, PA: Lippincott Williams & Wilkins; 2009: 3444–74.

44. Laura A, Strydom A. Intellectual disability across cultures. Psychiatry 2009;**8**(9):355–7.

45. Maulik PK, Mascarenhas MN, Mathers CD, Dua T, Saxena S. Prevalence of intellectual disability: a meta-analysis of population-based studies. Research in Developmental Disabilities 2011;**32**(2):419–36.

46. Forborne E. Editorial: the rising prevalence of autism. Journal of Child Psychology and Psychiatry 2018;**59**(7):717–20.

47. Elsabbagh M, Divan G, Koh YJ, Kim YS, Kauchali S, Marcín C, et al. Global prevalence of autism and other pervasive developmental disorders. Autism Research 2012;**5**(3):160–79.

48. Chiarotti F, Venerosi A. Epidemiology of autism spectrum disorders: a review of worldwide prevalence estimates since 2014. Brain Sciences 2020;**10**(5):274.

49. Tsai LY, Ghaziuddin M. DSM-5 ASD moves forward into the past. Journal of Autism and Developmental Disorders 2014;**44**(2):321–30.

50. **Idring S, Lundberg M, Sturm H, Dalman C, Gumpert C, Rai D,** et al. Changes in prevalence of autism spectrum disorders in 2001–2011: findings from the Stockholm youth cohort. Journal of Autism and Developmental Disorders 2015;**45**(6):1766–73.

51. **Delobel-Ayoub M, Saemundsen E, Gissler M, Ego A, Moilanen I, Ebeling H,** et al. Prevalence of autism spectrum disorder in 7–9-year-old children in Denmark, Finland, France and Iceland: a population-based registries approach within the ASDEU Project. Journal of Autism and Developmental Disorders 2020;**50**(3):949–59.

52. **Skonieczna-Żydecka K, Gorzkowska I, Pierzak-Sominka J, Adler G.** The prevalence of autism spectrum disorders in West Pomeranian and Pomeranian Regions of Poland. Journal of Applied Research in Intellectual Disabilities 2017;**30**(2):283–9.

53. **Bachmann CJ, Gerste B, Hoffmann F.** Diagnoses of autism spectrum disorders in Germany: time trends in administrative prevalence and diagnostic stability. Autism 2018;**22**(3):283–90.

54. **Baio** et al. 2014.

55. **Ouellette-Kuntz H, Coo H, Lam M, Breitenbach MM, Hennessey PE, Jackman PD,** et al. The changing prevalence of autism in three regions of Canada. Journal of Autism and Developmental Disorders 2014;**44**(1):120–36.

56. **Fombonne E, Marcin C, Manero AC, Bruno R, Diaz C, Villalobos M,** et al. Prevalence of autism spectrum disorders in Guanajuato, Mexico: the Leon survey. Journal of Autism and Developmental Disorders 2016;**46**(5):1669–85.

57. **Diallo FB, Fombonne É, Kisely S, Rochette L, Vasiliadis HM, Vanasse A,** et al. Prevalence and correlates of autism spectrum disorders in Quebec: Prévalence et corrélats des troubles du spectre de l'autisme au Québec. Canadian Journal of Psychiatry 2018;**63**(4):231–9.

58. **Maenner MJ, Shaw KA, Baio J, Washington A, Patrick M, DiRienzo M,** et al. Prevalence of autism spectrum disorder among children aged 8 years—Autism and Developmental Disabilities Monitoring Network, 11 Sites, United States, 2016. Morbidity and Mortality Weekly Report. Surveillance Summaries 2020;**69**(4):1–12.

59. **Qiu S, Lu Y, Li Y, Shi J, Cui H, Gu Y,** et al. Prevalence of autism spectrum disorder in Asia: a systematic review and meta-analysis. Psychiatry Research 2020;**284**:112679.

60. **Polanczyj G, de Lima MS, Horta BL, Biederman J, Rohde LA.** The worldwide prevalence of ADHD: a systematic review and metaregression analysis. American Journal of Psychiatry 2007;**164**(6):942–8.

61. **Edgerton RB.** Mental retardation in non-Western societies: toward a cross-cultural perspective on incompetence. In: **Haywood HC,** editor. Socio-Cultural Aspects of Mental Retardation. New York: Appleton-Century-Crofts; 1970: 227–37.

62. **McGrother CW, Bhaumik S, Thorp CF, Watson JM, Taub NA.** Prevalence, morbidity and service need among South Asian and white adults with intellectual disability in Leicestershire, UK. Journal of Intellectual Disability Research 2002;**46**(4):299–309.

63. **Raghavan R, Small N.** Cultural diversity and intellectual disability. Current Opinion in Psychiatry 2004;**17**(5):371–5.

64. **Marsh AA, Elfenbein HA, Ambady N.** Nonverbal 'accents': cultural differences in facial expressions of emotion. Psychological Science 2003;**14**(4):373–6.

65. Carter JA, Lees JA, Murira GM, Gona J, Neville BG, Newton CR. Issues in the development of cross-cultural assessments of speech and language for children. International Journal of Language & Communication Disorders 2005;**40**(4):385–401.

66. Yuki M, Maddux WW, Masuda T. Are the windows to the soul the same in the East and West? Cultural differences in using the eyes and mouth as cues to recognize emotions in Japan and the United States. Journal of Experimental Social Psychology 2007;**43**(2):303–11.

67. Coonrod EE, Stone WL. Early concerns of parents of children with autistic and nonautistic disorders. Infants & Young Children 2004;**17**(3):258–68.

68. de Leeuw A, Happé F, Hoekstra RA. A conceptual framework for understanding the cultural and contextual factors on autism across the globe. Autism Research 2020;**13**(7):1029–50.

69. Magaña S, Smith LE. The use of the Autism Diagnostic Interview-Revised with a Latino population of adolescents and adults with autism. Journal of Autism and Developmental Disorders 2013;**43**(5):1098–105.

70. Bello-Mojeed MA, Omigbodun OO, Bakare MO, Adewuya AO. Pattern of impairments and late diagnosis of autism spectrum disorder among a sub-Saharan African clinical population of children in Nigeria. Global Mental Health 2017;**4**:e5.

71. Hoekstra RA, Girma F, Tekola B, Yenus Z. Nothing about us without us: the importance of local collaboration and engagement in the global study of autism. BJPsych International 2018;**15**(2):40–3.

72. Lillard A, Pinkham A. Pretend play and cognitive development. In: Goswami U, ed. Blackwell Handbook of Childhood Cognitive Development, 2nd edition. Oxford: Blackwell; 2011: 285–311.

73. Weisberg DS. Pretend play. Wiley Interdisciplinary Reviews. Cognitive Science 2015;**6**(3):249–61.

74. Chen YW, Bundy AC, Cordier R, Chien YL, Einfeld SL. A cross-cultural exploration of the everyday social participation of individuals with autism spectrum disorders in Australia and Taiwan: an experience sampling study. Autism 2017;**21**(2):231–41.

75. Abubakar A, Ssewanyana D, Newton CR. A systematic review of research on autism spectrum disorders in sub-Saharan Africa. Behavioural Neurology 2016;**2016**:3501910.

76. Slobodin O, Masalha R. Challenges in ADHD care for ethnic minority children: a review of current literature. Transcultural Psychiatry 2020;**57**(3):468–83.

77. Stevens J, Harman JS, Kelleher KJ. Ethnic and regional differences in primary care for attention-deficit hyperactivity disorder. Journal of Developmental and Behavioral Pediatrics 2004;**25**(5):318–25.

78. Cooper SA, McLean G, Guthrie B, McConnachie A, Mercer S, Sullivan F, et al. Multiple physical and mental health comorbidity in adults with intellectual disabilities: population-based cross-sectional analysis. BMC Family Practice 2015;**16**:110.

79. Salvador-Carulla L, Rodríguez-Blázquez C, Martorell A. Intellectual disability: an approach from the health sciences perspective. Salud Publica de Mexico 2008;**50**(Suppl 2):142–50.

80. **Muskens JB, Velders FP, Staal WG.** Medical comorbidities in children and adolescents with autism spectrum disorders and attention deficit hyperactivity disorders: a systematic review. European Child & Adolescent Psychiatry 2017;**26**(9):1093–103.

81. **Zerbo O, Leong A, Barcellos L, Bernal P, Fireman B, Croen LA.** Immune mediated conditions in autism spectrum disorders. Brain, Behavior, and Immunity 2015;**46**:232–36.

82. **Tye C, Runicles AK, Whitehouse AJO, Alvares GA.** Characterizing the interplay between autism spectrum disorder and comorbid medical conditions: an integrative review. Frontiers in Psychiatry 2019;**9**:751. [Erratum in: Frontiers in Psychiatry 2019, **27**;10:438.]

83. **Laugesen B, Lauritsen MB, Færk E, Mohr-Jensen C.** Medical disorders in a Danish cohort of children with attention-deficit hyperactivity disorder. European Child & Adolescent Psychiatry 2002;**31**(2):349–59.

84. **Instanes JT, Klungsøyr K, Halmøy A, Fasmer OB.** Adult ADHD and comorbid somatic disease. Journal of Attention Disorders 2018;**22**(3):203–28.

85. **Fyson R, Cromby J.** Human rights and intellectual disabilities in an era of 'choice'. Journal of Intellectual Disabilities Research 2013;**57**(12):1164–72.

86. **United Nations.** Universal Declaration of Human Rights. United Nations; 1948. Available from: https://www.un.org/en/about-us/universal-declaration-of-human-rights

87. **United Nations.** Convention on the Rights of Persons With Disabilities. United Nations; 2006. Available from: https://www.un.org/development/desa/disabilities/convention-on-the-rights-of-persons-with-disabilities.html

88. **Fyson R, Cromby J.** Human rights and intellectual disabilities in an era of 'choice'. Journal of Intellectual Disabilities Research 2013;**57**(12):1164–72.

89. **Holt G, Costello H, Bouras N, Diareme N, Hillery J, Moss S,** et al. BIOMED-MEROPE* project: service provision for adults with intellectual disability: a European comparison. Journal of Intellectual Disability Research 2000;**44**(6):685–96.

90. **Autism Society.** Legal resources. n.d. Available from: https://www.autism-society.org/living-with-autism/legal-resources/

91. **Della Fina V, Cera R,** editors. Protecting the Rights of People With Autism in the Fields of Education and Employment: International, European and National Perspectives. Berlin: Springer Nature; 2015.

92. **Tyler MC.** The Disability Discrimination Act 1992: genesis, drafting and prospects. Melbourne University Law Review 1993;**19**:211.

93. **Buckmaster L.** The National Disability Insurance Scheme: A Quick Guide. Canberra: Parliamentary Library; 2016.

94. **Bakare MO, Munir KM.** Autism spectrum disorders (ASD) in Africa: a perspective. African Journal of Psychiatry 2011;**14**(3):208–10.

95. **Young S, Moss D, Sedgewick O, Fridman M, Hodgkins P.** A meta-analysis of the prevalence of attention deficit hyperactivity disorder in incarcerated populations. Psychological Medicine 2015;**45**(2):247–58.

96. **Rossen M, Clark GR, KIvrrz MS,** editors. The History of Mental Retardation: Collected Papers, Vol. I. Baltimore, MD: University Park Press; 1976.

97. **Dorman SS.** Pygmies and Bushmen of the Kalahari. Cape Town: Capetown Press; 1925.

98. **Jokinen N, Gomiero T, Watchman K, Janicki MP, Hogan M, Larsen F,** et al. Perspectives on family caregiving of people aging with intellectual disability affected by dementia: commentary from the International Summit on Intellectual Disability and Dementia. Journal of Gerontological Social Work 2018;**61**(4):411–31.

99. **Cox A, Marshall E, Mandleco B, Olsen S.** Coping responses to daily life stressors of children who have a disability. Journal of Family Nursing 2003;**9**(4):397–413.

100. **Duvdevany I, Abboud S.** Stress, social support and well-being of Arab mothers of children with intellectual disability who are served by welfare services in northern Israel. Journal of Intellectual Disability Research 2003;**47**(Pt 4–5):264–72.

101. **Shin JY.** Social support for families of children with mental retardation: comparison between Korea and the United States. Mental Retardation 2002;**40**(2):103–118.

102. **Craft M.** Classification, criteria, epidemiology and causation. In: **Craft M, Bicknell J, Hollins S,** editors. A Multi-Disciplinary Approach to Mental Handicap. London: Baillière Tindall; 1985: 75–88.

103. **Foucault M.** Madness and Civilization: A History of Insanity in the Age of Reason. London: Tavistock Publications; 1971.

104. **Soder M.** Housing integration of mentally retarded persons. Epilepsia 1972;**13**(1):249–51.

105. **Swenson S.** Neoliberalism and human services: threat and innovation. Journal of Intellectual Disability Research 2008;**52**(7):626–33.

106. **Braddock D, Hemp R, Rizzolo MC.** State of the states in developmental disabilities: 2004. Mental Retardation 2011;**42**(5):356–70.

107. **Carvalho CL, Ardore M, Castro R.** Family caregivers and the aging of the person with intellectual disabilities: implications to care. Revista Kairós Gerontologia 2015;**18**(3):333–52.

108. **Tossebro J, Bonfils IS, Teittinen A, Tideman M, Traustadóttir R, Vesala HT.** Normalization fifty years beyond—current trends in the Nordic countries. Journal of Policy and Practice in Intellectual Disabilities 2012;**9**(2):134–46.

109. **Roberts J, Ridley G.** Review of the Research to Identify the Most Effective Models of Best Practice in the Management of Children With Autism Spectrum Disorders. Sydney: University of Sydney, Centre for Development Disability Studies; 2004.

110. **Schreibman L, Dawson G, Stahmer AC, Landa R, Rogers SJ, McGee GG,** et al. Naturalistic developmental behavioral interventions: empirically validated treatments for autism spectrum disorder. Journal of Autism and Developmental Disorders 2015;**45**(8):2411–28.

111. **Green J, Charman T, McConachie H, Aldred C, Slonims V, Howlin P,** et al. Parent-mediated communication-focused treatment in children with autism (PACT): a randomised controlled trial. Lancet 2010;**375**(9732):2152–60.

112. **Divan G, Hamdani SU, Vajartkar V, Minhas A, Taylor C, Aldred C,** et al. Adapting an evidence-based intervention for autism spectrum disorder for scaling up in resource-constrained settings: the development of the PASS intervention in South Asia. Global Health Action 2015;**8**:27278.

113. Rahman A, Divan G, Hamdani SU, Vajaratkar V, Taylor C, Leadbitter K, et al. Effectiveness of the parent-mediated intervention for children with autism spectrum disorder in south Asia in India and Pakistan (PASS): a randomised controlled trial. Lancet Psychiatry 2016;3(2):128–36.

114. Divan G, Vajaratkar V, Cardozo P, Huzurbazar S, Verma M, Howarth E, et al. The feasibility and effectiveness of PASS Plus, a lay health worker delivered comprehensive intervention for autism spectrum disorders: pilot RCT in a rural low and middle income country setting. Autism Research 2019;12(2):328–39.

115. Manohar H, Kandasamy P, Chandrasekaran V, Rajkumar RP. Brief parent-mediated intervention for children with autism spectrum disorder: a feasibility study from South India. Journal of Autism and Developmental Disorders 2019;49(8):3146–58.

116. Flisher AJ, Sorsdahl K, Hatherhill S, Chehil S. Packages of care for attention-deficit hyperactivity disorder in low- and middle-income countries. PLoS Medicine 2010;7(2):e1000235.

117. Emerson E, McClonkey R, NoonanWalsh P, Felce D. Editorial. Intellectual disability in a global context. Journal of Policy and Practice in Intellectual Disabilities 2008;5(2):79–80.

118. Chiri G, Warfield ME. Unmet need and problems accessing core health care services for children with autism spectrum disorder. Maternal and Child Health Journal 2012;16(5):1081–91.

119. Ning M, Daniels J, Schwartz J, Dunlap K, Washington P, Kalantarian H, et al. Identification and quantification of gaps in access to autism resources in the United States: an infodemiological study. Journal of Medical Internet Research 2019;21(7):e13094.

120. Durkin MS, Maenner MJ, Meaney FJ, Levy SE, DiGuiseppi C, Nicholas JS, et al. Socioeconomic inequality in the prevalence of autism spectrum disorder: evidence from a US cross-sectional study. PloS One 2010;5(7):e11551.

121. Antezana L, Scarpa A, Valdespino A, Albright J, Richey JA. Rural trends in diagnosis and services for autism spectrum disorder. Frontiers in Psychology 2017;20(8):590.

122. Scheffler RM, Hinshaw SP, Modrek S, Levine P. The global market for ADHD medications. Health Affairs 2007;26(2):450–7.

123. Polanczyk G, Rohde LA, Szobot C, Schmitz M, Montiel-Nava C, Bauermeister JJ. ADHD treatment in Latin America and the Caribbean. Journal of the American Academy of Child and Adolescent Psychiatry 2008;47(6):721–2.

124. Manion ML, Bersani HA. Mental retardation as a western sociological construct: a cross-cultural analysis. Disability, Handicap & Society 1987;2(3):231–45.

125. Hughes J. Some selected attitudes to mental retardation in developed and developing countries. Teaching and Training 1983;21:9–18.

126. Hassiotis A. Clinical examples of cross-cultural work in a community learning disability service. International Journal of Social Psychiatry 1996;42(4):318–27.

127. Kromberg J, Zwane E, Manga P, et al. Intellectual disability in the context of a South African population. Journal of Policy and Practice in Intellectual Disabilities 2008;5:89–95.

128. **Skinner D, Weisner T.** Sociocultural studies of families of children with intellectual disabilities. Journal of Mental Retardation and Developmental Disabilities Research Reviews 2007;**13**(2):302–12.

129. **Doody O, Doody CM.** Intellectual disability nursing and transcultural care. British Journal of Nursing 2012;**21**(3):174–80.

130. **Gona JK, Newton CR, Rimba K, Mapenzi R, Kihara M, Van de Vijver FJ**, et al. Parents' and professionals' perceptions on causes and treatment options for autism spectrum disorders (ASD) in a multicultural context on the Kenyan Coast. PLoS One 2015;**10**(8):e0132729.

131. **Al-Dababneh KA, Al-Zboon EK, Baibers H.** Jordanian parents' beliefs about the causes of disability and the progress of their children with disabilities: insights on mainstream schools and segregated centres. European Journal of Special Needs Education 2017;**32**(3):362–76.

132. **Tilahun D, Hanlon C, Fekadu A, Tekola B, Baheretibeb Y**, Hoekstra RA. Stigma, explanatory models and unmet needs of caregivers of children with developmental disorders in a low-income African country: a cross-sectional facility-based survey. BMC Health Services Research 2016;**16**:152.

133. **Heys M, Alexander A, Medeiros E, Tumbahangphe KM, Gibbons F, Shrestha R,** et al. Understanding parents' and professionals' knowledge and awareness of autism in Nepal. Autism 2017;**21**(4):436–49.

134. **Shaked M, Bilu Y.** Grappling with affliction: autism in the Jewish ultraorthodox community in Israel. Culture, Medicine and Psychiatry 2006;**30**(1):1–27.

135. **Minhas A, Vajaratkar V, Divan G, Hamdani SU, Leadbitter K, Taylor C,** et al. Parents' perspectives on care of children with autistic spectrum disorder in South Asia—views from Pakistan and India. International Review of Psychiatry 2015;**27**(3):247–56.

136. **Shyu YI, Tsai JL, Tsai WC.** Explaining and selecting treatments for autism: parental explanatory models in Taiwan. Journal of Autism and Developmental Disorders 2010;**40**(11):1323–31.

137. **Ravindran N, Myers BJ.** Beliefs and practices regarding autism in Indian families now settled abroad: an internet survey. Focus on Autism and Other Developmental Disabilities 2013;**28**(1):44–53.

138. **Zakirova-Engstrand R, Hirvikoski T, Westling Allodi M, Roll-Pettersson L.** Culturally diverse families of young children with ASD in Sweden: parental explanatory models. PLoS One 2020;**15**(7):e0236329.

139. **Levy SE, Mandell DS, Merhar S, Ittenbach RF, Pinto-Martin JA.** Use of complementary and alternative medicine among children recently diagnosed with autistic spectrum disorder. Journal of Developmental and Behavioral Pediatrics 2003;**24**(6):418–23.

140. **Raven BH, Rubin JZ.** Social Psychology, 2nd edition. New York: John Wiley & Sons; 1983.

141. **Rees LM, Spreen O, Harnadek M.** Do attitudes towards persons with handicaps really shift over time? Comparison between 1975 and 1988. Mental Retardation 1991;**29**:81–6.

142. **Scior K.** Public awareness, attitudes and beliefs regarding intellectual disability: a systematic review. Research in Developmental Disabilities 2011;**32**(6):2164–82.

143. **Valentine D, McDermott S, Anderson D.** Mothers of adults with mental retardation: is race a factor in perceptions of burdens and gratifications? Families in Society 1998;**79**:577–84.

144. **Blacher J, Baker BL.** Positive impact of intellectual disability on families. American Journal of Mental Retardation: AJMR 2007;**112**(5):330–48.

145. **Blacher J, Begum GF, Marcoulides GA, Baker BL.** Longitudinal perspectives of child positive impact on families: relationship to disability and culture. American Journal on Intellectual and Developmental Disabilities 2013;**118**(2):141–55.

146. **Bywaters P, Ali Z, Fazil Q, Wallace LM, Singh G.** Attitudes towards disability amongst Pakistani and Bangladeshi parents of disabled children in the UK: considerations for service providers and the disability movement. Health & Social Care in the Community 2003;**11**(6):502–9.

147. **Gabel S.** South Asian Indian cultural orientations toward mental retardation. Mental Retardation 2004;**42**(1):12–25.

148. **Blacher J, Baker BL.** Positive impact of intellectual disability on families. American Journal of Mental Retardation 2007;**112**(5):330–48.

149. **McConkey R, Truesdale-Kennedy M, Chang M, Jarrah S, Shukri R.** The impact on mothers of bringing up a child with intellectual disabilities: a cross-cultural study. International Journal of Nursing Studies 2008;**45**(1):65–74.

150. **Blacher J, McIntyre LL.** Syndrome specificity and behavioural disorders in young adults with intellectual disability: cultural differences in family impact. Journal of Intellectual Disability Research 2006;**50**(Pt 3):184–98.

151. **Kim HU.** Autism across cultures: rethinking autism. Disability & Society 2012;**27**(4):535–45.

152. **Fox F, Aabe N, Turner K, Redwood S, Rai D.** 'It was like walking without knowing where I was going': a qualitative study of autism in a UK Somali migrant community. Journal of Autism and Developmental Disorders 2017;**47**(2):305–15.

153. **Burkett K, Morris E, Manning-Courtney P, Anthony J, Shambley-Ebron D.** African American families on autism diagnosis and treatment: the influence of culture. Journal of Autism and Developmental Disorders 2015;**45**(10):3244–54.

154. **Ilias K, Cornish K, Kummar AS, Park MS, Golden KJ.** Parenting stress and resilience in parents of children with autism spectrum disorder (ASD) in Southeast Asia: a systematic review. Frontiers in Psychology 2018;**9**:280.

155. **Chao KY, Chang HL, Chin WC, Li HM, Chen SH.** How Taiwanese parents of children with autism spectrum disorder experience the process of obtaining a diagnosis: a descriptive phenomenological analysis. Autism 2018;**22**(4):388–400.

156. **Desai MU, Divan G, Wertz FJ, Patel V.** The discovery of autism: Indian parents' experiences of caring for their child with an autism spectrum disorder. Transcultural Psychiatry 2012;**49**(3–4):613–37.

157. **Shu BC, Hsieh HC, Hsieh SC, Li SM.** Toward an understanding of mothering: the care giving process of mothers with autistic children. Journal of Nursing Research 2001;**9**(5):203–13.

158. **Ooi KL, Ong YS, Jacob SA, Khan TM.** A meta-synthesis on parenting a child with autism. Neuropsychiatric Disease and Treatment 2016;**12**:745–62.

159. **Grinker RR, Chambers N, Njongwe N, Lagman AE, Guthrie W, Stronach S**, et al. 'Communities' in community engagement: lessons learned from autism research in South Korea and South Africa. Autism Research 2012;**5**(3):201–10.

160. **Ha VS, Whittaker A, Whittaker M, Rodger S.** Living with autism spectrum disorder in Hanoi, Vietnam. Social Science & Medicine 2014;**120**:278–85.

161. **Timimi S, Taylor E.** ADHD is best understood as a cultural construct. British Journal of Psychiatry 2004;**184**(1):8–9.

162. **James A, Prout A,** editors. Constructing and Reconstructing Childhood: Contemporary Issues in the Sociological Study of Childhood, 3rd edition. London: Routledge; 2015.

Chapter 4

Mental health in intellectual disability across cultures

Jane McCarthy, Manji Daffi, Amala Jesu, and Michael McPartland

Introduction

People with intellectual disability (ID) have been recognized for many decades to be vulnerable to mental ill-health relative to their non-ID peers, due to an increased risk of a number of biological, psychological, and social factors (1). To date, the worldwide research has focused on prevalence rates and presentation of psychiatric disorders in people with ID. The presentation of psychiatric disorders in people with ID varies with severity of the intellectual impairment. More recent research has looked at aetiological factors (2) and the overlap with other neurodevelopmental conditions such as attention deficit hyperactivity disorder (ADHD) (3) and autism (4). This chapter will focus on prevalence and presentation of mental health conditions across different cultures and countries for people with ID. However, the evidence base is limited, even in European countries, so we have provided details only on countries in which evidence is reported.

Prevalence across cultures

Prevalence of intellectual disability

This topic has been dealt with in some detail in Chapter 1 of this book. We revisit some of the key points here. A meta-analysis by Maulik et al. (5) of studies published between 1980 and 2009 reported an overall prevalence of ID of 1.04% (10.37/1000 population) across the world. Changes in diagnostic practices, population characteristics, and exposure to known risk factors in recent years have placed this estimate in question, and led to the re-examination of prevalence, indicating the rates to be slightly higher. A systematic review in 2016 (6), while finding considerable heterogeneity in study settings, methodologies, age groups, and case definitions, reported a prevalence range of 0.05–1.55%. There were only two studies on incidence with one reporting a cumulative incidence to age 50 of 1.58% for males and 0.96% for females (7) and the other, where individuals were followed to a median of 14 years, reporting an incidence rate of 4.6 per 10,000 person-years (person-years is the sum of the number of years each individual contributed to the study) (8).

Despite large numbers of individuals with ID residing in low- and middle-income countries, population-based studies and reliable measures to identify people with ID are extremely limited, and therefore true prevalence estimates are difficult to obtain. Studies have suggested prevalence rates ranging from 0.09% to 18.3% (9) in low- and middle-income countries which are spread across Asia, Africa, Eastern Europe, and Latin America. More recently, there have been studies examining the age-adjusted prevalence of ID in rural and urban populations in India and its correlation with age in children and adults (10). They reported an overall prevalence of 1.05% (10.5/1000) in ID with higher rates in urban areas. The results of this study matched findings of the meta-analysis by Maulik and colleagues in 2011 (5).

Prevalence of psychiatric disorders

Studies on the prevalence of psychiatric disorders in adults with ID vary in rates for a number of reasons, including which study population is reported on; for example, a community-based sample, a clinic sample, including a defined geographical location, or which diagnostic tools were used, which may not be appropriate across all cultures. The trend over the past 25 years is to use validated diagnostic tools with trained professionals in studies of prevalence rates, which have improved the reliability of the findings (11). However, there has been very little research on evaluating the cross-cultural validity of diagnostic tools in people with ID, with the limited evidence indicating a variation in ratings across countries (12). Much of the data on prevalence rates comes from Europe and mainly the UK. Most reported studies to date are from ethnically homogeneous populations.

The past 20 years have seen the development of specific diagnostic systems such as the Diagnostic Criteria for Psychiatric Disorders for Use with Adults with Learning Disabilities (DC-LD) from the UK (13) and the *Diagnostic Manual—Intellectual Disability 2* (DM-ID-2) in North America (14), which have aided the understanding of how the presentation of psychiatric disorders may differ in people across the range of ID. The presentation of psychiatric disorders, especially of adults with severe ID, is very much dependent on third-party reports of the observed behaviours. DC-LD is adapted from the tenth revision of the International Classification of Diseases (ICD-10), so is more widely used in Europe, and DM-ID-2 is based on the fifth edition of the

Diagnostic and Statistical Manual of Mental Disorders (DSM-5) (15) which is the predominant diagnostic classification system used in North America. DC-LD includes challenging behaviour as mental disorders, whereas DSM does not, so this may impact reported rates of mental disorder.

A recent systematic review of prevalence of psychiatric disorders in adults with ID from 2003 to 2010 (16) examined 16 studies, reporting rates from 13.9% to 75.2%. This wide variation in reported prevalence rates was in part determined by the nature of the population samples enrolled in the constituent studies and also how diagnostic criteria were utilized. Of the 16 studies, ten were population based with six from Cooper and colleagues at the University of Glasgow in Scotland. These six studies based in Scotland included participants who were predominantly Caucasian (94.6%). These studies included those within a borderline range of intellectual functioning, and they may well be not representative of those with a clear diagnosis of ID.

The systematic review found no published work on prevalence rates in adult samples from either North or South America. There was a paucity of data on the cultural and linguistic variables of the participants in their presentation of coexisting psychiatric disorders.

Mental health, intellectual disability, and culture

United Kingdom

The UK population is 67.1 million according to the 2020 mid-year population estimates release (17). The following is the breakdown of the ethnic make-up in England and Wales from the 2021 census: White 81.7%; Asian, Asian British, Asian Welsh 9.3%; Black, Black British, Black Welsh, Caribbean or African 4%; mixed or multiple ethnic groups 2.9%, and other ethnic groups 2.1% (18). It has been recognized for some time that the prevalence of ID in non-White groups is likely to be at least as high as that in White groups (19). The UK has comprehensive health cover provided by the National Health Service, and some parts of the UK have established learning disability registers. Even in countries such as the UK with established health services there is under-recognition of mental health problems in people with ID. It has been recognized for nearly 40 years that the complexity of co-occurring conditions, communication deficits, and a lack of standardized assessment and diagnosis can lead to failure in the detection of mental disorder, which is compounded by diagnostic overshadowing (20) where presenting symptoms are attributed to the ID rather than a possible emerging and treatable mental or physical illness.

Studies have found that people with ID have higher rates of symptoms of common mental health problems (25%) compared to those with average

(17.2%) or above-average (13.4%) intellectual functioning (21). There is also a higher risk of mental health problems in children with an ID (22). The higher prevalence of mental health problems increases morbidity and mortality in this vulnerable group. Lifetime prevalence of mental illness in ID is 49.2% (2) and there is a two to three times higher prevalence of schizophrenia in people with ID (23). Similarly, in people with Down syndrome, the prevalence of dementia is much higher than general population (24). There are also high rates of associated developmental conditions such as autism and ADHD (25). Sheehan et al. (26) found that 21% of people with ID had a diagnosis of mental illness from studying their primary care records. As discussed previously, variations in prevalence rates are often attributed to the differences in the population studied, the diagnostic criteria used, and the diagnostic process.

Studies have found lower rates of schizophrenia diagnosis in people with ID of White ethnicity compared to other ethnic groups, but higher rates of diagnosis with personality disorder (27). A later study from South London of new referrals of adults with ID to a specialist mental health service also found that schizophrenia disorder was more likely in the Black group and other non-White groups (28). There is a higher rate of dementia in the White (4.2%) than in the Black (0.8%) or other non-White (0%) groups, which can be attributed to the demographics of the population with both the Black and other non-White groups being more likely to be younger than other ethnic groups. Another study based on data from a learning disability register found that those from ethnic minority communities (mainly South Asian) were less likely to have a clinical diagnosis of mental illness based on a psychiatric assessment than those in the White population (21.4% vs 35.4%) (29). This may be because the person with ID and their families are less likely to access psychiatric services. South Asian 16–19-year-olds with ID were less likely to be identified by family carers as having mental health problems and/or challenging behaviours (29%) than White people (63%), whereas the prevalence of other reported health problems was similar (30). For adults with ID living with family members, South Asian carers were less likely to report that the person they were caring for showed psychological symptoms of irrational fears or anxiousness (South Asian 9% vs White 16%, $p < 0.001$) (31).

People with ID from minority ethnic communities in the UK also experience significant inequalities in access to healthcare. A study in South London found that Black or Black British services users with ID using a Delphi consultation were less positive about a range of experiences in using mental health services compared to White British service users (32). The healthcare that is offered may be culturally inappropriate, unwelcoming, and discriminatory, with a culture-blaming attitude. Services may also have poor standards of communication and offer poor quality of care. Therefore, a person with an ID coming from a minority ethnic background is often put at a double disadvantage (33).

Other European countries

Like the UK, most of the other European countries have moved away from institutional models of care for people with ID and there has been greater emphasis on integration with community and normalization for people with ID. The BIOMED-MEROPE project (34) looked at service provision for adults with ID across five European countries. It identified significant gaps in services for people with ID and mental health needs being largely ignored in this population. There is also huge variation in how services for people with ID are organized and delivered between countries. There is often a separation between the disability needs and mental health needs by policymakers, which in turn makes the identification of mental health problems a challenge. In Poland, there is no specialist mental health services for people with ID and non-governmental organizations play a major role in the care of people with ID (35). The MEMENTA ('Mental healthcare provision for adults with intellectual disability and a mental disorder') study (36) has looked into the issue of the lack of services in Germany. There is growing agreement across Germany that mental healthcare for adults with ID and mental ill health has to be improved. Challenges, however, prevail due to the lack of robust scientific studies looking at the extent of mental health problems in ID. There is a paucity of evidence around cultural variation within the ID population across Europe.

Asia

Asia is the largest continent in the world, both in area and population, with over 4.75 billion people, or the equivalent of just under 60% of the world's population (37). Despite this vastness in size and population, there is a paucity of studies on ID in Asia (38,39). The prevalence of ID across Asia appears to be consistent with Western estimates at 0.06–1.3%, with the exception being China at 6.68% (this has to be interpreted with caution and could be secondary to the sample of study population) (40). Given the notable relationship between poverty and ID (41), the low reported prevalence rates in low-income countries, such as Nepal (0.06%) and Pakistan (0.09%), is surprising. Furthermore, one has to take into account the possibility of under-reporting, given the widespread stigma (42,43) and discrimination (41,44) associated with people with disability and their families in Asian cultures.

In the only two studies of mental health problems in ID conducted in Asia, the prevalence varied widely from 4.4% (45) to 48.3% (46). All Asian countries/territories have at least one law or policy that promotes the well-being of people with disabilities, with Japan being the only country that has a law spe-cifically enacted for people with ID. There is significant variation in the avail-ability of services across different Asian countries. Overall, there is a need for more robust epidemiological studies in order to develop the local knowledge and improve standards of care. Nonetheless, one must acknowledge that Asia is a diverse mix of countries with variable economic and political systems and understanding of ID is unlikely to have developed homogeneously throughout the region.

Asia: India

India has 17.5% of the world's population and the largest proportion of the world's population of children (47,48). The burden of chronic and infectious diseases, poverty, poor sanitation, poor access to healthcare, rapidly growing population, pollution, and exposure to harmful chemicals increase the risk of ID in the nation (49,50). Prevalence estimates of ID in India are often difficult to obtain due to the lack of robust population-based studies. There is signifi-cant variation in the reported prevalence of ID, ranging from 1.0% to 3.2% de-pending on the study method and study population (51). Variation can also be attributed to age, sex, population type, and place of residence (e.g. urban vs rural dwellings). Some of these factors have an impact on the level of awareness of ID and access to appropriate services where available (10).

The introduction of Person with Disabilities Act in 1996 (52) has provided impetus to improve the provision of basic facilities for individuals with ID, with a focus on education and early intervention services for children and young adults with ID. Mental health problems are often a hidden co-occurring condi-tion in people with ID and not studied often. There is a lack of culture-specific diagnostic tools and studies often rely on semi-structured interviews. The re-ported prevalence rates range from 50% to 56.7% (53), and the commonest diagnoses were attention deficits and disruptive behaviours (22.4%), followed by unspecified psychosis (13.9%) and other disorders of infancy and child-hood (11.1%). In the study by Khess and colleagues reported from 1998 (53) ($n = 60$), the majority of the study population had unspecified behavioural and emotional disorders (25%), followed by mood disorders (16.6%), hyperkinetic disorder (13%), autism (11.1%), and psychoses (11.1%). In a study by Kishore and colleagues in 2004 (46), unspecified psychosis was the commonest psy-chiatric diagnosis (16.7%) followed by bipolar affective disorder (13.3%) and schizophrenia (10%), which included both paranoid and undifferentiated sub-types. Three people (5%) had single-episode mania and two (3.3%) each had depression and autism. One person had delusional disorder, personality dis-order, conduct disorder, substance abuse and obsessive–compulsive disorder.

Further analysis revealed that in the mild and moderate ID groups, affective disorders and psychosis were common followed by behaviour disorder and other psychiatric disorders. In the group with severe ID the majority had behaviour problems.

The Americas: United States

The US has not taken a national approach to understanding mental health needs for adults with ID, though the research has grown in recent years (54). A recent study in the US found rates of a co-occurring psychiatric disorder of 55% in people with ID. This study was based on patient charts from 30 states, covering a population size of 13,466 individuals (55). A study on a representative sample of adolescents with ID reported that 65.1% met lifetime criteria for mental disorder. The presence of ID was associated with specific phobia, agoraphobia, and bipolar disorder (56). More recent research in the US has been on improving assessment and treatment of individuals with ID, with a strong focus on mental health outcomes rather than further studies of prevalence rates (57).

There has been very limited reporting of prevalence rates and presentation of mental disorder in those with ID across different cultures within the US. A study from South London, England, found those with ID and autism exhibit more challenging behaviour than those with ID alone (58). However, a study in the US found a significant interaction with race, autism, and challenging behaviour in adults with ID (59). Caucasian participants with autism exhibited more challenging behaviour than their African American peers, whereas the opposite holds true in those without autism. A study comparing Anglo and Latino young people with moderate to severe ID in South Carolina found that pattern of behaviour problems did not significantly differ between the two groups (60).

The Americas: Latin America and Caribbean

Latin America refers to all countries in South America, Central America, the Caribbean, and Mexico, with a total population size of nearly 655 million in 2021 (61). There is a paucity of scientific evidence on the health needs of people with ID across Latin America (62). The lack of health and educational resources along with high rates of poverty may lead to higher reported rates of ID across a number of Latin America countries. In addition, these risk factors also increase the risk for mental health problems. On the whole, there are few government policies on mental health and none specific for those with ID across Latin America. However, in 2015 the International Disability Alliance brought together over 100 participants for the first Regional Conference of Latin America and the Caribbean to promote the United Nations Convention on the Rights of Persons with Disabilities, with a report produced following the conference (63).

There is no published evidence following on from this convention regarding the mental health needs of people with ID across Latin America.

The Americas: Canada

Canada is a bilingual diverse population, with over 20% of the population born outside of Canada. It is a large country by landmass with a population size of over 38 million in 2021 (64). In 2013, Lunksy and colleagues (65) highlighted that research to date on the mental health needs of people with ID in Canada had focused on epidemiology, provision of secondary health services including forensic care, the development of skills in primary physicians, specific conditions such as autism, and the needs of families. The authors highlighted the need for future research in Canada to look at interventions and ensuring knowledge translates into practice.

Earlier studies within Canada focused on people with ID presenting with psychiatric disorders within inpatient services. Studies using administrative data of all hospitalizations of those with ID found one-third were for mental disorders, with depression (6.1%) and schizophrenia (10.4%) being the most common diagnoses (66). Another study of adults with ID in hospital care found they were more likely to display aggressive behaviours and exhibit higher rates of depression than their non-ID peers (67). People with ID do have access to community-based clinics in Canada, but those with serious mental illness are also likely to attend the emergency department (68). Those with ID accessing forensic services were more likely to have a diagnosis of psychotic disorder and also to stay in hospital longer than those without ID (69).

Research into the Indigenous population of Canada has mainly focused on those with fetal alcohol spectrum disorders (FASD) which describes a range of physical, cognitive, neurological, and behavioural impairments that result from prenatal exposure to alcohol with fetal alcohol syndrome (FAS) being the most severe presentation of FASD. Indigenous people in Canada include First Nations People, Métis, and Inuit, and made up 5% of the total population in 2021 (70) The rate of FAS is much higher in First Nations people than in the general population. A systematic literature search and meta-analysis found among the general population of Canada that the pooled prevalence was estimated to be 1/1000 for FAS and 5/1000 for FASD but the prevalence among the Indigenous population in Canada was estimated to be 38 times and 16 times higher, respectively (71).

Australia

The total population of Australia is just over 26 million as of 2023 (72). Australia does not collect data on race and ethnicity but asks about ancestry in the census

(72). In the 2021 National Census, Aboriginal people and Torres Strait Islander people, who are the Indigenous Australian People, represented 3.8% of the total population (73). In the same census, 51% identified their ancestry to be English, Scottish, or Irish and 30% as Australian (74).

The early research undertaken by Einfeld and colleagues published in 2006 (75) looked at rates of psychiatric disorders in young people with ID, and this work subsequently focused on the trajectory of psychopathology from childhood to adulthood with evidence of persistent psychopathology more so in those with severe or profound ID. More recent research in Australia has focused on health inequalities and access to specialist services (76,77).

One Australian study (78) used adapted data from a countrywide population-based sample of 37,580 individuals aged 15–64 years. Within the sample, 563 individuals were reported to have ID (1.3%), and the rate of psychiatric disorders in this subgroup was reported to be 23.3%. These disorders included anxiety, depression, and psychotic disorders. This was a large population-based sample size representing many geographical regions of Australia. A further study in Australia used secondary analysis of previously collected data from the records of 245,749 individuals using two registers, namely the ID Register and the Mental Health Information System of Australia (79). The prevalence rate of co-occurring ID and mental disorder was 31.7%, comparable to equivalent prevalence rates reported from UK-based study populations.

There is limited information regarding the mental health needs of people with ID in indigenous Australians, with rates of ID reported to be higher compared with non-indigenous Australians (80).

New Zealand

The population of New Zealand is predominantly bicultural by ethnic group, with the majority being of European descent and 16.5% as Maori. The Maori are the Indigenous people of Aotearoa New Zealand. Aotearoa is the current Maori name for New Zealand. There is very little research on prevalence and presentation of psychiatric disorders in people with ID in New Zealand (81). Studies to date have found significant overlap in the presentation of neurodevelopmental conditions, with levels of ADHD increasing with the severity of ID and autistic symptoms (82). The ethnicity or culture of a person with disability may influence access to services as has been found for autistic people within New Zealand (83).

Africa

Culture affects perspectives, interpretation, and understanding of behaviour (84). Similarly, our appreciation of normal boundaries, largely culturally determined, defines to an extent what is recognized as part of the symptomatology of mental illness. ID is not exempt from this proposition. Across the African continent, there is an under-representation of the typologies associated with ID (85) and ID may be dismissed as the clandestine work of spiritual forces. This results in fewer than the expected number of people with ID accessing healthcare facilities, and so they may use what may be considered unorthodox approaches such as 'prayer house' interventions (86).

The availability of very little, if any, data on health needs of people with ID in the African continent and virtually no information on the presentation of psychiatric illness needs further understanding. Mental health across Africa has very limited coverage in the scientific literature and this lack of research reflects the weakness of mental health services across the continent (87). The limited literature on needs of people with ID in Africa (88,89) is over 12 years old but highlighted the roles played by traditional healers and the many challenges for people with ID across Africa, such as high prevalence of ID, low priority for service development, and discrimination with poor access to education and justice. These challenges are set against the background of poverty, war, internal displacement, and the impact of HIV across Africa.

A useful, if not appropriate narrative would be to explore the reasons for the dearth of research on the needs of people with ID in the African continent. Using Nigeria as a case in point, it is hardly surprising why this trend is seen in Africa. The 2021 health sector budget of Nigeria was about £705 million (90). For an estimated population of 211 million people, this correlates with around £3.30 per person per year. To give context to these figures, the UK had a healthcare budget of £230 billion in 2021 (91) for a population of 67 million people in the same period of time, giving an approximate value of about £3400 being earmarked per person. The UK per capita healthcare budget being a thousand times greater than Nigeria's highlights the gulf in healthcare funding between the two countries. It would be too simplistic to assume that superstition and economic factors are the only reasons for the paucity of any appreciable work on ID in the continent; nevertheless, inadequate healthcare funding would translate to a disproportionately reduced allocation for mental health, and more so for ID. Therefore, it is not surprising that there has not been any significant work in field of ID in the continent. The African perspective on the mental health needs among people with ID leaves more questions than answers from a wider cultural perspective. It is therefore an area that requires a significant commitment in investment, research, and service development during the remainder of this century if we are to improve mental health outcomes and well-being of people with ID across the continent of Africa.

Culture-bound syndromes

A culture-bound syndrome is a disorder that occurs only in certain cultural contexts (92,93). In the period of Western colonization, Western physicians would come into contact with psychiatric conditions that they had not encountered at home, but were known to local people—amok was first described by early European travellers to the Malay Archipelago in the mid-sixteenth century (94). Through until 1970, European and North American psychiatrists described more than a dozen distinct 'exotic' psychiatric syndromes or disorders (95).

The term 'culture-bound syndrome' was introduced in the 1960s by Pow Meng Yap, a pioneer in cultural psychiatry working in Hong Kong (96–98). He initially classified these conditions as 'mental diseases peculiar to certain cultures', including koro, latah, amok, wihtigo psychosis, and the catatonic states of yogis. Culture-bound syndromes received a boost in their prominence by their inclusion albeit in the appendix of the DSM-IV of 1994 (99). Examples of culture-bound syndromes include the following:

- Amok—amok is a Malaysian word meaning to ferociously engage in battle. It is characterized by a period of brooding, followed by an outburst of unrestrained violence, ending with exhaustion and amnesia. It was first recognized in Malaysia, but has been described in other Southeast Asian countries as well (100).

- 'Brain fag'—first described in 1960, brain fag is a syndrome of difficulty concentrating, fatigue despite adequate rest, and pains around the head and neck. It was first described in Nigerian students, although it has been reported in other parts of Africa as well. Its name originates from what the students themselves called the condition, which they believed was due to brain fatigue (101).

- Koro—this was first referred to in 1865 in China. It is characterized by an overwhelming panic that the genitals (penis in males, vulva in females) will retract into the body. The affected individual may fear death should the genitals retract, and might seek out methods to stop retraction, such as by holding onto their penis, seeking help from family and friends, or using devices attached to the penis. It has been mainly observed in ethnically Chinese people (102). Koro can occur in epidemics, such as the one in Singapore in 1967 after rumours were spread that it could be caught from eating vaccinated pigs (103). Its name is thought to be Malay in origin, although it is often referred to by its Chinese name, shook yong.

- Dhat—a condition of non-specific symptoms (such as fatigue, low mood, sexual dysfunction, and poor appetite) attributed by the patient to a loss of semen, either in urine, through masturbation, or nocturnal emission (99). The name comes from the Sanskrit Dhatus, meaning 'elixir that constitutes the body'. It is thought to be related to the traditional Hindu belief that it takes 40 drops of blood to create a drop of bone marrow, and 40 drops of bone marrow to create a drop of sperm. It is prevalent in India, Sri Lanka, Nepal, Pakistan, Bangladesh, and some parts of South East Asia (104).

The current DSM-5 (2013) argues that the term 'cultural-bound syndrome' does not take into account that cultural differences may not always take the form of a distinct set of symptoms, but can involve ways of explaining or describing distress as well (15). As such, the DSM-5 has since reframed these syndromes as 'cultural concepts of distress', defined as 'ways cultural groups experience, understand, and communicate suffering, behavioural problems, or troubling thoughts and emotions'. It goes on to give us three cultural concepts:

- Cultural syndrome—clusters of symptoms that are recognized locally as a coherent pattern or syndrome.
- Cultural idioms of distress—shared ways of talking about personal or social concerns and distresses. The DSM-5 gives the example of talking about 'nerves' or 'depression' referring to a variety of forms of suffering.
- Cultural explanations—a cultural explanatory model for the cause or meaning of symptoms, illness, or distress.

Many other examples of culture-bound syndromes exist, and there is evidence to suggest that bulimia nervosa is culture bound as it does not appear to have been described in the absence of Western influence (105). Of course, each syndrome is likely to have its own risk factors, for example, brain fag has been shown to be more likely in those with above-average intelligence (101). Our understanding of culture-bound syndromes continues to develop, but unfortunately there does not appear to be any available evidence on the relationship between culture-bound syndromes and ID. There are cases of such syndromes being evident in those with ID, for example, two cases of Koro in two siblings with Laurence–Moon–Biedl syndrome during a 1969 Koro epidemic in India (102), but there is no evidence to allow conclusions with regard to any relationship between ID and culture-bound syndromes at present.

Conclusion

More research is needed to understand the variation in prevalence and presentation of psychiatric disorders in those with ID across cultures and countries.

The priority is to determine how the cultural identity of a person impacts presentation, access to healthcare, and treatment. In addition, we need to understand how best to address any cultural variations in health outcomes for those with ID who are at risk of developing psychiatric disorders. Future research on the presentation of psychiatric disorders should include an expansion of the geographical and cultural diversity of the participants recruited to studies.

References

1. Tsakanikos E, McCarthy J. Introduction: Part I. General issues and assessment of psychopathology. In: Tsakanikos E, McCarthy J, editors. Handbook of Psychopathology in Adults with Developmental and Intellectual Disabilities: Research, Policy and Practice. New York: Springer Science; 2014: 3–8.

2. Cooper S-A, Smiley E, Morrison J, Williamson A, Allan L. Mental ill-health in adults with intellectual disabilities: prevalence and associated factors. British Journal of Psychiatry 2007;**190**(1):27–35.

3. Royal College of Psychiatrists. Attention Deficit Hyperactivity Disorder (ADHD) in Adults With Intellectual Disability. College report 230. London: Royal College of Psychiatrists; 2021.

4. Bradley E, Caldwell P, Underwood L. Autism spectrum disorder. In: Tsakanikos E, McCarthy J, editors. Handbook of Psychopathology in Adults with Developmental and Intellectual Disabilities: Research, Policy and Practice. New York: Springer Science; 2014: 237–64.

5. Maulik PK, Mascarenhas MN, Mathers CD, Dua T, Saxena S. Prevalence of intellectual disability: a meta-analysis of population-based studies. Research in Developmental Disabilities 2011;**32**(2):419–36.

6. McKenzie K, Milton M, Smith G, Ouellette-Kuntz H. Systematic review of the prevalence and incidence of intellectual disabilities: current trends and issues. Current Developmental Disorders Report 2016;**3**(2):104–15.

7. Pedersen CB, Mors O, Bertelsen A, Waltoft BL, Agerbo E, McGrath JJ, et al. A comprehensive nationwide study of the incidence rate and lifetime risk for treated mental disorders. JAMA Psychiatry 2014;**71**(5):573–81.

8. Sandin S, Nygren KG, Iliadou A, Hultman CM, Reichenberg A. Autism and mental retardation among offspring born after in vitro fertilization. Journal of American Medical Association. 2013;**310**(1):75–84.

9. Maulik PK, Darmstadt GL. Childhood disability in low- and middle-income countries: overview of screening, prevention, services, legislation, and epidemiology. Pediatrics 2007;**120**(Suppl 1):182–5.

10. Lakhan R. An estimation of the prevalence of intellectual disabilities and its association with age in rural and urban populations in India. Journal of Neurosciences in Rural Practice 2015;**6**(4):523–8.

11. Moss S, Hurley A. Integrating assessment instruments within the diagnostic process. In: Tsakanikos E, McCarthy J, editors. Handbook of Psychopathology in Adults with Developmental and Intellectual Disabilities: Research, Policy and Practice. New York: Springer Science; 2014: 43–61.

12. **Sappok T, Brooks W, Heinrich M, McCarthy J, Underwood L.** Cross-cultural validity of the Social Communication Questionnaire for Adults with Intellectual Developmental Disorder. Journal of Autism and Developmental Disorders 2017;**47**(2):393–404.

13. **Royal College of Psychiatrists.** DC-LD: Diagnostic Criteria for Psychiatric Disorders for Use with Adults with Learning Disabilities/Mental Retardation. Occasional Paper OP48. London: Gaskell Press; 2001.

14. **Fletcher RJ, Barnhill J, Cooper SA,** editors. Diagnostic Manual—Intellectual Disability (DM-ID-2): A Textbook of Diagnosis of Mental Disorders in Persons with Intellectual Disability, 2nd edition. New York: NADD Press; 2016.

15. **American Psychiatric Association.** Diagnostic and Statistical Manual of Mental Disorders, 5th edition. Arlington, VA: American Psychiatric Association; 2013.

16. **Buckles J, Luckasson R, Keefe E.** A systematic review of the prevalence of psychiatric disorders in adults with intellectual disability. Journal of Mental Health Research in Intellectual Disabilities 2013;**6**(3):181–207.

17. **Office for National Statistics.** Overview of the UK population: 2020. 25 February 2022. Available from: https://www.ons.gov.uk/peoplepopulationandcommunity/populationa ndmigration/populationestimates/articles/overviewoftheukpopulation/2020

18. **Office for National Statistics. 2021.** https://www.ons.gov.uk/peoplepopulationandco mmunity/culturalidentity/ethnicity/bulletins/ethnicgroupenglandandwales/cen sus2021

19. **McGrother CW, Bhaumik S, Thorp CF, Watson JM, Taub NA.** Prevalence, morbidity and service need among South Asian and white adults with intellectual disability in Leicestershire, UK. Journal of Intellectual Disability Research 2002;**46**(Pt 4):299–309.

20. **Reiss S, Levitan GW, Szyszko J.** Emotional disturbance and mental retardation: diagnostic overshadowing. American Journal of Mental Deficiency 1982;**86**(6):567–74.

21. **Raj D, Stansfeld S, Weich S, Stewart R, McBride O, Brugha,T,** et al. Comorbidity in mental and physical illness. In: **McManus S, Bebbington P, Jenkins R, Brugha T,** editors. Mental Health and Wellbeing in England: Adult Psychiatric Morbidity Survey 2014. Leeds: NHS Digital.; 2016: 323–47.

22. **Berney T, Lovell M.** Children and adolescents with intellectual disabilities. In: **Bhaumik S, Alexander R,** editors. Oxford Textbook of the Psychiatry of Intellectual Disability. Oxford: Oxford University Press; 2020: 35–42.

23. **Humphries L, Desari M, Hassiotis A.** Schizophrenia and related psychoses in people with intellectual disability. In: **Bhaumik S, Alexander R,** editors. Oxford Textbook of the Psychiatry of Intellectual Disability. Oxford: Oxford University Press; 2020: 91–104.

24. **Strydom A, Dodd K, Uchendu N, Wilson S.** Dementia and other disorders associated with ageing in people with intellectual disability. In: **Bhaumik S, Alexander R,** editors. Oxford Textbook of the Psychiatry of Intellectual Disability. Oxford: Oxford University Press; 2020: 83–90.

25. **Allington-Smith P.** Mental health of children with learning disabilities Advances in Psychiatric Treatment 2006;**12**(2):130–40.

26. **Sheehan R, Hassiotis A, Walters K, Osborn D, Strydom A, Horsfall L.** Mental illness, challenging behaviour, and psychotropic drug prescribing in people with intellectual disability: UK population based cohort study. BMJ 2015;**351**:h4326.

27. **Cowley A, Holt G, Bouras N, Sturmey P, Newton JT, Costello H.** Descriptive psychopathology in people with mental retardation. Journal of Nervous and Mental Disease 2004;**192**(3):232–7.

28. **Tsakanikos E, McCarthy J, Kravariti E, Fearon P, Bouras N.** The role of ethnicity in clinical psychopathology and care pathways of adults with intellectual disabilities. Research in Developmental Disabilities 2010;**31**(2):410–15.

29. **Kiani R, Tyrer F, Hodgson A, Berkin N, Bhaumik S.** Urban–rural differences in the nature and prevalence of mental ill-health in adults with intellectual disabilities. Journal of Intellectual Disability Research 2013;**57**(2):119–27.

30. **Bhaumik S, Watson J, Barrett M, Raju B, Burton T, Forte J.** Transition for teenagers with intellectual disability: carers' perspectives. Journal of Policy and Practice in Intellectual Disabilities 2011;**8**(1):53–61.

31. **Devapriam J, Thorp CF, Tyrer F, Gangadharan SK, Raju LB, Bhaumik S.** A comparative study of stress and unmet needs in carers of South Asian and White adults with learning disabilities. Ethnicity and Inequalities in Health and Social Care 2008;**1**(2):35–43.

32. **Bonell S, Underwood L, Radhakrishnan V, McCarthy J.** Experiences of mental health service by people with intellectual disabilities from difference ethnic groups: a Delphi consultation. Journal of Intellectual Disability Research 2012;**56**(9):902–9.

33. **Mir G, Nocon A, Ahmad W, Jones L.** Learning Difficulties and Ethnicity. London: Department of Health; 2001.

34. **Holt G, Costello H, Bouras N, Diareme S, Hillery J, Moss S,** et al. BIOMED-MEROPE project: service provision for adults with intellectual disability: a European comparison. Journal of Intellectual Disability Research 2000;**44**(Pt 6):685–96.

35. Krysta K, Krysta J, Szczegielniak A, Krzystanek M. Services for patients with intellectual disability and mental health problems in Poland. Psychiatr Danub. 2019 Sep;31(Suppl 3):534–42. PMID: 31488787.

36. **Koch A, Vogel A, Holzmann M, Pfennig A, Salize HJ, Puschner B,** et al. MEMENTA—'Mental healthcare provision for adults with intellectual disability and a mental disorder'. A cross-sectional epidemiological multisite study assessing prevalence of psychiatric symptomatology, needs for care and quality of healthcare provision for adults with intellectual disability in Germany: a study protocol. BMJ Open 2014;**4**(5):e004878.

37. **Worldometer.** Asia Population (LIVE). May 2023. https://www.worldometers.info/world-population/asia-population/

38. **Parmenter T.** The present, past and future of the study of intellectual disability: challenges in developing countries. Salud Publica de Mexico 2008;**50**(Suppl 2):S124–31.

39. **Kwok HWM, Chui EMC.** A survey on mental healthcare for adults with intellectual disabilities in Asia. Journal of Intellectual Disability Research 2008;**52**(11):996–1002.

40. **Xie ZH, Bo SY, Zhang XT, Liu M, Zhang ZX, Yang XL,** et al. Sampling survey on intellectual disability in 0–6-year-old children in China. Journal of Intellectual Disability Research 2008;**52**(12):1029–38.

41. **Katz G, Lazcano-Ponce E.** Intellectual disability: definition, etiological factors, classification, diagnosis, treatment and prognosis. Salud Publica de Mexico 2008;**50**(Suppl 2):S132–41.

42. **Komardjaja I.** The place of people with intellectual disabilities in Bandung, Indonesia. Health and Place 2005;**11**(2):117–20.

43. **Gabel A.** South Asian Indian cultural orientations towards mental retardation. Mental Retardation 2004;**42**(1):12–25.

44. **Croot EJ, Grant G, Cooper CL, Mathers N.** Perceptions of the causes of childhood disability among Pakistani families living in the UK. Health and Social Care in the Community 2008;**16**(6):606–13.

45. **Jeevanandam L.** Perspectives of intellectual disability in Asia: epidemiology, policy, and services for children and adults. Current Opinion in Psychiatry 2009;**22**(5):462–8.

46. **Kishore MT, Nizamie A, Nizamie SH, Jahan M.** Psychiatric diagnosis in persons with intellectual disability in India. Journal of Intellectual Disability Research 2004;**48**(1):19–24.

47. **World Health Organization.** ECOSOC Meeting: 'Addressing non-communicable diseases and mental health: Major challenges to sustainable development in the 21st century'. Discussion paper: 'Mental health, poverty and development'. 2009. Available from: https://medbox.org/document/ecosoc-meeting-addressing-noncommunicable-diseases-and-mental-health-major-challenges-to-sustainable-development-in-the-21st-century#GO

48. **United Nations Children's Fund (UNICEF).** The situation of children in India. A profile. 2011. Available from: https://www.ecoi.net/en/file/local/1234700/1930_1386768757_sitan-india-may-2011.pdf

49. **Emerson E.** Poverty and people with intellectual disabilities. Mental Retardation and Developmental Disabilities Research Reviews 2007;**13**(2):107–13.

50. **Winkelstein W Jr.** Determinants of worldwide health. American Journal of Public Health 1992;**82**(7):931–2.

51. **Girimaji SC, Srinath S.** Perspectives of intellectual disability in India: epidemiology, policy, services for children and adults. Current Opinion in Psychiatry 2010;**23**(5):441–6.

52. **Ministry of Law, Justice and Company Affairs.** The Persons with Disabilities (Equal Opportunities, Protection of Rights and Full Participation) Act, 1995. New Delhi: Government of India; 1996.

53. **Khess CRJ, Dutta I, Chakrabarthy I, Bhattacharya P, Das J, Kothari S** Comorbidity in children with mental retardation. Indian Journal of Psychiatry 1998;**40**(3):289–94.

54. **Charlot L, Beesley J.** Intellectual disabilities and mental health: United States–based research. Journal of Mental Health Research in Intellectual Disabilities 2013;**6**(2):74–105.

55. **National Association of States United for Aging and Disabilities.** National Core Indicators for Aging and Disabilities for 2015–2016 (NCI-AD). Human Services Research Institute. 2017. Available from: https://nci-ad.org/upload/reports/NCI-AD_2015-2016_National_Report_FINAL.pdf

56. **Platt JM, Keyes KM, McLaughlin KA, Kaufman AS.** Intellectual disability and mental disorders in a US population representative sample of adolescents. Psychological Medicine 2018;**49**(6):952–61.

57. **Beasley JB, Kalb L, Klein A.** Improving mental health outcomes for individuals with intellectual disability through the Iowa START (I-START) Program. Journal of Mental Health Research in Intellectual Disabilities 2018;**11**(4):287–300.

58. McCarthy J, Hemmings C, Kravariti E, Dworzynski K, Holt G, Bouras N, et al. Challenging behaviour and co-morbid psychopathology in adults with intellectual disability and autism spectrum disorders. Research in Developmental Disabilities 2010;**31**(2):362–6.

59. Horovitz M, Matson JL, Hattier MA, Tureck K, Bamburg JW. Challenging behaviours in adults with intellectual disability: the effects of race and autism spectrum disorders. Journal of Mental Health Research in Intellectual Disabilities 2012;**6**(1):1–13.

60. Blacher J, McIntyre LL. Syndrome specificity and behavioural disorders in young adults with intellectual disability: cultural differences in family impact. Journal of Intellectual Disability Research 2006;**50**(3):184–98.

61. The World Bank. Latin America & Caribbean. 2021. Available from: https://data.worldb ank.org/country/ZJ

62. Mercadante MT, Evans-Lacko S, Paula CS. Perspectives of intellectual disability in Latin American countries: epidemiology, policy, and services for children and adults. Current Opinion in Psychiatry 2009;**22**(5):469–74.

63. International Disability Alliance. Advancement of the UN CRPD through the 2030 Agenda Towards Implementation in Latin America Conference report São Paulo, Brazil 22–24 October 2015. 2015. Available from: https://www.internationaldisabilityalliance. org/sites/default/files/documents/final_lac_report.pdf

64. The World Bank. Canada. 2021. Available from: https://data.worldbank.org/country/ canada

65. Lunsky Y, Lake JK, Balogh R, Weiss J, Morris S. A review of Canadian mental health research on intellectual and developmental disabilities. Journal of Mental Health Research in Intellectual Disabilities 2013;**6**(2):106–26.

66. Balogh RS, Hunter D, Ouellette-Kuntz, H. Hospital utilization among persons with an ID, Ontario, Canada, 1995–2001. Journal of Applied Research in Intellectual Disabilities 2005;**18**(2):181–90.

67. Martin L, Hirdes JP, Fries BE. Examining the characteristics of persons with intellectual disability receiving hospital services. Part 1—psychiatric hospitals/units. Journal of Developmental Disabilities 2007;**13**(3):89–103.

68. Lunsky Y, Balogh, RS, Cairney J. Predictors of emergency department visits in persons with intellectual disability experiencing a psychiatric crisis. Psychiatric Services 2012;**63**(3):287–90.

69. Raina P, Lunsky R. A comparison study of adults with intellectual disability and psychiatric disorder with and without forensic involvement. Research in Developmental Disabilities 2010;**31**(1):218–23.

70. Statistics Canada. First Nations people, Métis and Inuit in Canada. 2022. Available from: https://www150.statcan.gc.ca/n1/pub/11-627-m/11-627-m2022057-eng.htm

71. Popova S, Lange S, Charlotte P, Parunashvili N, Rehm J. Prevalence of alcohol consumption during pregnancy and fetal alcohol spectrum disorders among the general and Aboriginal populations in Canada and the United States. European Journal of Medical Genetics 2017;**60**(1):32–48.

72. Australian Bureau of Statistics. Population. 2023. Available from: https://www.abs.gov. au/statistics/people/population

73. Australian Bureau of Statistics. Estimates of Aboriginal and Torres Strait Islander Australians: preliminary 2021 census-based estimated resident population of

Aboriginal and Torres Strait Islander and non-Indigenous Australians. June 2021. Available from: https://www.abs.gov.au/statistics/people/aboriginal-and-torres-strait-islander-peoples/estimates-aboriginal-and-torres-strait-islander-australians/jun-2021

74. **Australian Bureau of Statistics.** Cultural diversity: census. Information on country of birth, year of arrival, ancestry, language and religion. June 2022. Available from: https://www.abs.gov.au/statistics/people/people-and-communities/cultural-diversity-census/2021

75. **Einfeld SL, Piccinin AM, Mackinnon A, Hofer SM, Taffe J, Gray KM,** et al. Psychopathology in young people with ID. JAMA 2006;**296**(16):1981–9.

76. **Torr, J.** Intellectual disability and mental ill health: a view of Australian research: Journal of Mental Health Research in Intellectual Disabilities 2013;**6**(2):159–78.

77. **Trollor J.** Making mental health services accessible to people with an intellectual disability. Australian and New Zealand Journal of Psychiatry 2014;**48**(5):395–8.

78. **White P, Chant D, Edwards N, Townsend C, Waghorn G.** Prevalence of intellectual disability and comorbid mental illness in an Australian community sample. Australian and New Zealand Journal of Psychiatry 2005;**39**(5):395–400.

79. **Morgan V, Leonard H, Bourke J, Jablensky A.** Intellectual disability co-occurring with schizophrenia and other psychiatric illness: population-based study. British Journal of Psychiatry 2008;**193**(5):364–72.

80. **Roy M, Balaratnasingam S.** Intellectual disability and Indigenous Australians: an overview. Asia-Pacific Psychiatry 2014;**6**(4):363–72.

81. **McCarthy J, Duff M.** Services for adults with intellectual disability in Aotearoa New Zealand. BJPsych International 2019;**16**(3):71–3.

82. **Matthews M, Bell E, Mirf-in-Veitch B.** Comparing psychopathology rates across autism spectrum disorders and intellectual disabilities. Advances in Mental Health and Intellectual Disabilities 2018;**12**(5/6):163–72.

83. **Broadstock M.** New Zealand Autism Spectrum Disorder Guideline Supplementary Paper on the Impact of Ethnicity on Recognition, Diagnosis, Education, Treatment and Support for People on the Autism Spectrum. Christchurch: INSIGHT Research; 2018.

84. **Spencer-Oatey H.** Culturally Speaking: Culture, Communication and Politeness Theory, 2nd edition. London: Continuum International Publishing Group; 2008.

85. **Blackie D.** Anomaly: Anthropology of Atypical Children. Unpublished PhD thesis, University of Witwatersrand, Johannesburg, Gauteng, South Africa, 2020.

86. **Aina OF.** Mental illness and cultural issues in West African films: implications for orthodox psychiatric practice. Medical Humanities 2004;**30**(1):23–6.

87. **Sankoh O, Sevalie S, Weston M.** Mental health in Africa. Lancet Global Health 2018;**6**(9):E954–5.

88. **Njenga F.** Perspectives of intellectual disability in Africa: epidemiology and policy services for children and adults. Current Opinion in Psychiatry 2009;**22**(5):457–61.

89. **Adnams CM.** Perspectives of intellectual disability in South Africa: epidemiology, policy, services for children and adults. Current Opinion in Psychiatry 2010;**23**(5):436–40.

90. **Budget Office of the Federation.** Budget documents. Federal Government of Nigeria; 2021. Available from: https://www.budgetoffice.gov.ng/index.php/resources/internal-resources/budget-documents/2021-budget

91. **Office for National Statistics**. Healthcare expenditure, UK health accounts provisional estimates. 2021. Available from: https://www.ons.gov.uk/peopl epopulationandcommunity/healthandsocialcare/healthcaresystem/bulletins/ healthcareexpenditureukhealthaccountsprovisionalestimates/2021

92. **Carel H, Cooper R**. Introduction: culture-bound syndromes. Studies in History and Philosophy of Biological and Biomedical Sciences 2010;**41**(4):307–8.

93. **Ventriglio A, Ayonrinde O, Bhugra D**. Relevance of culture-bound syndromes in the 21st century. Psychiatry and Clinical Neurosciences 2016;**70**(1):3–6.

94. **Kon Y**. Amok. British Journal of Psychiatry 1994;**165**(5):685–9.

95. **Tseng WS**. From peculiar psychiatric disorders through culture-bound syndromes to culture-related specific syndromes. Transcultural Psychiatry 2006;**43**(4):554–76.

96. **Yap PM**. Words and things in comparative psychiatry with special reference to exotic psychosis. Acta Psychiatrica Scandinavica 1962;**38**:157–82.

97. **Yap PM**. The culture bound syndromes. In: **Cahil W, Lin TY**, editors. Mental Health Research in Asia and the Pacific. Honolulu: East-West Centre Press; 1969: 33–53.

98. **Crozier I**. Introduction: Pow Meng Yap and the culture-bound syndromes. History of Psychiatry 2018;**29**(3):363–85.

99. **American Psychiatric Association**. Diagnostic and statistical manual of mental disorders, 4th edition, text revision. Washington, DC: **American Psychiatric Association**; 2000.

100. **Gaw AC, Bernstein RL**. Classification of amok in DSM-IV. Psychiatric Services 1992;**43**(8):789–93.

101. **Ola B, Morakinyo O, Adewuya A**. Brain fag syndrome—a myth or a reality. African Journal of Psychiatry 2009;**12**(2):135–43.

102. **Chowdhury AN**. The definition and classification of Koro. Culture, Medicine and Psychiatry 1996;**20**(1):41–65.

103. **Chong TM**. Epidemic Koro in Singapore. British Medical Journal 1968;**1**(5592):640–1.

104. **Udina M, Foulon H, Valdés M, Bhattacharyya S, Martín-Santos R**. Dhat syndrome: a systematic review. Psychosomatics 2013;**54**(3):212–18.

105. **Keel PK, Klump KL**. Are eating disorders culture-bound syndromes? Implications for conceptualizing their etiology. Psychological Bulletin 2003;**129**(5):747–69.

Chapter 5

Research in intellectual disability across cultures

Samuel J. Tromans, Kerim Munir,
Peter E. Langdon, and Regi T. Alexander

Introduction

Kirmayer and Ban (1) define cultural psychiatry as being 'concerned with the ways in which psychopathology and healing are shaped by cultural knowledge and practices'. While making comparisons across different cultures can be of significant clinical and academic value, it is important to recognize the substantial heterogeneity that exists within respective cultural groups, and avoid making fixed assumptions based upon a patient's cultural background (2). Cultural research can not only help us learn more about the distinctions between different cultures, as well as their commonalities (3), and represents an essential step in the development of cultural proficiency (4), but such research can lead to better global health outcomes. Such cultural knowledge is envisioned as an essential component in ensuring the provision of a truly biopsychosocial approach in patient care (1). Furthermore, with an increasingly globalized world (5), it is more important than ever before for clinicians to move away from predominantly ethnocentric models of care, towards care provision that is sensitive to the cultural needs of specific patients, as well as their wider family and/or professional carer units (6,7).

In general, when considering cultural research, a rule of thumb has been consideration of both emic and etic approaches. An emic approach relates to research focused on the study of observed phenomena within a specific culture, with negligible focus regarding how it relates to other cultures; in contrast, an etic approach is based on describing such phenomena in terms that can be applied across cultural boundaries. Most cross-cultural research intends to employ a combination of these approaches, to varying degrees (8).

With respect to cultural psychiatry research, it is also essential that any increased understanding of cultural influences among people with intellectual disability (ID) informs clinical practice. It is important to minimize the research-to-practice gap, to ensure that improved theoretical knowledge promptly leads to tangible benefits for patient care (9). However, such transfer of knowledge should not be a unidirectional process; researchers can equally learn a great deal from the cultural clinical practitioners, which, along with input from people with ID and their carers, can help inform subsequent research priorities (9). Furthermore, some individuals may have a dual researcher–practitioner role, which can help bridge the gap between research and clinical practice.

In this chapter, we discuss research priorities for transcultural ID research, international collaboration efforts, current gaps in the research literature, and barriers to conducting such research, as well as suggesting potential solutions.

Research priorities

Epidemiology

While ID is present across all cultural groups, it is difficult to accurately estimate cross-cultural prevalence, owing to differing definitions, as well as other confounding factors, such as educational opportunity and attainment (10). ID is now envisioned as a highly heterogeneous neurodevelopmental condition characterized by significant limitations in both intellectual functioning and adaptive behaviour that cover many everyday social and practical skills.

Intellectual functioning refers to general mental capacity including learning, problem solving, and reasoning and may be measured by means of an intelligence test and general intellectual quotient (IQ) scores. On tests with a standard deviation of 15 and a mean of 100, this involves a score of 70 ± 5. However, both the culturally adapted measures as well as clinical training and judgement are required to interpret the test results. Currently all the definitions of ID entail that three criteria are met: (i) deficits in intellectual functioning; (ii) deficits in adaptive functioning and behaviour (a collection of conceptual, social, and practical skills that are learned and performed by people in their everyday lives); and (iii) onset in the developmental period (although this is no longer specified by an age cut-off in both the 11th edition of the International Classification of Diseases of the World Health Organization, and the 5th edition of the *Diagnostic and Statistical Manual of Mental Disorders* (DSM-5) of the American Psychiatric Association definitions; the 12th edition of *Intellectual Disability*, by the American Association on Intellectual and Developmental Disabilities, has continued to specify an age of onset and extended this to before age 22).

Therefore, having an IQ score two standard deviations below the mean does not imply a person would have ID and therefore the statistically expected prevalence of ID on intellectual functioning measures alone, estimated to be 2.5%, is not necessarily accurate (10). Furthermore, such a determination based on intellectual functioning measures alone does not address variation by geography, availability of prenatal and postnatal care, as well as metabolic screening and other preventive interventions. The requirement of a co-presence of significant adaptive functional impairment (11,12) (known as Criterion B in DSM-5) is therefore critical in terms of a paradigm shift of defining ID not only as a neurodevelopmental disorder, but acknowledging that severity levels of ID based on mild, moderate, severe, and profound, are no longer dependent on IQ score ranges (i.e. statistical variation) but on co-measures of adaptive functioning. This has been an important step forward in addressing cross-cultural aspects of ID globally.

A prior meta-analysis of ID prevalence (13), based on intellectual functioning measures, including data from 52 studies published from 1980 to 2009, yielded an overall prevalence estimate of 1.04% (95% confidence interval 0.96–1.12). This composite estimate is consistent with more recent North American-based estimates from the National Health Interview Surveys, involving children aged 3–17 years (14). The 2009–2011 and 2015–2017 data yielded estimates of 0.9% and 1.2% respectively, representing a statistically significant (p <0.05) increase, which the authors suggested may be attributable to increased awareness and access to healthcare. The noted increase of mild ID among African American children adjusting for sex, maternal age, birth order, economic status, and maternal education (15) can also be attributable to demographic features of the population, such as referral patterns for intelligence testing and possible underrepresentation of White children, owing to them being more likely to have intelligence testing through private services and/or being placed in out-of-state long-term care facilities (15).

There is a paucity of epidemiological research pertaining to prevalence of ID in low- and middle-income countries (LMICs) (16,17). A study by Christianson et al. (16) including children aged 2–9 years across eight villages in rural South Africa, used a two-phase design, involving initial screening (n = 6692) followed by a comprehensive neurodevelopmental assessment of the children who screened positive (n = 722). A total of 238 children were diagnosed with ID, yielding a mild ID prevalence of 2.91%, and overall ID prevalence of 3.56%, though the authors strongly suspected that these values represented underestimates of the true figures. Nevertheless, these estimates are consistent with previously reported findings by Roeleveld et al. (18), who reported a mild ID prevalence of 2.98% among children in LMICs. The authors suggested potential contributory factors for the high reported rate of ID, including 'poor living conditions, malnutrition, limited intellectual stimulation, and unattended home births' (16), and suspected that many of these factors were potentially avoidable had the right resources been available at the right time.

High-quality epidemiological research pertaining to ID prevalence in different cultures is undoubtedly a research priority, as well as patterns of co-occurring conditions and other mental disorders among ID groups. Such data are essential in informing needs-based resource allocation for cultural groups, as well as potentially identifying preventable causes of ID (as envisioned in the neurodevelopmental classification in both the World Health Organization and American Psychiatric Association definitions) and developing public health interventions designed to equitably address them.

Barriers to accessing services

There is a general underutilization of health and social care services among minority ethnic groups, relative to the majority ethnic population (10,19). This may lead to people with ID from such groups not receiving care that would benefit both themselves as well as potentially their caregivers. Multiple factors underpinning such underutilization have been suggested, including a lack of awareness of the services available, language barriers, cultural belief systems (e.g. a mistrust of Western medical practices), and a lack of culturally sensitive service provision (2,20). There is a clear need for research in this area, to enhance understanding as to why certain cultural groups may underutilize health and social care services, and develop interventions to address such issues, with a view to ensuring equitable healthcare across cultural groups.

Cultural biases

Instruments used to assess and diagnose ID are prone to cultural bias and may not be equally valid across different cultural groups. This is indeed the case for other neurodevelopmental conditions that frequently co-occur with ID, such as autism (21). For example, a study by Carruthers et al. (22) investigated the performance of the child version of the Autism Quotient (AQ-Child) questionnaire (23) among children with autism and neurotypical children aged between 4 and 9 years from India, Japan, and the UK. They found that many of the items most predictive of an autism diagnosis overlapped across cultural groups, with five items demonstrating consistently excellent discriminatory power between the index children and their peers without autism. However, four items appeared to demonstrate cultural differences, including those related to spontaneity of behaviour, one-sided conversational style, sense of humour, and enjoyment of social occasions.

Similarly, application of major diagnostic criteria (11,12) across different cultures may be limited in their validity without due consideration of their meaning or appropriateness within the cultures under observation (24). Indeed, there may be locally derived categories that more effectively describe the experiences of specific cultural groups. Thus, it is essential to consider how different cultures describe their illness experiences in order to learn more about them and how they compare to conditions described in more mainstream diagnostic systems (11,12,25).

Furthermore, treatment approaches may not have equivalent efficacy across all cultural groups. Cross (4) asserts the importance of consideration of culture in the development of any new therapeutic approaches. Additionally, we would also suggest the importance of re-evaluating pre-existing approaches through a cultural lens. For example, cognitive behavioural therapy is a widely used psychological treatment approach, but it is generally described and delivered using Westernized concepts (26). Thus, a culturally adapted approach to cognitive behavioural therapy will likely be required for patients from other cultural groups. However, one should not assume that such adapted approaches would be as beneficial to patients as the treatment's original iteration is in Western groups, and related research would be required to establish their efficacy in cross-cultural contexts and populations.

Equally, when researching health in different cultures, there is a risk of viewing their experiences through the Euro-American lens that tends to predominate in academic mental health discourse (1). Indeed, some cross-cultural generalization may be appropriate, but through listening to the illness knowledge and experiences of indigenous people, new clinically relevant diagnostic entities may emerge (1). The inclusion of culture-bound syndromes in the fourth edition of the *Diagnostic and Statistical Manual of Mental Disorders* (DSM-IV) (27) represented a significant step forward in the acknowledgement of conditions that appear specific to a certain cultural group (5). Indeed, the DSM-IV introduced an appendix on 'cultural formulation' to assist clinicians in systematically evaluating and reporting the impact of a person's cultural context, as well as a person's cultural and ethnic reference group. For immigrants and ethnic minorities, the DSM-IV specified the need to indicate the 'degree of involvement with both the culture of origin and the host culture (where applicable)'. There is also a clear need for further research to improve understanding with respect to how different cultures conceptualize ID, in particular, co-occurring major mental disorders, with a greater focus on providing a voice to specific cultures rather than imposing the values and belief systems of prevailing predominant cultures, and/or the knowledge and assumptions of research team members (28). In the research setting, the cultural formulation entails assessment of the effect that cultural differences may have on the relationship between the person and the evaluating clinician. The DSM-5 continues the cultural formulation requirement in specification of the (i) cultural identity of the person; (ii) cultural conceptualization of distress; (iii) psychosocial stressors and cultural features of vulnerability and resilience; (iv) cultural features of the relationship between the person and the clinician; and (v) overall cultural assessment summarizing the implications of the components of the cultural formation and other clinically relevant problems and their suggested appropriate management.

Globally, in increasingly diverse societies, clinicians can not only reduce their propensity for cultural biases and become more culturally competent by actively engaging in training in cultural psychiatry, but cultural formulation ought to be a sine qua non of their clinical practice, with emphasis on strengths and weaknesses of what they are able to offer to cultural groups. In terms of research, Kirmayer (29) developed specific guidance for this purpose with detailed advice on conducting cultural psychiatry research. Furthermore, cultural psychiatry groups, such as the Royal College of Psychiatrist's Transcultural Psychiatry Special Interest Group in the UK (30), and journals, such as *Transcultural Psychiatry* (31), provide platforms for healthcare professionals to share knowledge and research among both their peers and further afield.

Stigma and discrimination

Sociologist Erving Goffman describes stigma as a discrediting attribute, whereby the stigmatized individual is viewed as having a spoiled identity (32,33). ID is often conceptualized as a stigmatized attribute that lies in the perceptions of others, making it likely for many affected individuals not to consider ID as part of their identity (34,35). The frequent evolution of the term used to describe psychiatry of ID as a 'Cinderella' subspecialty further supports the suggestion that not only having ID, but also working as a healthcare professional within the ID field, especially addressing mental health aspects of ID, carries a certain level of stigma (36). Furthermore, caregivers of people with ID, be they family or professional carers, also experience 'affiliate stigma', a form of self-stigmatization as a consequence of their association with a targeted index group, that is, people with ID (37).

Attitudes towards people with ID demonstrate variation across cultures. A study by Benomir et al. (38) compared the attitudes of three groups in the UK and in Libya: science students, psychology students, and professionals working in schools for people with ID. They used the Community Living Attitude Scales for Mental Retardation (CLAS-MR) (39), which measures attitudes across four subscales that include empowerment, exclusion, sheltering, and similarity. The researchers found that the Libyan sample demonstrated significantly less favourable scores on empowerment, exclusion, and similarity compared to their

UK peers, though there was no statistically significant difference with respect to sheltering (which assesses how much people with ID need to be supervised and protected). While the findings suggested that Libyan attitudes were less favourable relative to other Western countries too, they were similar to those found in Pakistan, a fellow Eastern country. Attitudes towards people with ID therefore demonstrate considerable variation across both cultures (40) and geographical regions (41). Research to improve understanding of attitudes in different cultures is essential in the development of any culturally sensitive anti-stigma interventions.

Healthcare organizations have been additionally culpable of discrimination directed towards certain ethnic groups, with Blanchett (42) describing ID as being a category predominantly reserved for the privileged white middle class, while minority groups with similar profiles of intellectual functioning and adaptive behaviour difficulties remain marginalized, without access to the same forms of support. Organizations need to be mindful of such institutional discrimination, and proactive in their approach to addressing it. A 2011 report by the Royal College of Psychiatrists (2) recommended embedding cultural competence into any healthcare organization's business plan and organizational activities, such as local policies and performance assessments. Furthermore, it recommended holding regular events that bring clinicians into contact with different cultural groups, to help foster a greater understanding of these communities.

Needs of caregivers

While some features are universal, the experiences of caregivers appear to demonstrate some differences across cultural boundaries. Chang and McConkey (43) interviewed 117 Taiwanese parents who had children with an ID, reporting that many of their findings were consistent with those among parents in different cultures. However, certain aspects of Taiwanese Chinese society, such as the expectation of sons to look after their parents in their old age, and on how children should behave around adults, further increased the impact of caregiving on mothers. The researchers recommended that any therapeutic approaches should be family based, involving supporting the family unit rather than the individual with ID in isolation.

A study by Chukwu et al. (44) focused on the different coping strategies employed by Nigerian families who had a member with a learning disability. Focus group discussions were held from which three main strategies were identified: problem-focused (involving information gathering to improve understanding), emotion-focused (involving 'letting off steam' and sometimes blaming other family members), and spiritual/religion-focused strategies. The latter approach included seeking support from their local spiritual/religious community, viewing their family member having ID ('learning disability') as a form of message from God, and sometimes visiting a native doctor, based on the belief that learning disability was a consequence of witchcraft.

Differences in the experiences of caregivers supporting people with ID are undoubtedly influenced by culture. In some instances, cultural distinctions may be subtle, in others, more readily apparent. Further research can help aid healthcare professionals by providing them with knowledge of different cultural groups and how they view ID. Despite this, healthcare professionals need to be flexible and respectful in their approach, using such knowledge as guidance rather than strict rules to be followed under all circumstances (45). Ultimately, it is essential for healthcare professionals to modify their approach according to the individual patient and caregivers with whom they are working.

People with intellectual disability as co-researchers

There needs to be an increasing role for people with ID serving as co-researchers, rather than their involvement being limited to the research participant role. All participatory research approaches empower and protect marginalized people. This is also important in empowering people with ID to be more involved in setting the agenda for ID research and funding priorities, and the general participatory framework of 'inclusion' and bringing the value of their lived experience to the fore (46,47). Current regulatory and ethical guidelines although necessary for their protection do not sufficiently ensure fair distributive justice. Additionally, St John et al. (48) reported that co-researchers with ID found the experience personally meaningful, as well as being able to establish an easy rapport with research participants, which appeared to elicit a greater wealth of information being obtained in related research interviews.

Despite this, a systematic review by Di Lorito et al. (46) reported that 'many current intellectual disability research projects still lack systematic involvement of patient and public involvement members', though also highlighted the importance of sufficient infrastructure to support such individuals. Relatedly, Tuffrey-Wijne and colleagues (49) developed a research skills training course for people with intellectual disabilities, citing both increased confidence and work opportunities among course attendees. Furthermore, where people with ID are involved as co-researchers, it is important to also ensure that their voices are heard in any resultant peer-reviewed journal articles, reports, or other forms of research output; this has often been lacking, as reported in a literature review by Strnadová and Walmsley (50).

International collaborations

Historically, the overwhelming majority of ID research has been conducted in higher-income countries (51), resulting in certain cultures being frequently overlooked, with a corresponding shallower research evidence base available to be referred to by healthcare professionals. Through advocating for LMICs, international groups can contribute towards redressing this balance.

An effective cross-cultural approach to care for people with ID benefits greatly from international collaboration. The International Association for the Scientific Study of Intellectual and Developmental Disabilities (IASSIDD), originally founded in 1964, is perhaps the best known ID research group (52), and has frequently collaborated with the World Health Organization, including on the *World Report on Disability* (53).

Other organizations promoting international collaboration in the field of ID research include the European Association for Mental Health in Intellectual Disability (54), the World Psychiatric Association Scientific Section on ID and the Work Group on ID (in collaboration with many national organizations including the American Psychiatric Association, and the American Association of Child and Adolescent Psychiatry Committee on Autism and Intellectual Disability), and the National Association of Dually Diagnosed (NADD) in the US. The NADD has been influential in its sponsorship of the *Diagnostic Manual—Intellectual Disability*, 2nd edition (DM-ID-2) (55). These bodies have organized regular meetings and publish newsletters, and play a key role in promoting international research.

Summary

In general, there is limited research pertaining to the interaction of ID across cultures globally with a specific paucity of understanding of the impact of culture on ID, and vice versa, in LMICs. There is a clear need to pursue avenues of research likely to yield the greatest benefit for the greatest number of people per unit of research funding. Furthermore, people with ID and their carers should be involved throughout the research process, from identifying research priorities through to the dissemination of findings and their impact on health and social care policy. Biomedical research involving people with ID can contribute greatly to improvements in their quality of life, and the major ethical violations of the past ought not to be a pretext for their exclusion from research due to convenience-related factors involving difficulty in obtaining informed consent (47). Active procedures ought to be in place in institutional review boards to ensure equitable participation.

Furthermore, in order to provide equitable care for all people with ID, a culturally competent workforce is required, with respect to healthcare professionals, researchers, and clinical academics. This requires not just members of the aforementioned groups to have knowledge and expertise with respect to different cultural groups, but also for such groups to be represented in the professional workforce, where they can play an essential role (2). A 'colour-blind' approach to healthcare provision, based upon treating all individuals the same, fails to recognize the needs of specific cultural groups, and has likely contributed to inequalities in care provision (2,56).

Research involving people with ID should always consider cultural factors, as this influences both their own and their caregiver's narratives pertaining to mental health, whether diagnostic criteria for certain conditions are met, and the response to various treatment approaches, as well as expression of choice and acceptability in their implementation. It is essential that people with ID are given a voice in any research involving them and are active participants not just as study subjects but as co-researchers.

References

1. **Kirmayer LJ, Ban L.** Cultural psychiatry: research strategies and future directions. Advances in Psychosomatic Medicine 2013;**33**:97–114.
2. **Royal College of Psychiatrists**. Minority Ethnic Communities and Specialist Learning Disability Services. Report of the Faculty of the Psychiatry of Learning Disability Working Group. London: Royal College of Psychiatrists; 2011.
3. **Ember CR.** Cross-Cultural Research Methods. Lanham, MD: AltaMira Press; 2009.
4. **Cross TL.** Towards a Culturally Competent System of Care: A Monograph on Effective Services for Minority Children Who Are Severely Emotionally Disturbed. Washington, DC: Child and Adolescent Service System Program; 1989.
5. **Baig BJ.** Social and transcultural aspects of psychiatry. In: **Johnstone EC, Cunningham Owens D, Lawrie SM, McIntosh AM, Sharpe M**, editors. Companion to Psychiatric Studies, 8th edition. Edinburgh: Churchill Livingstone; 2010: 109–19.
6. **Doody O, Doody CM.** Intellectual disability nursing and transcultural care. British Journal of Nursing 2012;**21**(3):174–80.
7. **Gerrish K.** Preparation of nurses to meet the needs of an ethnically diverse society: educational implications. Nurse Education Today 1997;**17**(5):359–65.
8. **Cheung FM.** Cross-cultural psychopathology. In: **Butcher JN**, editor. Oxford Handbook of Personality Assessment. Oxford: Oxford University Press; 1998: 44–56.
9. **Artiles AJ, Thorius KK, Bal A, Neal R, Waitoller F, Hernandez-Saca D.** Beyond culture as group traits: future learning disabilities ontology, epistemology, and inquiry on research knowledge use. Learning Disability Quarterly 2011;**34**(3):167–79.
10. **Allison L, Strydom A.** Intellectual disability across cultures. Psychiatry 2009;**8**(9):355–7.

11. **American Psychiatric Association**. Diagnostic and Statistical Manual of Mental Disorders: DSM-5. Arlington, VA: American Psychiatric Publishing; 2013.
12. **World Health Organization**. ICD-11 for Mortality and Morbidity Statistics. Geneva: World Health Organization; 2018.
13. **Maulik PK, Mascarenhas MN, Mathers CD, Dua T, Saxena S**. Prevalence of intellectual disability: a meta-analysis of population-based studies. Research in Developmental Disabilities 2011;**32**(2):419–36.
14. **Zablotsky B, Black LI, Maenner MJ, Schieve LA, Danielson ML, Bitsko RH**, et al. Prevalence and trends of developmental disabilities among children in the United States: 2009–2017. Pediatrics 2019;**144**(4):e20190811.
15. **Murphy CC, Yeargin-Allsopp M, Decoufle P, Drews CD**. The administrative prevalence of mental retardation in 10-year-old children in metropolitan Atlanta, 1985 through 1987. American Journal of Public Health 1995;**85**(3):319–23.
16. **Christianson A, Zwane M, Manga P, Rosen E, Venter A, Downs D**, et al. Children with intellectual disability in rural South Africa: prevalence and associated disability. Journal of Intellectual Disability Research 2002;**46**(2):179–86.
17. **Munir KM**. The co-occurrence of mental disorders in children and adolescents with intellectual disability/intellectual developmental disorder. Current Opinion in Psychiatry 2016;**29**(2):95–102.
18. **Roeleveld N, Zielhuis GA, Gabreëls F**. The prevalence of mental retardation: a critical review of recent literature. Developmental Medicine & Child Neurology 1997;**39**(2):125–32.
19. **Alegría M, Chatterji P, Wells K, Cao Z, Chen C, Takeuchi D**, et al. Disparity in depression treatment among racial and ethnic minority populations in the United States. Psychiatric Services 2008;**59**(11):1264–72.
20. **Raghavan R, Waseem F**. Services for young people with learning disabilities and mental health needs from South Asian communities. Advances in Mental Health and Learning Disabilities 2007;**1**(3):27–31.
21. **Tromans S, Chester V, Gemegah E, Roberts K, Morgan Z, Yao GL**, et al. Autism identification across ethnic groups: a narrative review. Advances in Autism 2020;**7**(3):241–55.
22. **Carruthers S, Kinnaird E, Rudra A, Smith P, Allison C, Auyeung B**, et al. A cross-cultural study of autistic traits across India, Japan and the UK. Molecular Autism 2018;**9**(1):52.
23. **Auyeung B, Baron-Cohen S, Wheelwright S, Allison C**. The Autism Spectrum Quotient: Children's Version (AQ-Child). Journal of Autism and Developmental Disorders 2008;**38**(7):1230–40.
24. **Kirmayer LJ**. Ethno-and cultural psychiatry. In: **Callan H**, editor. The International Encyclopedia of Anthropology. Hoboken, NJ: Wiley Blackwell; 2018: 1–11.
25. **Callan H**, editor. The International Encyclopedia of Anthropology. Hoboken, NJ: Wiley Blackwell; 2018.
26. **Rathod S, Kingdon D**. Cognitive behaviour therapy across cultures. Psychiatry 2009;**8**(9):370–1.
27. **American Psychiatric Association**. Diagnostic and Statistical Manual of Mental Disorders: DSM-IV. Washington, DC: American Psychiatric Association; 1994.

28. **Kamaldeep B, Jankovic Gavrilovic J.** Cultural psychiatry. In: **Wright P, Stern J, Phelan M**, editors. Core Psychiatry. London: WB Saunders; 2012: 105–13.

29. **Kirmayer LJ, Fung K, Rousseau C, Lo HT, Menzies P, Guzder J**, et al. Guidelines for training in cultural psychiatry. Canadian Journal of Psychiatry 2021;**66**(2):195–246.

30. **Royal College of Psychiatrists.** Transcultural (TSIG). 2021. Available from: https://www.rcpsych.ac.uk/members/special-interest-groups/transcultural

31. **SAGE Journals.** Transcultural Psychiatry. 2021. Available from: https://journals.sage pub.com/home/tps

32. **Goffman E.** Stigma: Notes on the Management of Spoiled Identity. New York: Simon and Schuster; 1963.

33. **Ahmedani BK.** Mental health stigma: society, individuals, and the profession. Journal of Social Work Values and Ethics 2011;**8**(2):4-1-4-16.

34. **Dorozenko KP, Roberts LD, Bishop B.** The identities and social roles of people with an intellectual disability: challenging dominant cultural worldviews, values and mythologies. Disability & Society 2015;**30**(9):1345–64.

35. **McVittie C, Goodall KE, McKinlay A.** Resisting having learning disabilities by managing relative abilities. British Journal of Learning Disabilities 2008;**36**(4):256–62.

36. **Hassiotis A.** Clinical examples of cross-cultural work in a community learning disability service. International Journal of Social Psychiatry 1996;**42**(4):318–27.

37. **Mak WW, Cheung RY.** Affiliate stigma among caregivers of people with intellectual disability or mental illness. Journal of Applied Research in Intellectual Disabilities 2008;**21**(6):532–45.

38. **Benomir AM, Nicolson RI, Beail N.** Attitudes towards people with intellectual disability in the UK and Libya: a cross-cultural comparison. Research in Developmental Disabilities 2016;**51**:1–9.

39. **Henry D, Keys C, Jopp D, Balcazar F.** The Community Living Attitudes Scale, Mental Retardation Form: development and psychometric properties. Mental Retardation 1996;**34**(3):149–58.

40. **Scior K, Addai-Davis J, Kenyon M, Sheridan J.** Stigma, public awareness about intellectual disability and attitudes to inclusion among different ethnic groups. Journal of Intellectual Disability Research 2013;**57**(11):1014–26.

41. **Scior K, Hamid A, Hastings R, Werner S, Belton C, Laniyan A**, et al. Intellectual disability stigma and initiatives to challenge it and promote inclusion around the globe. Journal of Policy and Practice in Intellectual Disabilities 2020;**17**(2):165–75.

42. **Blanchett WJ.** Telling it like it is: the role of race, class, & culture in the perpetuation of learning disability as a privileged category for the white middle class. Disability Studies Quarterly 2010;**30**(2):1230–77.

43. **Chang M, McConkey R.** The perceptions and experiences of Taiwanese parents who have children with an intellectual disability. International Journal of Disability, Development and Education 2008;**55**(1):27–41.

44. **Chukwu NE, Okoye UO, Onyeneho NG, Okeibunor JC.** Coping strategies of families of persons with learning disability in Imo state of Nigeria. Journal of Health, Population and Nutrition 2019;**38**(1):1–9.

45. **Crotty G, Doody O.** Transcultural care and individuals with an intellectual disability. Journal of Intellectual Disabilities 2016;**20**(4):386–96.

46. **Di Lorito C, Bosco A, Birt L, Hassiotis A.** Co-research with adults with intellectual disability: a systematic review. Journal of Applied Research in Intellectual Disabilities 2018;**31**(5):669–86.

47. **Yan EG, Munir KM.** Regulatory and ethical principles in research involving children and individuals with developmental disabilities. Ethics & Behavior 2004;**14**(1):31–49.

48. **St John B, Mihaila I, Dorrance K, DaWalt LS, Ausderau KK.** Reflections from co-researchers with intellectual disability: benefits to inclusion in a research study team. Intellectual and Developmental Disabilities 2018;**56**(4):251–62.

49. **Tuffrey-Wijne I, Lam CKK, Marsden D, Conway B, Harris C, Jeffrey D,** et al. Developing a training course to teach research skills to people with learning disabilities: 'It gives us a voice. We CAN be researchers!'. British Journal of Learning Disabilities 2020;**48**(4):301–14.

50. **Strnadová I, Walmsley J.** Peer-reviewed articles on inclusive research: do co-researchers with intellectual disabilities have a voice? Journal of Applied Research in Intellectual Disabilities 2018;**31**(1):132–41.

51. **Thurston R, Tromans S, Chester V, Cooper SA, Strydom A, Bhaumik S,** et al. Current and future research priorities in the psychiatry of intellectual disability. In: **Bhaumik S, Alexander R,** editors. Oxford Textbook of the Psychiatry of Intellectual Disability. Oxford: Oxford University Press; 2020: 275–88.

52. International Association for the Scientific Study of Intellectual and Developmental Disabilities. Homepage. 2023. Available from: https://www.iassidd.org/

53. **World Health Organization.** World report on disability. 2011. Available from: https://apps.who.int/iris/handle/10665/44575

54. **European Association for Mental Health in Intellectual Disability.** History. Available from: https://eamhid.eu/about-eamhid/history/

55. **Fletcher RJ, Barnhill J, Cooper SA.** Diagnostic Manual—Intellectual Disability: A Textbook of Mental Disorders in Persons with Intellectual Disability, 2nd edition. Kingston, NY: NADD Press; 2016.

56. **Mir G, Nocon A, Ahmad W, Jones L.** Learning Difficulties and Ethnicity. London: Department of Health; 2001.

Part 2

Social and cultural perspectives

Chapter 6

Anthropology and intellectual disability

Patrick McKearney and Tyler Zoanni

Introduction

The fifth edition of the *Diagnostic and Statistical Manual of Mental Disorders* (DSM-5) defines intellectual disability, in part, as the inability to meet development and sociocultural standards for personal independence and social responsibility. This recognition of the cultural aspect of the condition leads directly into questions about nurture and sociality that go beyond the remit of biology alone, and into those that anthropology concerns itself with. Anthropology demonstrates the central role that socialization plays in shaping people's capacities—most notably by showing how people diagnosed with intellectual disabilities are frequently 'socialised for incompetence' by the care they receive in families, institutions, and communities (1). The idea that the resulting incompetence is somehow the inevitable product of their biology is hard to maintain in the light of such evidence.

Anthropology also shows us that the 'personal independence' the DSM-V refers to means very different things across cultures, and also varies in its importance. The conditions that people must 'adapt' to, as the DSM-V puts it, also depend on how people in a society communicate, organize relationships, and manage to live independently—if, indeed, living independently is required at all. Social life in different places requires very different kinds of competencies from people, offers very different imaginations of what it means to be one's own person, and increases or reduces the emphasis on autonomy in the first place.

Anthropology's long tradition of ethnographic research encourages us to look beyond professional contexts and interactions where intellectual disability is an established psychiatric category. Ethnography in community settings enables us to see how people navigate their everyday lives in other kinds of relationships, and thus to see what role professional interactions actually play in a wider story. Anthropology's methodological innovations enable us to get closer to the experiences, lives, and self-narrations of these individuals themselves;

enabling us to see what it is like to live as someone classified as intellectually disabled, as well as what such classifications leave out about them as rich, rounded, and feeling humans.

Anthropology especially focuses our attention on societies that conduct social life very differently from the Euro-American countries in which the category of intellectual disability was developed. The kind of social life that people need to adapt to in these contexts is different in unexpected and even unimaginable ways. What constitutes an intellectual disability in these contexts is therefore similarly variable. This work reveals the particularity of the cultural conditions that support the psychiatric framing of intellectual disability, and its limitation in framing the lives of such individuals in other contexts.

Anthropology is yet to conduct extensive ethnographic research on intellectual disability. There is a robust body of anthropological literature on cross-cultural variation within mental health, and an emerging one on physical disability and sensory conditions like blindness and deafness (2,3). But there is not a parallel tradition in relation to intellectual disability (4,5). There is a small but important strand of anthropological work on intellectual disability in the latter half of the twentieth century. In this chapter, we explore how that tradition combines with wider anthropological work on dependence, disability, and the mind to offer us alternative perspectives on intellectual disability.

We start by focusing on the most developed anthropological conversation about intellectual disability—a conversation stemming from a major collaborative and longitudinal research project at the University of California, Los Angeles (UCLA) in the US. We also discuss a different tradition of research on North America and Europe that emerges out of feminist concerns with reproduction, care, and dependence. We also place the different themes of these diverse research traditions into dialogue with social constructionist arguments and the limited anthropological research that has been conducted on people with intellectual disabilities living outside of Euro-America.

Anthropology's tradition of studying intellectual disability

Anthropology's first engagement with people with intellectual disabilities emerged in the 1960s alongside wider social scientific responses to the professional treatment of those classed as having mental conditions within North Atlantic welfare states.

Robert Edgerton's (6) monograph *The Cloak of Competence* presents extensive data on the lives of disabled people in urban California who had been discharged from a residential institution. Edgerton's work demonstrates the incredible efforts these individuals undertook to confront 'the shattering stigma' of being regarded as 'retarded' by working to conceal, through a 'cloak of competence' their own intellectual impairments and difficulty understanding how to navigate life outside of institutions (6). This, in turn, entailed confronting the psychological scars of humiliation, loss, and fear left by their former confinement. It included, also, finding ways to navigate the structural poverty they faced. They often did so through constructing ad hoc relationships of support, such as with romantic partners; though many people in Edgerton's study were also forcibly sterilized and felt undermined by their inability to have children.

Edgerton treats 'mental retardation' not purely as a biological condition but also a social status that has its own stigmatizing effects on people quite apart from their mental capacities (6,7). This approach aims also to 'see people through their own eyes and to hear them through their own words' by exploring disabled people's thoughts, actions, and feelings (6). These are characteristics of the subsequent works produced by the large research group he headed at UCLA. The team conducted a series of thorough longitudinal ethnographic studies tracking many of Edgerton's original cohort of informants, and others besides, into diverse settings and into their older years. They published their findings in volumes that Edgerton edited with his colleagues (8,9). One of this research group's key findings was that, over the life course, these individuals ended up significantly improving their capacity to navigate everyday life despite a relative fixity in their cognitive ability (8,10).

L. L. Langness and Harold Levine's (1) *Culture and Retardation* is particularly notable among this tradition for its systematic focus on life history. It departs from standard parentally focused life histories that present a person with disabilities as 'aspects of a man who might have been' rather than the person in and of him- or herself (11). By contrast with that tradition, the book's detailed portraits of the complexity of people's lives turn them from 'a background influence' on the foregrounded family into main characters with agency, individuality, and richness. It challenges the clinical reduction of such individuals to their mental impairments, and thus of 'mental retardation' more generally as 'a single homogenous group best characterised as an IQ range' (1).

This volume builds on Edgerton's demonstration of the social implications of being treated as intellectually disabled. Edgerton had showed how poorly living in an institution had prepared people for life outside, how far they had to hide their resulting incompetence to avoid being stigmatized, and how much work it took for them to learn the new social skills required of them. Langness and Levine's book further demonstrates how difficult it is for those with intellectual disabilities even to access the contexts in which others learn social roles. They describe this as being actively socialised into 'incompetence'. So, for instance, they found that young Black men with intellectual disabilities would tend to remain in households, or in friendships with female friends or service workers, rather than with men their age who would enable them to learn the behaviours expected of them (12). The volume presents another example of a father warning his disabled son off drinking by getting him blind-drunk, while he offers his non-disabled son a range of social contexts in which he can experiment with his limits (13). This is even more the case for those who have only ever lived in institutions:

> Once one has lived as retarded, been systematically denied information about the everyday world, provided with false information, his or her chances for subsequent normal development are slim. (1)

Demonstrating the effects of socialization reveals how problematic it is to take a person's capacities at a given moment as a read-out of their innate abilities. A long-term perspective on their development over the life course is required (11).

This ties in directly with Edgerton's own arguments about the necessary role ethnography plays in looking beyond simple casual relationships between single factors in people's lives, and thus facile quantitative measures of 'success' for people with intellectual disabilities. He argues that standard measurements of the causes and effects of disability on people's lives are not only narrow, but also attempt to stabilize a picture that is constantly 'in process' (8). Edgerton also argues against interviews and fleeting diagnostic snapshots, contending that avoiding any simplistic picture of this sort can only be done through long-term ethnography crucially embedded in the relevant, naturalist context of that person's life, rather than in contrived experimental or research-driven situations.

Critique and methodological innovation

The subsequent tradition of ethnographic inquiry influenced by Edgerton's work was not uncritical of it. Several anthropologists argued that Edgerton reproduced a pathologizing psychiatric perspective—as seen in his acceptance of the category of 'mental retardation'. They developed the work of Edgerton's research group by innovating new ways ethnographically and analytically to centre the lives, perspectives, and voices of intellectually disabled people themselves, challenging the assumptions underlying the category itself.

Bogdan and Taylor's (14) landmark study describes Ed Murphy and Pattie Burt, two people labelled 'retarded' as they moved through various kinds of institutions and independent living arrangements over their life courses. The book is grounded in first-person life stories that are assembled from multiple, extensive, and wide-ranging interviews in which Ed and Pattie emerge as articulate, thoughtful, human beings. This challenges dominant professional and research perspectives on their lives. Ed, for instance, remarks that to understand people like him 'you need experts': that is, 'people who have lived it' (14,15).

Indeed, Bogdan and Taylor are critical of the very category of 'mental retardation', which they take to be a sociopolitical construct that is not only scientifically vague but also has devastating effects on people's lives. They contribute to a wider argument that labelling someone as having an 'intellectual disability' is a performative act that does not so much describe a neutral biological condition, but rather socially *makes* someone 'intellectually disabled' (16–18). As David Goode argues of a man with Down syndrome called Bobby:

> What most persons would call Bobby's competence (with emphasis on the possessive) is actually part of his socially produced, organisationally adequate identity. Any clinician's assessment of Bobby's competence reflects as much about the social organisation of clinical work, the clinician's training, and a particular clinic's instruments and procedures as it does about Bobby per se. (19)

Bogdan and Taylor follow Edgerton in demonstrating the often-considerable difficulties of Ed's and Pattie's lives as 'stories of lost opportunity brought about by institutional confinement' (14). But they take Edgerton to task for what they regard as his dismissive portrayals of such people, arguing that he had internalized dominant discourses about disability and naturalized the category of mental retardation (14). Ed's and Pattie's lives come across as much fuller and richer than the brief sketches of misery that defined the first publication of Edgerton's monograph. Bogdan and Taylor end with a strong concluding plea to abandon stigmatizing labels and to ask both what is wrong with society, rather than disabled people, and what can be done to make it more accommodating and indeed dignifying (10,14).

Michael Angrosino similarly sought ways to narrate the lives of people with intellectual disabilities from their own perspective by asking 'What does it feel like to *be* mentally disabled and to make one's way in the world with that condition?' (20). He draws inspiration from Edgerton's work but critiques its framework for beginning with 'the acceptance of clinically defined disorder, such that the contextualised life history serves mainly to illustrate the process of "adjustment" to a presumed mainstream norm' (21). Angrosino develops, against the aspirations to objectivity in Edgerton's work, the *auto*biographical potential of the 'life-history' approach.

Angrosino (1994) describes how Vonnie Lee, a resident of a group home with a 'mental condition', narrates his life story through snatched, seemingly incoherent, and insignificant comments while on the bus. Using the bus, it emerges, is an important change in the way Lee experiences, navigates, and describes his life. And when we take this context into account, and let Lee tell his story in it, we see that there is nothing 'disordered' about it (21). In *Opportunity*

House (20), Angrosino goes further by writing ethnographically based semi-fictional narratives. The characters are fictionalized composites of people he met volunteering at a non-profit residential community for people with an intellectual disability and a psychiatric disorder (20).

Angrosino contends that anthropology's resourcefulness at deciphering seemingly 'exotic' symbols ought to be applied to understand forms of disabled activity that might otherwise seem meaningless (21). A later chapter in an edited volume, for instance, explores the self-presentations of individuals with intellectual disabilities as strategies for managing their dependency upon others (22). People's way of presenting themselves, he argues, are neither innocent facts nor ways to cover up who they really are (20). They are 'extended metaphors of the self', produced by feeling, thinking, and interactional agents (22). People with 'mental conditions' hold these as much as anyone else—to the point that we ought to question the position from which we are attributing 'mental retardation' to them in the first place.

The methodological innovations of this research tradition as a whole offer a range of distinctively anthropological ways of studying intellectual disability (23). By combining scepticism of official categories with detailed ethnographic work, they reveal how many seemingly 'pathological' or 'disabled' forms of action are, in fact, frequently strategies for negotiating complex social worlds (19,24–27).

The construction and contingency of 'intellectual disability'

Subsequent anthropological work on intellectual disability contributes to our understanding of how intellectual disability is shaped in the Global North by its particular economic, political, and institutional arrangements. This is especially evident with anthropological work on autism, where the scholarship is particularly robust (28,29). Here we highlight some of the contributions of the less consolidated conversation on intellectual disability.

R. P. McDermott (30) contributes to a rich stream of work on education by provocatively reversing the causality of diagnosis (31–34). McDermott argues that a young man is identified as having a disability only because of the existence of 'social arrangements' that foreground and stigmatize 'differential rates of learning' (30: p 272). Specifically, it is only in a variety of classroom tasks and, most of all, during tests that Adam fully appears as a disabled person (33,35,36).

Contemporary work on professional care in Euro-American settings reinforces this line of argument. Kelly Johnson's (37) ethnography of the closure of a long-stay and large-scale home in Australia contributes to a long tradition of work on institutions (14,38). She demonstrates how interpreting a group of women through the pathologizing lens of 'challenging behaviour' has devastating effects upon them— shaping them into the abject, asocial, and at times violent beings that they are expected to be. But Johnson demonstrates how this perspective is formed through, often quite random, demands of institutional organization; not expertise, let alone anything specific to the actual women. Jack Levinson and McKearney build on similar arguments to demonstrate how the particular pressures of care in contemporary Britain and the US similarly leads individuals to be classified as dependent, violent, and in need of intervention in ways that are conspicuously contingent (39–41).

Scholars also demonstrate the ways such individuals become caught within tensions in contemporary forms of welfare. Intellectual disability, it turns out, has two quite different uses as a category in practice (42). On the one hand, it marks out particularly dependent individuals as legitimate recipients of state welfare. On the other, it identifies them as subjects whose rights are in danger of being overridden. Even if it might be possible to resolve this tension in theory, anthropologists demonstrate that these two aspirations go in quite different directions on the ground—leading carers and people with disabilities themselves into conflicts they cannot resolve (26,39,43–48).

Anthropology enables us to see beyond the policies, attitudes, or cultures that so much social policy focuses on. In practice, it is frequently the relationship between potentially infinite demands, and finite resources, that leads carers to distinguish between legitimate and illegitimate needs—even if, in another welfare regime, it might be perfectly possible to take such concerns seriously (39,49). Don Kulick and Jens Rydström's (50) *Loneliness and Its Opposite* demonstrates how these kind of tensions shape the ways in which people's sexual desires, identities, and needs are responded to in Denmark and Sweden. The countries have similarly permissive attitudes when it comes to sexuality in general. But, in practice, the way Sweden legislates and regulates care work makes it practically impossible for carers to take the risks necessary to facilitate the sexual desires of many disabled people. And the result is that, while the Danish structuring of care innovatively supports disabled people's sexual lives, there is practically no engagement with sexuality on the ground in Swedish care.

Reconfiguring dependence in Euro-America

This work raises the question as to whether and how intellectual disability might manifest quite differently in arrangements that place less emphasis on individual capacity and personal independence. Bogdan and Taylor call for a 'sociology of acceptance', to accompany a social science of exclusion, to examine just what it is that enables some disabled people to have 'moral careers that lead to inclusion' (51). Anthropological work in intellectual disability has explored these issues by drawing upon a tradition of feminist scholarship that critiques the value placed on autonomy, capacity, and independence in Western societies (see especially 52,53). By focusing, instead, on relationships of care, we can ask: what becomes of intellectual disability in situations more accommodating of dependence?

A range of ethnography focuses on families with an intellectually disabled member through biography and auto-ethnography on the transformations that parenting a disabled child brings (54–64). In laying the ground for this kind of work, Rayna Rapp's (57) *Testing Women, Testing the Fetus* explored how amniocentesis allows an assessment of the risk of severe impairments in a pregnancy, and thus prompts difficult decisions about abortion or carrying the pregnancy to term. Rapp portrays the North American mothers in her study as everyday 'moral philosophers' insofar as they struggle with questions about the nature of the good life and decisions about life and death. She also discovered that these parents often become activists who work to support their and other families through peer groups, national advocacy, and using media to expand the horizons of people's understandings of good lives and good families. Though intellectual and other disabilities are often viewed as diminishments of human life from a professional or philosophical perspective, in the lives of families, these lives lay the ground for personal and collective transformations and innovations (65).

Gayle Landsman (61), in *Reconstructing Motherhood and Disability in the Age of Perfect Babies*, likewise focuses on mothers of, often intellectually, disabled children in the US. She describes how the everyday expectations for children to develop in ideal ways, as well as wider societal discourses about the worthlessness of an intellectually disabled life, produce impairment as a problem that they are blamed for as mothers. In this context, they learn to reimagine their own lives and that of their children in order to work out new familial futures with integrity, meaning, and value. Similarly, Ginsburg and Rapp move from looking at the moment of reproductive decision-making (57) to the ways in which an intellectually disabled person's development has wider 'reverberations'; producing 'cultural innovation' of new models of kinship, education, the life course, and citizenship (58,59).

Other work explores how these hopeful possibilities can take shape in professional caring relationships. Jeanette Pols, Brigitte Alhoff, and Els Bransen (66) describe how carers in the Netherlands respond to people with intellectual disabilities who engage in substance abuse. The ideal of autonomy that carers are meant to pursue presumes that those with cognitive disabilities are able to 'govern their own lives' (66). But, in practice, carers think these individuals sometimes take choices that are 'not good for their own well-being' (66). In these instances, the ideal of autonomy will only guide carers towards neglect. So, carers engage, instead, in persuasion—attempting to lead care recipients away from worse decisions towards better ones. Such care assumes, unlike demanding ideals of independence in liberal societies, that minds are relational rather than self-sufficient, not closed systems but rather open to 'influence' (44,66).

This focus on the possibilities latent within professional care is explored ethnographically in Angrosino's, Zoanni's and McKearney's ethnographic work on the L'Arche communities (67–71). L'Arche is an originally French and Catholic venture (now ecumenical, interfaith, and spread across the world) to form small-scale groups in which those with and without intellectual disabilities share life together. McKearney (2017), for instance, argues that in L'Arche homes in the UK, the dependence of those with intellectual disabilities is transformed from a barrier to intimacy, belonging, and interaction into the foundation of it (72–74).

Is intellectual disability a social construct?

This work raises the question as to whether there might be whole societies, and not just minority communities, where things might be this way. Anthropology has long attended to the possibility that other societies might enact relationality and dependence quite differently from the West, with pivotal works and debates centring on this question (75–81). Might people with intellectual disabilities struggle not only on certain psychometric tests, but also with a specific kind of Euro-American adult life that requires a high degree of individual autonomy?

That has been the argument of certain social constructionists who claim that 'intellectual disability' does not refer to anything other than a way in which certain Euro-American institutions apprehend people (27,82). At the most general level, scholars argue that disability in general, and intellectual disability in particular, is the product of the demands of modern industrial capitalism, while positing that in other cultures and in 'pre-modern' Europe people with cognitive impairments led relatively normal lives (83,84).

Actual anthropological evidence of those diverse other societies, rather unsurprisingly, does not conform to such neat generalizations. In a significant literature review, Edgerton (4) argues that the extant cross-cultural ethnographic research by no means demonstrates that intellectual disability is always inconspicuous, better accommodated, or less stigmatized outside of the institutions of the industrialized West (85). Cross-cultural research has only occasionally been gathered together in comparative fashion since his intervention (5,86,87). But what has been done offers us some routes into building a more complex and diverse picture of the way that intellectual impairment is responded to outside of the industrial and institutional context of the West.

In the absence of significant state support, care is often organized at the margins of existing kinship structures. In Christine Sargent's work in Jordan (88–91), Helena Fietz's research in Brazil (92,93), and McKearney's ongoing fieldwork in India, mothers who are primarily responsible for their children's care are desperately worried about who, after they die, will look after their offspring. Although this is also a common worry in the Global North, there is little state welfare in Jordan, Brazil, or India to provide residence or ongoing care. And even for those families that have the resources, paying for private residential care to be provided by non-kin is a 'relatively uncommon and unpopular option'—indeed, it is one that is often highly stigmatized (91,93). Mothers are also uncertain that their other children or the child's potential spouses will take on such a responsibility.

In some cases, people look to work or new forms of voluntary institutions for care beyond parents' lives (93,94). In stark contrast to societies in which care is expected to be separated from romance or eroticism, marriage is often practised as a way of creating new relationships of dependence—with the spouse or their parents (50,91,95). Indeed, in a context in which everyone remains within hierarchical kinship relations and frequently in complex webs of dependence within the home, it is rare for a person with intellectual disabilities to become conspicuous *only* because they cannot operate totally autonomously.

A small body of work on Africa explores how intellectual disability manifests only in interaction between a non-typical mind and wider fabric of social life. Zoanni demonstrates the ways in which understandings of intellectual disability in Uganda are forged at the intersection of local models of the mind, long-standing patterns of kinship care, and newer forms of Christian charity (65,71,96). He demonstrates that a person only stands out as 'disabled' when they break particular social expectations about key features of personhood, such as by lacking the ability to speak or being socially and biologically reproductive. This leads to different arrangements of care; in which, for example, a person with cerebral palsy (which entails no intellectual disability) is offered care in a group home, while someone with Down syndrome works as a taxi driver (96). Outside kinship relations, dedicated care for people with intellectual disabilities is only available within a handful of Christian institutions, which in turn reproduce kinship models of highly paternalistic care that renders the cared-for as 'children'. At the same time, the category of the 'child' provides a socially legible status that affirms disabled people as deserving of care and resources.

Julie Livingston (97) and Benedicte Ingstad's (98) research on Botswana sheds light on *mopakwane*—a term that refers to severe and multiple disabilities (including mental ones) or the condition of being severely malnourished and dehydrated (99,100). *Mopakwane* are typically cared for by their families, and their arrival thus involves a significant rearrangement of expectations for the life course and the kinship group. Parents will likely be blamed for the child's condition, but typically try to move responsibility away from themselves; by claiming that it is something that naturally happens, that it was the result of witchcraft, or that *mopakwane* are, in fact, a gift from God (98).

In these forms of social life, the specific way of parsing intelligence behind the psychiatric definition of 'intellectual disability' gives way to alternative categories for comprehending differences, such as people's capacity to care for children, to marry, to do certain kinds of work, to speak, or to comport themselves properly (87). This research in Africa suggests, in particular, that the colonial and postcolonial demands for the creation of school systems, new expectations of literacy, and new regimes of testing have created conditions that render children disabled in a way that was not true for earlier living conditions, especially in rural settings (96,97). These works also demonstrate that alternative social forms of social organization can create opportunities for those with intellectual disabilities: to be less conspicuously incompetent (to the point that their categorization as 'disabled' ought to be called into question), to remain within relations of care, and to access relationships in which they are recognized as full persons.

It is important to note that these are also significant findings from anthropological research in Euro-America outside of institutional contexts. That scholarship demonstrates just how complex people with intellectual disabilities' relational lives are—involving parents, social workers, lovers, and much more (12,26,54,95,101). The way intellectual disability manifests in Euro-America may have more to do with classic anthropological themes such as kinship and dependence than the heavily professionalized and psychologized scientific literature leads us to imagine. Anthropology research, within and beyond Euro-America, reveals a complexity to the social life of intellectual disability that is rarely comprehended from the perspective of biomedicine or professional care. It shows forms of relationship, activity, and experience that the aims of 'prevention' and 'cure' or 'inclusion' and 'independence' tend to miss (11,87).

Conclusion

None of this anthropological research confirms the 'utopian' hopes of strong social constructionist arguments (102). The reliance of people with intellectual disabilities upon others troubles expectations about work in Jordan, Uganda, and Kerala. Economic forms other than capitalism can also require such capacities. And 'manual' or 'menial' work can rely on complex forms of thinking that not everyone in a society is capable of (4,85). Intellectual disability troubles the kinship systems for distributing care in these contexts, and thus the expectations about personhood that they rely on.

Even if such societies expect people to be dependent, they tend also to expect changes over the life course in how that dependence manifests and interacts with that of others. Nothing suggests people in these societies, for instance, are obviously less concerned than they are in Euro-America about those they see as disabled raising children (95,103). The sense, also, that intellectual disability is a significant enough problem that people need to distribute responsibility for it is a surprising continuity across many ethnographies within and beyond Euro-America (60,64,90,104–106).

This is of a piece with the evidence we have on lay perceptions of cognitive disability outside of professional settings in Euro-American societies as well. Edgerton's research group was able to show that people can be regarded as 'slow' for their difficulty in performing tasks beyond those mandated by educational and professional institutions (107). They demonstrated how some young adults in California are regarded as impaired outside of school, for instance, when people notice their incapacity to tell the time, to count money, or to comprehend the stakes of their decisions (108,109).

Anthropology offers us a more empirical way to go about social constructionism—and to fill in the critical cultural gaps left by psychiatric universals. Of particular help on this front is the concept of 'competence', as developed by Richard Jenkins' volume (86). Chapters from field sites in South America, Africa, North America, and Europe shift the emphasis from a theoretical debate about the condition's cultural construction into an empirical investigation into the cultural expectations, political–economic demands, histories of classification, and environmental and material conditions in particular places. The volume demonstrates that these all play a central, yet not easily predictable, role in the way intellectual disability manifests, is experienced, and plays out in practice.

Competence has three key advantages over a purely universal frame. First, by approaching disabled people in terms of their competence, rather than limitation, impairment, or diagnosis, it allows research to escape still-dominant cultural assumptions which frame disabled people solely in terms of inherent deficit. Second, its focus on particularity allows us to investigate the gaps left by the DSM-5's vague references to a potential diversity of sociocultural expectations of mental maturity—gaps that a universalizing science will never fill. Third, competence is a question, not an answer.

The DSM-5 defines intellectual disability with certainty in relation to a limitation in someone's ability to take personal responsibility and the ability to function 'independently'. The idea of competence, by contrast, leaves open the question as to whether individual responsibility and personal independence are universal prerequisites of social interaction and a meaningful life—or whether social variation might also make a difference at this level too. What kind of common-sense, reasoning, and judging capacities do people actually rely on in practice? What social differences actually make a difference to the lives of people with intellectual disabilities—that is, to the kinds of capacities they need, to their ability to develop them, and to the importance of being capable in the first place?

This furthers puts into social perspective the individualized concept of mental development that underwrites psychiatric approaches to intellectual disability. The DSM-5 defines intellectual disability in terms of a lack of progress towards expected milestones, and the failure to attain full mental maturity. But we ought to stop seeing that as exclusively about a person's individual ability. It is also a question about the culturally variable expectations of how an individual life ought to progress.

> The lives of mentally retarded persons seem to get increasingly out of synchronisation with what might be regarded as the 'normal' life course. This comes about as a result of natural maturation and aging in conflict with cultural expectations about the 'normal' course of development. It is also, we believe, a result of faulty and incomplete socialisation. (1)

This approach is more precise than imagining a 'relationship between some ill-defined (and ever-changing) state of retardation as a cause and "retarded" behaviour as effect' (11). Instead, it requires us to investigate ethnographically the particular normative trajectories in a given setting, the forms of learning that enable people to follow them, and how precisely people end up departing from them. It allows us to view such individuals in diachronic perspective and thus to attend more accurately to what pulls them away from expected developmental paths, as well as how those departures come to be imagined, classified, and responded to (11).

References

1. **Langness LL, Levine HG**, editors. Culture and Retardation: Life Histories of Mildly Mentally Retarded Persons in American Society. Dordrecht: D. Reidel; 1988.
2. **Devlieger C.** Disability. In: Cambridge Encyclopedia of Anthropology. 14 June 2018. Available from: https://www.anthroencyclopedia.com/entry/disability

3. **Ginsburg F, Rapp R.** Disability worlds. Annual Review of Anthropology 2013;**42**:53–68.

4. **Edgerton RB.** Mental retardation in non-Western societies: toward a cross- cultural perspective on incompetence. In: **Haywood HC**, editor. Social-cultural aspects of mental retardation. New York: Appleton-Century-Crofts; 1970: 227–37.

5. **McKearney P, Zoanni T.** Introduction: for an anthropology of cognitive disability. Cambridge Journal of Anthropology 2018;**36**(1):1–22.

6. **Edgerton RB.** The Cloak of Competence, 1st edition. Berkeley, CA: University of California Press; 1967.

7. **Goffman E.** Stigma: Notes on the Management of Spoiled Identity. Harmondsworth, Middlesex: Penguin Books; 1968.

8. **Edgerton RB**, editor. Lives in Process: Mildly Retarded Adults in a Large City. Washington, DC: American Association on Mental Deficiency; 1984.

9. **Edgerton RB, Gaston MA.** 'I've Seen It All!': Lives of Older Persons with Mental Retardation in the Community. Baltimore, MD: Paul H. Brookes; 1991.

10. **Edgerton RB.** The Cloak of Competence, 2nd edition. Berkeley, CA: University of California Press; 1993.

11. **Langness LL, Levine HG.** Introduction. In: **Langness LL, Levine HG**, editors. Culture and Retardation: Life Histories of Mildly Mentally Retarded Persons in American society. Dordrecht: D. Reidel Pub. Co.; 1988: ix–xv.

12. **Mitchell-Kernan C, Tucker MB.** The social structures of mildly mentally retarded Afro-Americans: gender comparisons. In: **Edgerton RB**, editor. Lives in Process: Mildly Retarded Adults in a Large City. Washington, DC: American Association on Mental Deficiency; 1984: 173–92.

13. **Koegel P.** You are what you drink: evidence of a socialized incompetence in the life of a mildly retarded adult. In: **Langness LL, Levine HG**, editors. Culture and Retardation: Life Histories of Mildly Mentally Retarded Persons in American Society. Dordrecht: D. Reidel; 1988: 47–64.

14. **Bogdan R, Taylor SJ.** Inside Out: The Social Meaning of Mental Retardation. Toronto: University of Toronto Press; 1982.

15. **Hartblay C.** Disability expertise: claiming disability anthropology. Current Anthropology 2020;**61**(Suppl 21):S1–140.

16. **Dexter LA.** The Tyranny of Schooling: An Inquiry Into the Problem of 'Stupidity'. London: Basic Books; 1964.

17. **Lungren N.** Learning to become (in)competent: children in Belize speak out. In: **Jenkins R**, editor. Questions of Competence: Culture, Classification and Intellectual Disability. Cambridge: Cambridge University Press; 1999: 194–221.

18. **Ferguson PM, Ferguson DL, Taylor SJ**, editors. Interpreting Disability: A Qualitative Reader. New York: Teachers College Press; 1992.

19. **Goode DA.** Who is Bobby?: ideology and method in the discovery of a Down syndrome person's competence. In: **Ferguson PM, Ferguson DL, Taylor SJ**, editors. Interpreting Disability: A Qualitative Reader. New York: Teachers College Press; 1992: 197–212.

20. **Angrosino MV.** Opportunity house: ethnographic stories of mental retardation. Walnut Creek, CA: Altamira Press; 1998.

21. **Angrosino MV.** On the bus with Vonnie Lee: explorations in life history and metaphor. Journal of Contemporary Ethnography 1994;**23**(1):14–28.

22. **Angrosino MV.** Mental disability in the United States: an interactionist perspective. In: **Jenkins R**, editor. Questions of Competence: Culture, Classification and Intellectual Disability. Cambridge: Cambridge University Press; 1999: 25–53.

23. **Cascio MA, Racine E.** Research Involving Participants with Cognitive Disability and Differences: Ethics, Autonomy, Inclusion, and Innovation. Oxford: Oxford University Press; 2019.

24. **Koegel P.** Social support and individual adaptation. In: **Langness LL, Levine HG,** editors. Culture and Retardation: Life Histories of Mildly Mentally Retarded Persons in American Society. Dordrecht: D. Reidel; 1988: 127–54.

25. **Whittemore RD.** Theodore V. Barrett: an account of adaptive competence. In: **Langness LL, Levine HG,** editors. Culture and Retardation: Life Histories of Mildly Mentally Retarded Persons in American Society. Dordrecht: D. Reidel; 1988: 155–90.

26. **Todis B.** 'Nobody helps!': lack of perceived support in the lives of elderly people with developmental disabilities. In: **Ferguson PM, Ferguson DL, Taylor SJ,** editors. Interpreting Disability: A Qualitative Reader. New York: Teachers College Press; 1992: 61–77.

27. **Rapley M.** The Social Construction of Intellectual Disability. Cambridge: Cambridge University Press; 2004.

28. **Grinker RR.** Unstrange Minds: A Father Remaps the World of Autism. Thriplow, UK: Icon; 2008.

29. **Belek B.** Autism and the proficiency of social ineptitude: probing the rules of 'appropriate' behavior. Ethos 2018;**46**(2):161–79.

30. **McDermott RP.** The acquisition of a child by a learning disability. In: **Chaiklin S, Lave J,** editors. Understanding Practice, 1st edition. Cambridge: Cambridge University Press; 1993: 269–305.

31. **Gleason JJ.** Special Education in Context: An Ethnographic Study of Persons with Developmental Disabilities. Cambridge: Cambridge University Press; 1989.

32. **Mercieca DP.** Living Otherwise: Students with Profound and Multiple Learning Disabilities as Agents in Educational Contexts (Studies in Inclusive Education, Volume 17). Rotterdam: SensePublishers; 2013.

33. **Avery JD.** An Ethnography of Severe Intellectual Disability: Becoming 'Dirty Little Freaks'. Cham: Palgrave Macmillan; 2020.

34. **Rapp R, Ginsburg F.** The paradox of recognition: success or stigma for children with learning disabilities. In: **McLaughlin J, Phillimore P, Richardson, D,** editors. Contesting Recognition. London: Palgrave Macmillan; 2011: 166–86.

35. **McDermott R, Varenne H.** Culture as disability. Anthropology & Education Quarterly 1995;**26**(3):324–48.

36. **McDermott R, Goldman S, Varenne H.** The cultural work of learning disabilities. Educational Researcher 2006;**35**(6):12–17.

37. **Johnson K.** Deinstitutionalising Women: An Ethnographic Study of Institutional Closure. Cambridge: Cambridge University Press; 1998.

38. **Goffman E.** Asylums: Essays on the Social Situation of Mental Patients and Other Inmates. Harmondsworth: Penguin; 1968.

39. **Levinson J.** Making Life Work: Freedom and Disability in a Community Group Home. Minneapolis, MN: University of Minnesota Press; 2010.

40. **McKearney P.** What escapes persuasion: why intellectual disability troubles 'dependence' in liberal societies. Medical Anthropology 2021;**40**(2):155–68.

41. **McKearney P.** Disabling violence: intellectual disability and the limits of ethical engagement. Journal of the Royal Anthropological Institute. 2022;28(3):956–74.

42. **Redley M.** Full and equal equality. Tizard Learning Disability Review 2018;**23**(2):72–7.

43. **Redley M, Weinberg D.** Learning disability and the limits of liberal citizenship: interactional impediments to political empowerment. Sociology of Health & Illness 2007;**29**(5):767–86.

44. **McKearney P.** Challenging care: professionally not knowing what good care is. Anthropology and Humanism 2020;**45**(2):223–32.

45. **McKearney P.** Between dependence and freedom: on the impossibility of liberal care. *forthcoming*. Current Anthropology.

46. **Banks C.** Everyday ethnography interpreting and 'doing' empowerment and protection care imperatives in a supported-living environment for intellectually disabled adults. Findings from experiences as a support worker. Suomen Antropologi: Journal of the Finnish Anthropological Society 2012;37(3):75–88.

47. **Davies CA.** Caring communities or effective networks?: Community care and people with learning difficulties in South Wales. In: **Edgar I**, **Russell A**, editors. The Anthropology of Welfare. London: Routledge; 2002: 120–36.

48. **Davies CA.** Constructing other selves: (in)competences and the category of learning difficulties. In: **Jenkins R**, editor. Questions of Competence: Culture, Classification and Intellectual Disability. Cambridge: Cambridge University Press; 1999: 102–24.

49. **Hudson B.** Michael Lipsky and street-level bureaucracy: a neglected perspective. In: **Barton L**, editor. Disability and Dependency. London: Palmer Press; 1989: 41–52.

50. **Kulick D, Rydström J.** Loneliness and Its Opposite: Sex, Disability, and the Ethics of Engagement. Durham, NC: Duke University Press; 2015.

51. **Bogdan R, Taylor SJ.** The social construction of humanness: relationships with severely disabled people. In: **Ferguson PM, Ferguson DL, Taylor SJ**, editors. Interpreting Disability: A Qualitative Reader. New York: Teachers College Press; 1992: 135–48.

52. **Kittay EF.** Love's Labor: Essays on Women, Equality, and Dependency. New York: Routledge; 1999.

53. **Kittay EF.** Learning From My Daughter: The Value and Care of Disabled Minds. New York: Oxford University Press; 2019.

54. **Hubert J.** Home-bound: Crisis in the Care of Young People with Severe Learning Difficulties; A Story of Twenty Families. London: King's Fund Centre; 1991.

55. **Hubert J, Hollins S.** Working with elderly carers of people with learning disabilities and planning for the future. Advances in Psychiatric Treatment 2000;**6**(1):41–8.

56. **Hubert J.** 'My heart is always where he is'. Perspectives of mothers of young people with severe intellectual disabilities and challenging behaviour living at home. British Journal of Learning Disabilities 2011;**39**(3):216–24.

57. **Rapp R.** Testing Women, Testing the Fetus: The Social Impact of Amniocentesis in America. New York: Routledge; 1999.

58. **Rapp R, Ginsburg F.** Reverberations: disability and the new kinship imaginary. Anthropological Quarterly 2011;**84**(2):379–410.

59. **Rapp R, Ginsburg F.** Worlding the 'new normal' for young adults with disabilities. In: **Thomas GM, Sakellariou D,** editors. Disability, Normalcy, and the Everyday. London: Routledge; 2018: 100–20.

60. **Landsman G.** Does God give special kids to special parents? Personhood and the child with disabilities as gift and giver. In: **Layne L,** editor. Transformative Motherhood: On Giving and Getting in a Consumer Culture. New York: NYU Press; 1999: 133–66.

61. **Landsman G.** Reconstructing Motherhood and Disability in the Age of Perfect Babies. New York: Routledge; 2008.

62. **Jackson AJ.** Worlds of care: the emotional lives of fathers caring for children with disabilities. Oakland, CA: University of California Press; 2021.

63. **Rutherford D.** Proximity to Disability. Anthropological Quarterly 2020;**93**(1):1453–81.

64. **Mattingly C.** Moral Laboratories: Family Peril and the Struggle for a Good Life. Berkeley, CA: University of California Press; 2014.

65. **Zoanni T.** The possibilities of failure: personhood and cognitive disability in urban Uganda. Cambridge Journal of Anthropology 2018;**36**(1):61–79.

66. **Pols J, Althoff B, Bransen E.** The limits of autonomy: ideals in care for people with learning disabilities. Medical Anthropology 2017;**36**(8):772–85.

67. **Angrosino MV.** L'Arche: the phenomenology of Christian counterculturalism. Qualitative Inquiry 2003;**9**(6):934–54.

68. **McKearney P.** L'Arche, learning disability, and domestic citizenship: dependent political belonging in a contemporary British city. City & Society 2017;**29**(2):260–80.

69. **McKearney P.** Receiving the gift of cognitive disability: recognizing agency in the limits of the rational subject. Cambridge Journal of Anthropology 2018;**36**(1):40–60.

70. **McKearney P.** The weight of living: autonomy, care, and responsibility for the self. Journal of Disability and Religion 2019;**22**(3):223–32.

71. **Zoanni T.** Appearances of disability and Christianity in Uganda. Cultural Anthropology 2019;**34**(3):444–70.

72. **Lancaster-Gaye D,** editor. Personal Relationships, the Handicapped and the Community: Some European Thoughts and Solutions. London: Routledge; 1972.

73. **Siebers T.** Disability and the right to have rights. Disability Studies Quarterly 2007;**27**(1/2): 4–19.

74. **Jackson R.** Discovering Camphill: New Perspectives, Research and Developments. Edinburgh: Floris Books; 2011.

75. **Wagner R.** The Invention of Culture. Chicago, IL: University of Chicago Press; 1975.

76. **Dumont L.** Homo Hierarchicus: The Caste System and Its Implications. Chicago, IL: University of Chicago Press; 1980.

77. **Dumont L.** Essays on Individualism: Modern Ideology in Anthropological Perspective. Chicago, IL: University of Chicago Press; 1986.

78. **Strathern M.** The Gender of the Gift: Problems with Women and Problems with Society in Melanesia. Berkley, CA: University of California Press; 1990.

79. **Mahmood S.** Politics of Piety: The Islamic Revival and the Feminist Subject. Princeton, NJ: Princeton University Press; 2012.

80. **Ferguson J.** Declarations of dependence: labour, personhood, and welfare in southern Africa. Journal of the Royal Anthropological Institute 2013;**19**(2):223–42.

81. **Robbins J.** Beyond the suffering subject: toward an anthropology of the good. Journal of the Royal Anthropological Institute 2013;**19**(3):447–62.

82. **Goodley D.** 'Learning difficulties', the social model of disability and impairment: challenging epistemologies. Disability & Society 2001;**16**(2):207–31.

83. **Ginzberg E.** The mentally handicapped in a technological society. In: **Osler S, Cooke R**, editors. The Biosocial Basis of Mental Retardation. Baltimore, MD: Johns Hopkins University Press; 1965: 1–15.

84. **Oliver M.** Disability and dependency: a creation of industrial societies. In: **Barton L**, editor. Disability and Dependency. London: Palmer Press; 1989: 6–22.

85. **Groce NE.** Everyone Here Spoke Sign Language. Cambridge, MA: Harvard University Press; 2009.

86. **Jenkins R**, editor. Questions of Competence: Culture, Classification and Intellectual Disability. Cambridge: Cambridge University Press; 1999.

87. **McKearney P, Zogas A.** Mentally fit: negotiating the boundaries of cognitive disability. Medical Anthropology 2021;**40**(2):111–15.

88. **Sargent C.** Ambivalent Inheritance: Down Syndrome and Kinship Futures in Jordan. PhD Thesis, University of Michigan; 2018. Available from: https://deepblue.lib.umich.edu/bitstream/handle/2027.42/145926/casarge_1.pdf

89. **Sargent C.** Situating disability in the anthropology of the Middle East. International Journal of Middle East Studies 2019;**51**(1):1–4.

90. **Sargent C.** The stakes of (not) knowing. Medicine Anthropology Theory 2020;**7**(2):10–32.

91. **Sargent C.** Kinship, connective care, and disability in Jordan. Medical Anthropology 2021;**40**(2):1–13.

92. **Fietz H.** The work of care. Somatosphere; 2019. Available from: http://somatosphere.net/2019/the-work-of-care.html/

93. **Fietz H.** Negotiating care: living arrangements and adults with cognitive disabilities in South Brazil. Développement Humain, Handicap et Changement Social 2020;**26**(1):37.

94. **Aydos V, Fietz H.** When citizenship demands care: the inclusion of people with autism in the Brazilian labour market. Disability Studies Quarterly 2017;**37**(4):6807.

95. **Craft A, Craft MJ.** Handicapped Married Couples: A Welsh Study of Couples Handicapped from Birth by Mental, Physical, or Personality Disorder. London: Routledge & Kegan Paul; 1980.

96. **Zoanni T.** The ecology of disabled minds in urban Uganda. Medical Anthropology 2021;**40**(2):169–81.

97. **Livingston J.** Debility and the Moral Imagination in Botswana: Disability, Chronic Illness, and Aging. Bloomington, IN: Indiana University Press; 2005.

98. **Ingstad B.** Mpho ya Modimo—a gift from God: perspectives on 'attitudes' toward disabled persons. In: **Ingstad B, Whyte SR**, editors. Disability and Culture. Berkeley, CA: University of California Press; 1995: 246–63.

99. **Ingstad B, Whyte SR**, editors. Disability and Culture. Berkeley, CA: University of California Press; 1995.

100. **Ingstad B, Whyte SR.** Disability in Local and Global Worlds. Berkeley, CA: University of California Press; 2007.

101. **Kaufman S.** Friendship, coping systems and community adjustment of mildly retarded adults. In: **Edgerton RB,** editor. Lives in Process: Mildly Retarded Adults in a Large City. Washington, DC: American Association on Mental Deficiency; 1984: 73–92.

102. **Shakespeare T.** Disability Rights and Wrongs Revisited. London: Routledge; 2013.

103. **Booth T, Booth W.** Risk, resilience and competence: parents with learning difficulties and their children. In: **Jenkins R,** editor. Questions of Competence: Culture, Classification and Intellectual Disability. Cambridge: Cambridge University Press; 1999: 76–101.

104. **Mehrotra N, Vaidya S.** Exploring constructs of intellectual disability and personhood in Haryana and Delhi. Indian Journal of Gender Studies 2008;**15**(2):317–40.

105. **Gammeltoft T.** Haunting Images: A Cultural Account of Selective Reproduction in Vietnam. Berkeley, CA: University of California Press; 2014.

106. **Orsi RA.** 'Mildred, is it fun to be a cripple?' The culture of suffering in mid-twentieth century American Catholicism. In: Between Heaven and Earth: The Religious Worlds People Make and the Scholars Who Study Them. Princeton, NJ: Princeton University Press; 2013: 19–47.

107. **Edgerton RB.** A case of delabeling: some practical and theoretical implications. In: **Langness LL, Levine HG,** editors. Culture and Retardation: Life Histories of Mildly Mentally Retarded Persons in American Society. Dordrecht: D. Reidel; 1988: 101–26.

108. **Kogel P, Edgerton RB.** Black 'six-hour retarded children' as young adults. In: **Edgerton RB,** editor. Lives in Process: Mildly Retarded Adults in a Large City. Washington, DC: American Association on Mental Deficiency; 1984: 145–71.

109. **Kernan KT, Sharon S.** Getting there: directions given by mildly retarded and nonretarded adults. In: **Edgerton RB,** editor. Lives in Process: Mildly Retarded Adults in a Large City. Washington, DC: American Association on Mental Deficiency; 1984: 9–26.

A previous version of this text has been published as: McKearney, Patrick, and Tyler Zoanni. 2023. "Intellectual disability". In The Open Encyclopedia of Anthropology, edited by Felix Stein. Online: http://doi.org/10.29164/22intellectualdisability

Chapter 7

Perception of intellectual disability across cultures

Shweta Gangavati, Chandanie G. Hewage, Arjun Nayar, and Santosh K. Chaturvedi

Introduction

Culture can be conceptualized as an amalgamation of religious beliefs, societal practices, educational and socioeconomic factors, and other influences that shape people's thinking and behaviours. This makes it difficult to clearly describe, predict, or understand these behaviours based on one aspect of a culture, as there can be a unique mix of many factors contributing to this. Moreover, with the advent of the internet and improved accessibility to information in the digital world, people have access to information other than what is commonly shared within their own cultures. The increasing popularity and use of virtual reality are creating a type of digital culture which is likely to become prominent in times to come (1). Although many people with intellectual disability (ID) experience inequalities in digital access (2), the digital world is bound to exert its influence on the attitudes and behaviours of society. In comparison to the pre-digital era, this is beginning to challenge the boundaries of geography. This chapter explores the perception of ID as shaped by some of these factors.

Perception of intellectual disability

On the one hand, the label of ID continues to attract stigma, which can lead to social isolation and lack of support, and on the other hand, a diagnosis of ID can open doors to services and support from health, social, and voluntary care services. Perception of ID varies across different cultures and this perception in turn influences the response of the community to their members with ID. Knowledge of the various factors that influence the perception of ID is therefore useful in the support of individuals with ID as well as in choosing appropriate public health interventions. The key frames by which we look at the perception of ID in this chapter are time, religion, socioeconomics, geographical region, and media. The phenomenon of stigma, which is closely related to perception, is also discussed.

Perception of intellectual disability over time periods

The terms used to describe individuals with ID may shed some light on how these people were perceived by communities during different periods. The terms used in the past are now perceived to be 'value laden', with negative connotations. In the Middle Ages, people with ID were generally thought to be influenced by satanic and demonic forces with reports of people with ID being feared and treated cruelly (3). Monasteries and convents in medieval Europe looked after their basic needs while at the same time keeping them away from mainstream society.

In 1905, Alfred Binet suggested the need for special education for children who lacked success in normal classrooms. However, as Parmenter (4) stated, 'terms such as "morons", "idiots", and "imbeciles" were used to classify people according to scores on intelligence tests devised by Binet'. Between 1850 and 1940, the terminology used included 'fools', 'cretins', 'feeble minded', and 'mentally defective'. Between 1940 and 1970 the terms used were 'mentally retarded' and 'mentally handicapped'. The term "mental retardation," which was introduced as a progressive measure to combat stigma and prejudice, would gradually become unacceptable itself. Dan Barry, a *New York Times* reporter and columnist, describes in his article titled 'Giving a name, and dignity, to a disability', 'each succeeding term that enters the lexicon for this group invariably develops a pejorative connotation as the years go by' (5).

While significant leaps were being made in medicine, philosophy, and literature, it appears that even some of the pioneers of these movements failed to give attention to people with ID. Hippocrates and Aristotle classed people with ID as "barely human". As Dan Barry puts it, even a commission on "idiocy" led by an early disability rights advocate, wrote that "it appeared to us certain that the existence of too many idiots, in every generation, must be the consequence of some violation of the natural laws; that, where there was so much suffering, there must have been sin" (5).

John Locke, a British philosopher who lived between 1623 and 1704, wrote about the value of education for people with ID, and it was described as the 'Age of Enlightenment' within the European context (3). The French physician, Edouard Seguin, advocated for the role of education in improving the lives of people with ID (6). Despite such positive initiatives, the social acceptance of people with ID has been a very gradual process, with much work still to be done.

From 1970 to 1990, people became more aware of the stigma that these terms and connotations caused to people with ID. These terms were replaced by alternative ones such as 'developmentally handicapped' and 'developmentally disabled'. In 2010, Rosa's Law was passed in the US, whereby the term 'mental retardation' was replaced with 'intellectual disability' (7). In the UK, the terms ID and learning disability are used in both research and clinical practice. History teaches us that, over time, the perception of disability will change, and we will be judged by future generations on our approach to disability and disabled people. It is possible that the current terms we use could be viewed as pejorative in future. To cite an example, there is an effort in India to replace the word 'viklang' (meaning disability) with 'divyang' (meaning divine body) (8).

Perception of intellectual disability and religions

There is very limited literature on how people from different religions perceive and respond to people with ID. Religious texts make reference to people with disabilities which may be interpreted as being inclusive of people with ID. There is, however, no specific reference to ID. In this section, we therefore use the reference to disabilities in its general meaning from religious texts to explore how people with ID have been viewed by religions. In addition, we use limited current literature on how families or carers use their religious beliefs to draw strength in caring for people with ID.

We acknowledge that there could be variations in perception of ID within the same religion based on other factors such as location, country of origin, or ethnic background. As there is another chapter on religion and spirituality in this textbook (see Chapter 13), this chapter focuses specifically on how the perception of ID is influenced by religious beliefs.

Eastern religions including Hinduism, Buddhism, Jainism, and Sikhism

We have included these Eastern religions together, as there are many concepts and beliefs shared extensively by them. In the ancient religious texts of Eastern religions, there is no direct reference to people with ID. Therefore, what is discussed in this section applies to a variety of disabilities, including ID. There is variability in how disability or people with disability are perceived even within the context of a single religion and often religious textbooks or beliefs are interpreted differently by people over time.

Eastern religions have used the concept of 'karma' or 'karma-phala' to make sense of the cause of disability. The notion of karma is reflected in most of the Eastern religions including Hinduism, Buddhism, Jainism, and Sikhism.

However, there are some differences in how this is interpreted and acted upon. Karma is a Sanskrit word for action and is explained as 'deeds done in the past (including one's previous life) affecting the current life'. Negative karma is a result of wrong things a person has done in the past, whereas a person accumulates positive karma by practising right and good things (9). The belief that disability is caused by the negative karma of the individual with a disability or that of the family can evoke feelings of guilt and social isolation of people from families with a disabled person. This can create stigmatization leading to the social isolation of families and barriers to accessing appropriate services at the right time (10).

Many Hindus believe in the concept of reincarnation or rebirth, and they also believe that collecting positive karmas in the present life ensures the betterment of their next life. Caring for those with disabilities is regarded as a righteous and ethical duty of normal people. The person with the disability, and those who care, get an opportunity to gain positive karma by doing good deeds (11).

Buddhists believe that the effects of karma can be influenced by performing righteous, moral, ethical, and good acts (12). Buddha's teachings reiterate that caring for the sick and the disabled is a supreme act and is like caring for Buddha himself. Hence Buddhists believe one can acquire good or positive karma by taking care of the disabled. Most of the time disabled people are also considered as those who need supportive care like the sick. As a result, Buddhists willingly care for the sick and the disabled. Not only families, but unrelated wealthy people also willingly and generously contribute to the caring of the disabled, including people with ID. It is not uncommon to see people with ID being overprotected and receiving excessive support depriving them of the opportunity to develop as much independence as they potentially can.

Belief in the concept of karma has both negative and positive aspects. On the one hand, karma is seen as the consequence of one's action which could contribute to stigma and neglect or ill-treatment of people with disability. On the other hand, believers of the Eastern religions draw on the same belief to come to terms with the disability and cope with it. The belief that one can achieve positive karma by supporting someone with a disability leads to a positive attitude to caring for someone with a disability. Interpretation of religious beliefs when combined with a lack of understanding of disability, can lead to negative beliefs against disability. One of the authors has come across an incident in a Buddhist community that shows that this negative reaction to people with disability is not always influenced by religion but by the ignorance of people. In this incident, the parents of a child with Down syndrome in a primary school were requested by the class teacher to remove the child from her class, as the teacher was pregnant and believed that seeing this child daily may cause problems to her unborn fetus. This belief is not related to the religion, but perhaps a belief shared by a few people in the local community.

Belief systems of Eastern religions also have a close link with astrology. Karma is believed to influence the person through the planetary constellation at the time of birth (11). When a baby is born, it is common practice for a horoscope to be prepared by an astrologer. Astrologers predict and forecast the future of the newborn according to the horoscope. An astrologer may predict problems in children with ID at birth and attribute them to certain planetary placements. Various religious activities may be prescribed to compensate for the planetary placements. Although this explanation may help the family cope with the situation initially, this could contribute to delay in seeking the right support and missing the opportunity for early assessment and intervention.

Judaism and intellectual disability

According to Judaism, Moses was sent by God and is considered the most important prophet. The Torah (the first five books of the Hebrew Bible) gives the 'law of the God' as revealed to Moses. According to the Torah, disability is caused by 'Yahweh' (meaning the God of the Israelites). Disability is viewed as a punishment for acts that go against the law, rule, or code of conduct laid down according to God's revelations.

At the same time, God commands people in Judaism 'not to insult the deaf or place a stumbling block before the blind'. 'Halakha', the collective body of Jewish religious laws, states that people should support sick people. Detailed exploration of documentary evidence of Judaism and disability reveals that there are many instances of recommending giving equal respect and rights to people with disabilities. There are examples of Jewish communities across the world providing special approaches for supporting students with ID (13). A paper by Kandel et al. (14) discusses the marriage of people with ID from the perspectives of Jewish law and comments that some of the principles are more accommodative and liberal.

Christianity, Catholicism, and intellectual disability

There is no specific reference to ID in the Bible, although physical disability is documented in the New Testament. The causes of the disability are described in different ways. While there is some reference to disability being a punishment for a person's sins, it is also considered a way of portraying God's power to people and there is an incident where Jesus was able to miraculously heal a blind man and revealed to his disciples that 'the work of God might be displayed in him'.

In Christian beliefs during the Middle Ages, people viewed disabilities mainly in two ways. Some believed that disability was God's punishment for a person's sins, leading to a negative attitude towards and ill-treatment of those with disability, including ID. At the same time, disabled people were believed by some to be more devoted to God and to possess special gifts (15).

In contemporary Christianity, people with disabilities are viewed as God's will or wish and it is agreed to accept them in society as for any other person. Evidence suggests that although parents may use religions for 'meaning making' either positively or negatively at the beginning, they eventually would often put aside the negative feelings to accept their child while holding on to their faith (16). Disabled individuals are considered spiritually equal and people with disabilities are included in the community and all the activities of the Church like any non-disabled person. Some believe that having a disabled child born to them is because they are the chosen ones by God to do a special role by caring for the special child. Hence, they consider it a privilege and very faithfully look after the disabled child well.

Islam and intellectual disability

Although disability is not directly mentioned in the Quran, the religious text of Islam, the term 'disadvantaged people' is considered to include people with special needs. It is considered a challenge given by Allah. Muslims are expected to care for and protect disabled people. Muslims who are capable of earning are expected to give part of their earnings regularly to care for the needy, which include the poor, sick, and disabled. Disabled people to some extent are exempted from the compulsory engagement of prayers. In the community, they are included in all activities like any other person without discrimination. Although sharing the same belief system, within the Muslim religion, attitude to disability can vary based on socioeconomic status, education, geographical, or cultural contexts (17).

Socioeconomic factors and perception of intellectual disability

Traditional religion is only one of many factors which influence how people live. Other factors that could influence the perception of ID include urban–rural backgrounds and socioeconomic backgrounds.

Urban–rural locations have been linked with differences in how people with ID are perceived and how these perceptions affect access to support and services. A Scottish study showed that people with ID living in rural areas have better access to daytime activities, including employment (18), but this is not reflected in other parts of the world, particularly in developing countries. The overall prevalence of ID in the developing world is reported to be higher in rural areas (18). While there is some evidence indicating better acceptance and better integration of people with ID in farming communities of rural backgrounds this is not universally true. Acceptance is better if the person with ID has a milder level of disability and is in a large extended family. An extended family setting provides opportunities for all family members to share the tasks of supporting the person with ID. Rural communities at the same time have lesser access to healthcare, are comparatively less educated, and have less access to the latest information about healthcare. Lack of information and alternative sociocultural explanations for the disability could lead to carers using alternative systems of support such as faith healing. This can, in turn, delay access to appropriate services to treat health conditions, as well as providing support for the person's development. Therefore, in countries such as India, several family-focused interventions and community-based rehabilitation interventions have been implemented to provide much-needed support for families who have children with ID (19). Culturally acceptable parent associations to provide advocacy services, awareness, and support in policymaking have also been set up.

One of the authors of this chapter conducted a study in India which concluded that rejection, hostility, neglect, and other negative attitudes were significantly higher in families from urban areas and those with higher education (20). It is possible that the urban middle-class communities that highly value the intellectual (and productive) abilities of a person tend to marginalize, shame, and discriminate against those who are unable to compete intellectually and thrive financially. This problem is worsened by the fact that they live in nuclear families and have fewer children in each family. Due to the stigma, children with ID from middle social class families are sometimes kept hidden and may not receive necessary care. The experience of some of the authors who have worked and researched in the Indian subcontinent suggests that educated and affluent parents, as well as others around them, often set up services training themselves to provide better care for people with ID like their children. Some may also choose to migrate to bigger cities where they have better access to services.

Perception of intellectual disability and stigma across the world

Stigma is a significant issue faced by people with ID from around the world but has not received the same attention as the stigma of mental illness (21). An international survey across ten countries involving 8000 people from the mainstream population found that most people have a low expectation of what people with ID can achieve. Just over half believed that the negative attitude of the society posed an obstacle to the inclusion of people with ID in the community (22). A study on social acceptance and stigma towards people with ID found that there are variations even in developed countries (23). People from Austria and Germany were significantly less likely to identify symptoms of someone with ID and likely to be more hostile towards social contacts than people from the UK. Caregivers' and parents' explanatory models of ID in Khayelitsha, Cape Town, South Africa were explored by Swartz and Mkbile (24). Participants showed a high level of discomfort, shame, and embarrassment when asked about the words they used to describe ID. There were also a variety of causative explanations for ID which varied from life events during pregnancy and maternal health to witchcraft, and spirits or ancestors being unhappy. Understanding the cause of ID could have a significant effect on how it is perceived. A significant level of stigma is reported in studies from India, China, Vietnam, and Nigeria (20,25–27). The level of stigma and how it affects carer stress can vary based on the level of disability and associated behaviours. A study from Israel suggests a more positive attitude to mild than severe ID (28).

Differentiation between ID and mental illness can also vary in different parts of the world. There is also a variation in the level of stigma attached to these conditions. Langness and Levine (29) noted that in the US, some people with mild ID pretended to have a psychiatric illness, as this carries a lower degree of public delegitimization than does ID. This shows that the understanding and perception of society can influence the presentation and how people seek support. Different communities across the world over time have struggled to understand ID and differentiate it from other conditions affecting behaviour, such as mental illness. In Trinidad, the popular concept of *doltishness* includes both ID ('you're born with it') and dementia ('you become like a child a second time') and is distinguished as a whole from *madness* (30). There is no implication of the involvement of spirits in doltishness and the aetiology is naturalistic.

Beliefs about ID could also vary based on parents' country of origin. A cross-cultural study by Fatimilehin and Nadirshaw (31) reported that the differences in attitudes and beliefs between British Asian and British White families were more linked to the differences in religious and cultural differences than the other characteristics of the child with a disability or their parents. Asian British families had more contact with a 'holy' person, were less aware of what their child's problem was called, unsure of the cause of their child's disability, and believed in a religious or spiritual explanation of the cause. Their faith helped them to cope, but they had limited practical support within their communities. There was an expectation that one of the relatives would continue to provide care when the current carers (usually parents) were unable to provide this. In contrast, most White British families had a medical explanation and did not rely on spiritual explanation.

Depiction of intellectual disability in media, books, and films across cultures

Books, films, and social media have a two-way relationship with society. The stories that are narrated in these media are influenced by the sociocultural context of society. At the same time, these stories in turn influence the perspectives of society. Therefore, the representation of diversity within these stories has a significant influence in shaping society's views of conditions like ID. If the story is told as close as possible to the real lived experience of people with ID, this could reduce stigma and improve the perception of society towards people with ID (32).

As Iyer (33) stated, 'knowledge of fictional images can enhance a professional's understanding of individual lives'. It could also highlight the unspoken stereotypes that exist in popular culture regarding people with disabilities. This may prove to be a valuable tool for reasoned and informed advocacy when clinicians speak for or about people with ID. Iyer (33) explored the depiction of ID and autism through various characters in fiction, including those depicted in William Faulkner's *The Sound and Fury*, Salman Rushdie's *Shame*, and Charles Dickens' *Barnaby Rudge*. Drawing a parallel between the two groups who are often misrepresented in fiction, namely people with mental illness and people with ID, she highlights how first-person accounts from people with mental illness themselves changed the perception of mental illness, while the situation for people with ID continues to be the same. She argues that the fictional representation of people with ID by others which people with ID themselves cannot contest presents an ethical challenge. Characters with ID are seldom the main characters in fiction. They are portrayed as passive victims of exploitation as in *Such a Long Journey*, an award-winning novel written by Rohinton Mistry, targets of ridicule and cruelty as in *Of Mice and Men* by John Steinbeck, or as violent, as in *To Kill a Mockingbird*, written by Harper Lee. Descriptions of physical appearances and behaviours in fiction often contrast people with ID as distinct from the readers, making them 'the others'. The distance created by emphasizing the lack of normative functioning inevitably affects the lives of these individuals, and of those people who care for them.

As stated already generally about media, films reflect the society in which they are made and give an overview of cultural values and norms. Films have been used to understand the sociocultural aspects of mental illness (34). History is a testament to the fact that films influence fashion, lifestyle, attitudes, and behaviour and can have a deep bearing on our perceptions about several aspects of our lives—be it romantic liaisons (portrayed relentlessly in Bollywood films), violence, extraterrestrial life, or a perfect hero like James Bond.

Several films have been made regarding people with ID/other developmental disorders like autism and some have people with ID or autism starring in them. The film *Like Normal People*, released in 1979, depicts the struggle of two people with ID who wish to get married and the opposition they face. *Rain Man*, released in 1988, has a gifted autistic individual as the central character. In 2018, a documentary named *Intelligent Lives* followed the lives of three people with ID and how they beat all odds to achieve qualifications in sports and academics. *I am Sam* shows the struggle of a father with ID to keep his daughter with him. There are films made in different countries and cultures like India, Israel, and France depicting the lives of people with ID. Bollywood films like *Ahaan* and *Eshwar* have touched upon ID. *My Four Children* is a documentary about an Israeli mother who fosters four children with Down's syndrome. *Swathi Mutthu* (White Pearl), a Kannada (South Indian) film describes a man with subnormal intelligence and his relationship with a widow. In the film, the hero raises important issues such as why a widow cannot remarry, and finally gets married to her. Another Kannada film *Gurushishyaru* (Master and the Disciples), depicts a group of men with ID and their interactions with their teacher.

While characters with ID played by popular actors like Dustin Hoffman (in *Rain Man*) and Tom Hanks (in *Forrest Gump*) led to increased awareness of the respective conditions in the population, there have been debates about how realistic such representations of people with ID are (35). The two films mentioned above shows gifted individuals with autism which is not the reality with the rest of the population. Infantilization of behaviours or making the tasks they do simple and monotonous in many of the films create an image that people with ID are childlike or not capable of undertaking meaningful social roles. When female characters are portrayed as intellectually challenged in films, they end up being sexually abused or exploited in various other ways. In contrast, the attribution of special abilities like the character's phenomenal visual memory in *Rain Man* can make the person feel superhuman. Both could create an unrealistic picture of the situation of people with ID and other developmental disorders like autism for the general public. Moreover, these simplifications take out the sociocultural contexts of these individuals and the reality of the two-way relationship between the impairment in an individual and the environment in defining the disability. The approaches taken by the films seem to focus on the cognitive impairment of the individuals with no acknowledgement of socially created disabling barriers (36). It is very rare to see creative artists highlighting the strengths of people with ID, which will influences the perception of ID in the public sphere. Telling stories drawn from real-life experiences, providing multiple perspectives, and involvement of people with ID themselves in the creation of films are essential to change this.

It is quite heartening to note that there have been a few films that have not only explored ID but that people with ID acted in them. In *Peanut Butter Falcon*, the main character is played by an actor with Down syndrome. The film *My Brother* released in 2006 had two individuals with ID who starred in it.

People with ID are making their presence felt on the small screen as well. In the UK, recent TV advertisements have featured people with Down's syndrome. A girl with Down syndrome appeared in advertisements for well-known brands like Marks and Spencer, River Island, and Aveeno (37). A YouTube video positively portrayed people with ID and their journey into making a rock music band. Delta 7 (38) is a music band comprising people with ID, who describe how music helped shape their life. It is indeed heartening to watch some of the popular Ted Talks being delivered by people with ID (39,40).

We hope that there will be continued efforts at portraying people with ID in a realistic and inclusive way which then will further help change people's perceptions for the better, as well as reducing the stigma and abuse of this vulnerable population.

Conclusion

In summary, the perceptions of people with ID across cultures are varied and multifaceted, being influenced by religious beliefs, societal attitudes, educational status of parents, and socioeconomic backgrounds. Identifying these themes is essential as it helps healthcare workers, policymakers, educationalists, and often community leaders to address these issues, to ensure that help and support is available for people with ID and their families. This will improve access to care and support, which will hopefully translate into better health and social outcomes for people with ID.

From a sociocultural perspective, the role of religious healers in this context is often unrecognized and underestimated. Often, they are the ones who are the first point of contact for many families as per their religious customs and beliefs, and if these community leaders can then dispel some myths and signpost the families to appropriate healthcare settings, families might be more inclined to seek medical support.

Traditionally, fiction played a role in shaping how society viewed people with ID, but the increasing influence of new media such as YouTube and other similar platforms is providing opportunities as well as challenges. Involvement of people with ID themselves as actors, narrators, or models in these media is likely to have a positive impact.

Finally, it is hoped that the concerted effort of professionals, families, and society as well as the media will enhance the uptake of services in this marginalized group of individuals. This would allow people with ID to lead fulfilling lives and pave the way for a paradigm shift in societal attitudes towards them.

References

1. **Schlemmer E, Backes L.** Digital virtual culture in metaverse. In: **Schlemmer E, Backes L**, editors. Learning in Metaverse: Co-Existing in Real Virtuality. Hershey, PA: IGI Global; 2015: 278–93.

2. **Glencross S, Mason J, Katsikitis M, Greenwood KM.** Internet use by people with intellectual disability: exploring digital inequality—a systematic review. Cyberpsychology, Behavior, and Social Networking 2021;**24**(8):503–20.

3. **Sanfilios-Rothschild C.** The sociology and social psychology of disability and rehabilitation. Australian Journal of Occupational Therapy 2010;**19**(3):147.

4. **Parmenter TR.** The present, past and future of the study of intellectual disability: challenges in developing countries. Salud Publica de Mexico 2008;**50**(Suppl 2):S124–31.

5. **Barry D.** Giving a name, and dignity, to a disability. The New York Times 7 May 2016. Available from: https://www.nytimes.com/2016/05/08/sunday-review/giving-a-name-and-dignity-to-a-disability.html

6. **Stainton T.** Reason, value and persons: the construction of intellectual disability in western thought from antiquity to the romantic age. In: **Hanes R, Brown I, Hansen NE**, editors. The Routledge History of Disability. New York: Routledge; 2017: 11–34.

7. **Educational Department.** Rosa's law. Federal Register of the United States Government; 2017. Available from: https://www.federalregister.gov/documents/2017/07/11/2017-14343/rosas-law

8. **Venugopal V.** PM Narendra Modi suggests use of 'divyang' for persons with disability in his 'Mann Ki Baat'. The Economic Times 28 December 2015. Available from: https://economictimes.indiatimes.com/news/politics-and-nation/pm-narendra-modi-suggests-use-of-divyang-for-persons-with-disability-in-his-mann-ki-baat/articleshow/50341878.cms

9. **White CJM, Norenzayan A, Schaller M.** The content and correlates of belief in karma across cultures. Personality and Social Psychology Bulletin 2019;**45**(8):1184–201.

10. **Wilson A.** Barriers and enablers provided by Hindu beliefs and practices for people with disabilities in India. Christian Journal for Global Health 2019;**6**(2):12–25.

11. **Gupta VB.** How Hindus cope with disability. Journal of Religion, Disability & Health 2011;**15**(1):72–8.

12. **Lin CT, Yen WH.** On the naturalization of karma and rebirth. International Journal of Dharma Studies 2015;**3**(1):6.

13. **Merrick J, Gabbay Y, Lifshitz H.** Judaism and the person with intellectual disability. Journal of Religion, Disability & Health 2001;**5**(2–3):49–63.

14. **Kandel I, Bergwerk K, Merrick J.** Marriage and parenthood among persons with intellectual disability in Jewish Law. Journal of Religion, Disability & Health 2007;**10**(3–4):207–16.

15. **Cusack CM.** Graciosi: medieval Christian attitudes to disability. Disability and Rehabilitation 1997;**19**(10):414–19.

16. **Baines S, Hatton C.** The impact of the birth of a child with intellectual disabilities on pre-existing parental Christian faith from the perspective of parents who have parented their child to adulthood. Journal of Applied Research in Intellectual Disabilities 2015;**28**(6):524–35.

17. **Al-Aoufi H, Al-Zyoud N, Shahminan N.** Islam and the cultural conceptualisation of disability. International Journal of Adolescence and Youth 2012;**17**(4):205–19.

18. **Nicholson L, Cooper SA.** Social exclusion and people with intellectual disabilities: a rural-urban comparison. Journal of Intellectual Disability Research 2013;**57**(4):333–46.

19. **Girimaji SC, Srinath S.** Perspectives of intellectual disability in India: epidemiology, policy, services for children and adults. Current Opinion in Psychiatry 2010;**23**(5):441–6.

20. **Chaturvedi SK, Malhotra S.** A follow-up study of mental retardation focussing on parental attitudes. Indian Journal of Psychiatry 1984;**26**(4):370–6.

21. **Ditchman N, Werner S, Kosyluk K, Jones N, Elg B, Corrigan PW.** Stigma and intellectual disability: potential application of mental illness research. Rehabilitation Psychology 2013;**58**(2):206–16.

22. **Siperstein Gary N, Norins J, Corbin S, Shriver T.** Multinational study of attitudes toward individuals with intellectual disabilities. Special Olympics Committee Report; 2003. Available from: https://dotorg.brightspotcdn.com/22/87/ce42454e460cb0d609ab8adb6098/attitudes-toward-id-english.pdf

23. **Zeilinger EL, Stiehl KAM, Bagnall H, Scior K.** Intellectual disability literacy and its connection to stigma: a multinational comparison study in three European countries. PLoS One 2020;**15**(10):e0239936.

24. **Mkabile S, Swartz L.** Caregivers' and parents' explanatory models of intellectual disability in Khayelitsha, Cape Town, South Africa. Journal of Applied Research in Intellectual Disabilities 2020;**33**(5):1026–37.

25. **Feaster D, Franzen A.** From stigma to acceptance: intellectual and developmental disabilities in Central China. Journal of Intellectual Disabilities 2021;**25**(4):507–26.

26. **Ngo H, Shin JY, Nhan NV, Yang LH.** Stigma and restriction on the social life of families of children with intellectual disabilities in Vietnam. Singapore Medical Journal 2012;**53**(7):451–7.

27. **Okoh G.** Mental handicap in Nigeria: a study of attitudes in Bendel State. Journal of the British Institute of Mental Handicap (APEX) 2009;**15**(1):35–6.

28. **Weller L, Aminadav C.** Attitudes towards mild and severe mental handicap in Israel. British Journal of Medical Psychology 1989;**62**(Pt 3):273–80.

29. **Langness L, Levine HG,** editors. Culture and Retardation: Life Histories of Mildly Mentally Retarded Persons in American Society. Dordrecht: D. Reidel; 1986.

30. **Littlewood R.** Mental health and intellectual disability: culture and diversity. Journal of Intellectual Disability Research 2006;**50**(8):555–60.

31. **Fatimilehin IA, Nadirshaw Z.** A cross-cultural study of parental attitudes and beliefs about learning disability (mental handicap). Mental Handicap Research 2010;**7**(3):202–27.

32. **Schwartz D, Blue E, McDonald M, Giuliani G, Weber G, Seirup H**, et al. Dispelling stereotypes: promoting disability equality through film. Disability and Society 2010;**25**(7):841–8.

33. **Iyer A.** Depiction of intellectual disability in fiction. Advances in Psychiatric Treatment 2007;**13**(2):127–33.

34. **Bhugra D.** Mad Tales from Bollywood. Hove: Psychology Press; 2013.

35. **Conn R, Bhugra D.** The portrayal of autism in Hollywood films. International Journal of Culture and Mental Health 2012;**5**(1):54–62.

36. **Renwick R, Schormans AF, Shore D.** Hollywood takes on intellectual/developmental disability: cinematic representations of occupational participation. OTJR: Occupation, Participation and Health 2014;**34**(1):20–31.

37. **Shaw M.** Sheffield little girl with Down Syndrome stars in new M&S advert. YorkshireLive; 2 March 2021. Available from: https://www.examinerlive.co.uk/news/local-news/sheffield-little-girl-down-syndrome-19950486

38. **Youtube**. The rock band with learning disabilities—Delta 7. 2020. Available from: https://www.youtube.com/watch?v=EdA_WMdaF6w

39. **Schwab M.** How I know including people with Down syndrome is a good thing. TEDx Talks; 2019. Available from: https://www.ted.com/talks/matthew_schwab_how_i_know_including_people_with_down_syndrome_is_a_good_thing

40. **Gaffney K.** I have one more chromosome than you. So what? TEDx Talks; 2015. Available from: https://www.youtube.com/watch?v=HwxjoBQdn0s

Chapter 8

Safeguarding the rights of people with intellectual disability across cultures

Sreeja Sahadevan, Kamalika Mukherji, Thomas John Kuttichirayil, and Inyang Takon

Power is no blessing in itself, except when it is used to protect the innocent.
Jonathan Swift.

The evolution of the concept of safeguarding

Humanity has evolved considerably from the days of our ancient ancestors, and no trait distinguishes us more from other creatures than our ability to display empathy. It is a mark of our progress and refinement. How well we protect the lives and rights of the vulnerable among us thus undoubtedly is a measure of the advancement of our species.

However, it has not always been the case that people have been considerate of those who are weaker than them. History is replete with instances of excesses against women, children, disabled people, and ethnic and religious minorities as they are perceived by some as weaker sections of society. The mentally ill have faced persecution at the hands of various agencies over centuries, and it has only been from the middle of the last century onwards that the situation began to perceptibly improve (1). The annihilation of the 'unfit' had been a policy of the Nazi era in the early twentieth century which promoted sterilization, experimentation, and euthanasia of mentally and physically disabled people, curtailing their fundamental right to life (2). The inhumane cruelties of the Second World War still haunt us, and it is of great concern and contradiction that such human rights violations occurred at a time when humanity was witnessing paradigm shifts in science (1).

What does safeguarding mean to different cultures?

Across the globe, the terms mental retardation, learning disability, and developmental disability refer to people with intellectual disability (ID). The meaning of the term safeguarding is coloured by the cultural aspects of different regions, similar to the nosological difference in conceptualizing ID around the world (3).

According to the UK Royal College of Psychiatrists (4), safeguarding is regarded as a measure to protect the rights of people, especially the vulnerable, from any kind of abuse harm or neglect.

The rights of people with intellectual disability

The United Nations Convention on the Rights of Persons with Disabilities (UN CRPD) promotes a human rights-based approach to disability rather than a charity- or medical-based approach (5,6). The right to non-discrimination and equality has been emphasized in the Convention. It points out that disability-based discrimination has been marked in multiple domains, including education, employment, transport, housing, social life, and accessibility to public places and services.

Regarding the rights of people with ID, acceptance, integration, and inclusion into mainstream society are still challenges in many countries (7,8). The denial of legal capacity has been implicated in preventing a person from their right to vote, to engage in married life, own property, sign contracts, and decide on their own healthcare and treatment (9). Often medical research fails to take consent from intellectually disabled individuals, and at times their carers fail to act in their best interests. Deprivation of liberty on the basis of disability has been an outcome of considering disability as a lawful ground to either institutionalize the person or to isolate at home, by treating them as unsafe to themselves or others (9,10).

Sex and gender-based bias and discrimination also exist among people with ID (11). Across cultures there have been advocacies for gender equality and representation for all ages. Perhaps the most prominent discrimination based on gender, even in people with ID, is the right to education. An intellectually disabled girl is seldom sent to a school in many communities, especially in developing nations, either due to parental fear of sexual exploitation or not being prioritized due to lack of resources (12).

The right to education for intellectually disabled children is now being recognized across the world, and many countries are trying to incorporate inclusive educational policies for them along with mainstream national curricula (13). Worldwide, people struggle to provide inclusive education due to lack of resources, as well as prejudices that intellectually disabled children cannot be trained in a school and that they could hinder the education of other children (14). There are many special education schools to cater for the training of people with ID both in developing and developed countries, and there is an ongoing debate on whether mainstream education should be inclusive or exclusive for intellectually disabled children.

The need for safeguarding the rights of people with intellectual disability

According to the World Health Organization, middle- and low-income countries lack robust data regarding safeguarding the rights of people with ID (15). As per available data, an adult with a mental health disorder or ID might be four times more vulnerable than their non-disabled peers, whereas people with other disabilities are one-and-a-half times more vulnerable (15). Regarding children with ID and severe mental health issues, they form the most vulnerable group for exploitation and abuse in any modality. The risk of sexual abuse is almost 4.6 times higher for children with ID and severe mental impairment, when compared with the vulnerability of their non-ID peers (15). In reality, the available statistics could be the tip of the iceberg, as many such incidents are not reported or recorded across the world due to a variety of reasons such as stigma, and a lack of awareness or support (16).

These finding should alert us regarding the need for safeguarding of one of the most vulnerable groups of people across the world. Even though the numbers are alarming, unfortunately the perceived need for safeguarding the rights of people with ID across cultures differs. In many geographical areas, the society needs to become more sensitive towards the rights of people with ID.

Vulnerability

There are many facets to the vulnerability of people with ID, as this can vary across regions, religions, ethnicities, and cultures. For instance, in many parts of the world, for years people believed that abuse, especially sexual abuse, did not occur among people with ID (16) when, in fact, victims of sexual abuse are disproportionately higher among people with ID, across age, sex, or socioeconomic class (16).

Some aspects like religion and faith-related factors might be protective; in contrast, some of those beliefs can potentially expose the vulnerable towards abuse (17). For example, in some communities in Asia and Africa, a member of the family with an ID is considered as both a blessing to the family, and an icon of fortune and good luck to their family and the community. Those people are given respect, dignity, love, and care within the family and the community, which together act as a protective factor against neglect and abuse. Many Western countries value human rights and dignity, they treat people with ID with concern, and try and protect their rights as well (18).

Much of the time, the victims of abuse with ID lack the ability to express themselves, even if they can verbalize their experience; largely, the abusers are their caregivers, upon whom the victim might be physically, economically, and socially dependent. Moreover, the society and even the legal system would not usually rely on the testimony of a person with ID due to their lack of mental capacity or their ability to produce the evidence of the abuse, unless it is obvious. Another important aspect of the vulnerability of people with ID is their inability to understand when they are subjected to discrimination, neglect, or abuse. This could not only act as a barrier for the issue to come to the surface, but also as a predisposing as well as perpetuating factor for being abused by the society.

In many cultures, getting married is common among people with ID and they might have children (19). Literature shows that the rights of intellectually disabled people to rear children are widely disregarded by the society. Many cultures across the world, especially among the developed countries during the eugenics movement, advocated for sterilization of people with ID, hence controlling their ability to procreate (2). After many decades, the focus on sterilization has shifted to legal restrictions on marriage in many countries (1). Today, we have many parents with ID across the globe; promisingly, many of their children are brought up well with appropriate and adequate social support within their families (20).

Mental health issues often co-occur with ID (15), leading to a 'double disability', and increasing the person's vulnerability. Studies have reported that the risk of violence is highest among people with ID compared to both the general population as well as people with other types of disabilities (15). According to prison studies, especially from countries like the UK, a pooled prevalence 6.1% (95% CI 2.5–11.1) of the imprisoned population have ID (15). In many parts of the world, violence can lead to manhandling of the offender and other cruel physical punishments given by the family and society alike. Co-occurring mental illness can be a trigger in committing offences and ultimately making the individual vulnerable as well.

Similarly, physical disabilities including sensory impairments, epilepsy, and deformities can be co-occurring conditions in a large number of people with

ID, which also increase the risk of vulnerability. The precise nature of this vulnerability again varies with the culture or the society.

Individuals at extremes of age, as in any other group, are vulnerable to exploitation and might need active involvement to safeguard their rights. Children have always been at risk of exploitation and abuse, and those with ID exceedingly so. From being bullied and ostracized in school to suffering abuse and exploitation, such children are the ones most in need of safeguarding.

Stigma and safeguarding

Communities differ in the practice and perception of stigma associated with ID, and pose a challenge in identifying the vulnerability and implementing safeguarding measures (13,17). In many regions, including within Asia, parents try to hide their children with ID from mainstream society as stigma might affect the social dignity, acceptance, marriage prospects, and social inclusion of other children within the family unit (20). The society might not be largely accommodative towards a disabled person and some societies might see people with ID as a bad omen at an auspicious function or gathering (21).

The stigma might act as a barrier for becoming involved in training and education, disability certification, rehabilitation programmes, and being enrolled in social support and security schemes of the government and other welfare agencies (22). In some cases, the society is not aware that mental health issues in people with ID are medically treatable with conventional medicines and therapies.

Migration and safeguarding

Across the globe, the cultural differences of migrant populations in a particular country are potential barriers for effective safeguarding of the rights of people with ID (17). For instance, in most Asian communities, the role of family and community in deciding a person's prospects is more pronounced, while independence and autonomy are less valued compared to Western communities. Moreover, they differ in the perception and understanding of a disability and the need of seeking support for the same. Some families from South-East Asia may not accept support from others as families believe it is inappropriate to accept support from strangers even if they offer to provide this. The reluctance of people to seek help due to reasons like stigma, fear of financial burden, language barriers, and hospitalization is also a major concern. Many of the migrants to Western countries, especially newcomers, may not be aware about the services available in the new country or the pathways of care (23).

Online victimization and safeguarding

The internet has intruded more and more into the daily life of ordinary people, crossing cultural barriers across the world, transforming it into a global village. Nowadays, the internet is accessible and affordable to all social classes and this does not exclude people with ID. However, the digital inclusion of people with ID on online platforms and social media has its own disadvantages in terms of vulnerability to victimization and perpetration (24). The major risk factors identified for people with ID include exposure to harmful, manipulative, or exploitative content like sexual violence and pornography, experience of negative online experiences like being bullied, grooming for sexual behaviour, radicalization, and engagement in criminal activities.

Legal frameworks available for safeguarding the rights of people with intellectual disability

Living a life free from harm and abuse is a fundamental human right and an essential requirement for good health and inclusion in society (25). Safeguarding ensures that additional measures are in place for those less able to protect themselves from harm or abuse which includes people with physical and intellectual disabilities.

In the UK, the Care Act 2014 (26) made safeguarding a legal responsibility for statutory organizations. The Care Act 2014 defines who is a vulnerable adult and has six key principles which govern the process:

1. *Empowerment*, leading to person-led decisions.
2. *Prevention* of harm, including proactive action before harm occurs.
3. *Proportionality* stops protections going too far; any intervention should be appropriate to the risk presented.
4. *Protection* provides support and representation for those in greatest need.
5. *Partnership* encourages local solutions working with their communities; communities have a part to play in preventing, detecting, and reporting neglect and abuse.
6. *Accountability* ensures that decisions are made transparently, and with clear reasoning.

Although everyone has a responsibility to report if they suspect that a vulnerable person is being abused, the primary legal responsibility lies with local government or local authorities.

Each local authority area, or councils as they are called in the UK, has a Safeguarding Adults Board, which comes together in local areas with representation from health and social care, police, charities, and the third sector to find the best way to safeguard the rights of vulnerable people. There are a number of other areas of UK legislation that should be considered by those reporting, investigating, or dealing with the outcome when safeguarding the rights of a person with ID:

◆ Consent and capacity: Mental Capacity Act 2005 (27)—it is important to establish the capacity of the person to understand the concerns raised and how far they can engage in the process.

◆ Disclosure and information sharing for safeguarding a vulnerable person or in the public interest: Data Protection Act 2018 (28).

◆ The Deprivation of Liberty Safeguards (DoLS) (29) are an amendment to the Mental Capacity Act 2005 and came into force in 2009. They provide a legal framework to protect those who lack the capacity to consent to the arrangements for their treatment or care and where levels of restriction or restraint used in delivering that care for the purpose of protection from risk/harm are so extensive as to potentially be depriving the person of their liberty. The test of DoLS has now been revised into a 'acid test' by the Supreme Court: is the person under continuous supervision and control *and* is the person not free to leave? Every element of these must be satisfied and continue to be tested in law (29).

The UN CRPD (5) is an international human rights treaty intended to protect the rights and dignity of all people with disabilities. The UN CRPD specifically aligns the importance of international development in addressing the rights of people with disabilities.

The UN CRPD is underlined by eight guiding principles:

1. Respect for dignity, individual autonomy, including the freedom to make one's own choices, and independence of persons with disabilities.

2. Non-discrimination.

3. Full and effective participation and inclusion in society.

4. Respect for difference and acceptance of persons with disabilities as part of human diversity and humanity.

5. Equality of opportunity.

6. Accessibility.

7. Equality between men and women.

8. Respect for the evolving capacity of children with disabilities and respect for the right of children with disabilities to preserve their identities.

When a state ratifies a treaty, it takes on legal obligations under international law. Not all countries have adopted the UN CRPD. As international law, the convention is to be followed by public bodies and should be referred to by courts, tribunals, and other administrative processes when making decisions that affect disabled people. This means that the UN CRPD can be referred to in courts, tribunals, and administrative proceedings such as case conferences, reviews, and school/work exclusion decisions.

The UN 2030 Agenda for Sustainable Development (30) states that disability cannot be a reason for lack of access to development programmes and the realization of human rights. The Sustainable Development Goals framework (30) includes seven targets, which explicitly refer to people with disabilities, and six further targets for people in vulnerable situations, which include people with disabilities.

Cultural competence for health workers in the assessment for safeguarding

The cross-cultural competence of healthcare and social care workers plays a pivotal role in understanding the situation and safeguarding the rights of people with ID (31). Lack of awareness and respect for cultural attributes of migrants' beliefs, values, language, and nuance might result in serious deficits in the assessment and delivery of safeguarding services. The main components of a culturally competent assessment of the needs of people with ID in safeguarding their rights according to the Newcastle Safeguarding Adults Board, UK (32) could be summarized under the following aspects:

1. The assessment of needs in terms of safeguarding against the background of complex family or supported home circumstances.

2. Impact of religion or spirituality practised by the family members or carers.

3. Assessment of strengths and resilience of the immediate family or carers and community.

4. A proportionate assessment involving professionals from multidisciplinary agencies utilizing their full potential and including the opinion of the person with ID for a holistic evaluation.

5. Partnership with governmental and other agencies promoting safeguarding and welfare of people with ID.

6. Professionals involved in safeguarding should follow informed practice by educating and updating themselves about the cultural aspects and the current legislations and support systems involved in safeguarding people with ID.

What could be done or achieved globally to protect the rights of people with intellectual disabilities?

Despite the existing legal framework and knowledge of the rights of people with ID, existing literature and anecdotal information have shown that current practices in the developing and the developed world still fall short of what is desired (31).

In determining what could be done to protect the rights of people with ID, we need to understand why these challenges exist. Existing literature has shown difficulties at an individual level, with family members/carers of people with ID not acknowledging that they have the capacity to make decisions for themselves (33). Focus group interviews with staff working with people with ID reported that only 20% of family carers considered that individuals with ID should be involved in the decision to engage in a relationship, compared to 79% among staff carers (34). People with ID are also less informed of what they are entitled to do, and many already see themselves as not eligible to access certain services or activities that more able people could access or participate in (35).

Challenges can also exist at the community level, with attitudes towards the person with ID sometimes resulting in them being stigmatized or isolated (7,17). Organizations can also act in ways that could be discriminatory towards people with ID, with a lack of policies in place to protect them (36).

We need to go beyond having frameworks like the UN CRPD (5) and should ensure that we have practical solutions that can protect the rights of people with ID in different cultural contexts. Many countries have signed up to the Convention without the accompanying evidence to show the rights of people with ID are being protected. There need to be objective measures to help document if these rights are being protected.

Moving forward, we can look at approaches towards achieving the rights in the following categories.

Individual

People with ID need to be given access to information involving them and choices they have to make using methods they can understand. This might involve using appropriate visual communication tools (including the use of braille for the visually impaired), auditory technology for the hearing impaired, and the use of relevant equipment/technology to take into account people's different disabilities. Information needs to be broken down into small chunks and be culturally sensitive. The information also needs to consider the individual's particular cognitive abilities and how they process information. The emphasis should be on society making it possible for the person with ID to access the relevant information needed to make an informed decision.

Protecting the rights of the individual is important in choice of healthcare, treatments, and consent for procedures and research. Family members and carers who have been appointed to support the person with ID will need to understand the importance of the rights of the person with ID, and there should be legal frameworks protecting these decisions. The increasing emphasis on person-centred care does highlight the need for individuals with ID to have the relevant information to enable them to make these choices (37).

Community

Hosting educational events is a good way of engaging the community on the rights of people with ID. Such events need to be adapted to different cultures, but maintain the core message of observing the rights of people with ID. Training will need to address the subjects of stigma, segregation, poverty, and isolation, all of which are common experiences among people with ID (38).

In communities or countries where there are no established systems to monitor this process, consideration should be given to working with core groups of people within that community to act as stakeholders and to develop pathways to ensure the rights of people with ID can be protected.

Non-governmental organizations that support people with ID within the local community should be supported to be involved with protecting the rights of people with ID. Family members and carers can seek support from such organizations to help with their understanding of what is required or have a support worker from the organization to provide representation for the person with ID when needed.

Organization

Academic and employment organizations have a role in protecting the rights of people with ID; however, review of their input in some countries remains substandard (39). Studies that have reviewed the content of educational curricula for medical professionals have shown that the emphasis is on medical causation and rehabilitation, with very little information on the holistic care and rights of people with ID (40). Subspecialty training programmes outside developmental paediatrics and ID psychiatry have very little content on the comprehensive needs of people with ID (41). It is not surprising that clinicians in most medical specialties lack confidence in communicating and understanding the needs of people with ID (41). People with ID access care in all medical subspecialties and need to be confident that their rights are being protected.

Training in ID should be incorporated into the training curricula for medical students and all postgraduate medical training. Nurses and non-medical personnel such as therapists, other hospital and community workers, teachers, and social workers should be exposed to training on the rights of people with ID.

Academics should also conduct local research and develop outcome measures that explore the different rights discussed in the UN CRPD (5). These activities will help with providing information that is required to make relevant changes needed to ensure the rights of people with ID are protected.

Employment organizations should have mandatory training on protection of the rights of people with ID as part of their regular training events. Organizations should also be benchmarked on their ability to meet this requirement. Organizations should ensure that information is available and accessible to people with ID and that they have explored different opportunities to ensure they meet this requirement. Organizations should ensure they do not put pressure on people with ID to make decisions that they have not chosen themselves.

Human rights organizations in all countries should be actively involved in monitoring, if the rights of people with ID are not being protected. The services for people with ID should be preferably based on the human rights approach as it would improve the acceptance as well as accessibility (42).

Country

Countries should ensure they have systems that monitor compliance with the rights of people with ID. Specific monitoring can be set up for the different rights as referred to in the UN CRPD. Countries need to make sure that people with ID have legal capacity in order to ensure all the rights described under the UN CRPD are being followed.

While some countries, particularly in the Western world, have legal structures to monitor if legal capacity is taken into account in people with ID (26,29), many less developed countries do not have these in place. Those countries which are lacking formal monitoring systems to safeguard the rights of people with ID should be encouraged to establish laws to ensure these rights are protected. Countries should be also encouraged to carry out regular audits to show how people with ID access the different services and have their rights protected.

Media

The media should be encouraged to hold governments as well as societies accountable in protecting the rights of people with ID. The media could feature documentaries and reports on the different aspects of rights of people with ID, how their rights are safeguarded, and flaws in the systems and highlighting the legal aspects would help in sensitizing the society regarding this.

Conclusion

In conclusion, with the advent of the social model of disability, there have been welcome changes in the way that people with disability are treated. From looking upon the illness suffered by the disabled as the cause for disability, to understanding and accepting the role that society plays in improving the quality of life of the affected individuals, this concept has brought about policy changes and legislation which have improved the scenario considerably. Although this is reflected in the way that people with a disability are looked after in developed countries, there is unfortunately a large disparity when compared with attitudes and policy in developing nations. There is thus a pressing need to improve legislation, mindsets, and opportunities across the world to ensure that the rights of people with ID are safeguarded.

References

1. **Annas GJ, Grodin MA.** Reflections on the 70th anniversary of the Nuremberg doctors' trial. American Journal of Public Health 2018;**108**(1):10–12.
2. **Grodin MA, Miller EL, Kelly JI.** The Nazi physicians as leaders in eugenics and 'euthanasia': lessons for today. American Journal of Public Health 2018;**108**(1):53–7.
3. **Salvador-Carulla L, Saxena S.** Intellectual disability: between disability and clinical nosology. Lancet 2009;**374**(9704):1798–9.
4. **Royal College of Psychiatrists.** College safeguarding policy and procedures. 2021. Available from: https://www.rcpsych.ac.uk/docs/default-source/about-us/safeguarding/rcpsych-safeguarding-policy---hr-december--2020.pdf
5. **Department of Economic and Social Affairs.** Convention on the Rights of Persons with Disabilities (CRPD). United Nations; 2021. Available from: https://www.un.org/development/desa/disabilities/convention-on-the-rights-of-persons-with-disabilities.html
6. **Steinert C, Steinert T, Flammer E, Jaeger S.** Impact of the UN Convention on the Rights of Persons with Disabilities (UN-CRPD) on mental health care research—a systematic review. BMC Psychiatry 2016;**12**(16):14.
7. **Benomir AM, Nicolson RI, Beail N.** Attitudes towards people with intellectual disability in the UK and Libya: a cross-cultural comparison. Research in Developmental Disabilities 2016;**51–52**:1–9.
8. **Simpson MK.** Power, ideology and structure: the legacy of normalization for intellectual disability. Social Inclusion 2018;**6**(2):12–21.
9. **Hemmings C.** Advances in research and safeguarding for people with intellectual disabilities. Current Opinion in Psychiatry 2012;**25**(5):339–41.

10. **Devi N.** Supported decision-making and personal autonomy for persons with intellectual disabilities: Article 12 of the UN Convention on the Rights of Persons with Disabilities. Journal of Law, Medicine & Ethics 2013;**41**(4):792–806.

11. **Cunningham JK, De La Rosa JS, Quinones CA, McGuffin BA, Kutob RM.** Gender, psychiatric disability, and dropout from peer support specialist training. Psychological Services 2020;**19**(1):103–10.

12. **Tefera B, van Engen ML, Schippers A, Eide AH, Kersten A, van der Klink J.** Education, work, and motherhood in low and middle income countries: a review of equality challenges and opportunities for women with disabilities. Social Inclusion 2018;**6**(1):82–93.

13. **Okyere C, Aldersey HM, Lysaght R.** The experiences of children with intellectual and developmental disabilities in inclusive schools in Accra, Ghana. African Journal of Disability 2019;**8**:542.

14. **Forlin C.** Teachers' personal concerns about including children with a disability in regular classrooms. Journal of Developmental and Physical Disabilities 1998;**10**(1):87–106.

15. **Hughes K, Bellis MA, Jones L, Wood S, Bates G, Eckley L,** et al. Prevalence and risk of violence against adults with disabilities: a systematic review and meta-analysis of observational studies. Lancet 2012;**379**(9826):1621–9.

16. **Willott S, Badger W, Evans V.** People with an intellectual disability: under-reporting sexual violence. Journal of Adult Protection 2020;**22**(2):75–86.

17. **Edwardraj S, Mumtaj K, Prasad JH, Kuruvilla A, Jacob KS.** Perceptions about intellectual disability: a qualitative study from Vellore, South India. Journal of Intellectual Disability Research 2010;**54**(8):736–48.

18. **McCrudden C.** Human dignity and judicial interpretation of human rights. European Journal of International Law 2008;**19**(4):655–724.

19. **Clawson R, Patterson A, Fyson R, McCarthy M.** The demographics of forced marriage of people with learning disabilities: findings from a national database. Journal of Adult Protection 2020;**22**(2):59–74.

20. **Feldman MA, Aunos M.** Recent trends and future directions in research regarding parents with intellectual and developmental disabilities. Current Developmental Disorders Reports 2020;7(3):173–81.

21. **Rohwerder B.** Disability Stigma in Developing Countries. K4D Helpdesk Report. Brighton: Institute of Development Studies; 2018. Available from: https://assets.publishing.service.gov.uk/media/5b18fe3240f0b634aec30791/Disability_stigma_in_developing_countries.pdf

22. **Munyi CW.** Past and present perceptions towards disability: a historical perspective. Disability Studies Quarterly 2012;**32**(2):3068.

23. **Bhayana A, Bhayana B.** Approach to developmental disabilities in newcomer families. Canadian Family Physician 2018;**64**(8):567–73.

24. **Chadwick DD.** Online risk for people with intellectual disabilities. Tizard Learning Disability Review 2019;**24**(4):180–7.

25. **Garratt H, Garratt H.** Safeguarding. NHS England; 2021. Available from: https://www.england.nhs.uk/safeguarding/about/

26. **Legislation.gov.uk.** Care Act 2014. 2014. Available from: https://www.legislation.gov.uk/ukpga/2014/23/contents

27. **Legislation.gov.uk.** Mental Capacity Act 2005. 2021. Available from: https://www.legislation.gov.uk/ukpga/2005/9/contents

28. **GOV.UK.** Data protection. 2021. Available from: https://www.gov.uk/data-protection

29. **Social Care Institute for Excellence.** Deprivation of Liberty Safeguards (DoLs) at a glance. 2021. Available from: https://www.scie.org.uk/mca/dols/at-a-glance

30. **Department of Economic and Social Affairs.** #Envision2030: 17 goals to transform the world for persons with disabilities. United Nations; 2021. Available from: https://www.un.org/development/desa/disabilities/envision2030.html

31. **Bhaumik S, Tromans S, Gangadharan SK, Kapugama C, Michael DM, Wani A**, et al. Intellectual disability psychiatry: a competency-based framework for psychiatrists. International Journal of Culture and Mental Health 2017;**10**(4):468–76.

32. **Newcastle Safeguarding Adults Board.** Vision and priorities 2016–2018. Letstalknewcastle.co.uk; 2021. Available from: https://letstalknewcastle.co.uk/files/3._Newcastle_Safeguarding_Adults_Board_Vision_and_Priorities_2016-2018_-_Final_.pdf

33. **Saaltink R, MacKinnon G, Owen F, Tardif-Williams C.** Protection, participation and protection through participation: young people with intellectual disabilities and decision making in the family context. Journal of Intellectual Disability Research 2012;**56**(11):1076–86.

34. **Wickström M, Larsson M, Höglund B.** How can sexual and reproductive health and rights be enhanced for young people with intellectual disability?—focus group interviews with staff in Sweden. Reproductive Health 2020;**17**(1):86.

35. **Wark S, MacPhail C, McKay K, Müller A.** Informed consent in a vulnerable population group: supporting individuals aging with intellectual disability to participate in developing their own health and support programs. Australian Health Review 2016;**41**(4):436–42.

36. **Barnes C.** Institutional discrimination against disabled people a case for legislation. British Council of Organisations of Disabled People; 2021. Available from: https://disability-studies.leeds.ac.uk/wp-content/uploads/sites/40/library/Barnes-bcodp.pdf

37. **Watchman K, Mattheys K, McKernon M, Strachan H, Andreis F, Murdoch J.** A person-centred approach to implementation of psychosocial interventions with people who have an intellectual disability and dementia—a participatory action study. Journal of Applied Research in Intellectual Disabilities 2021;**34**(1):164–77.

38. **Faculty of Psychiatry of Intellectual Disability.** Community-based services for people with intellectual disability and mental health problems Literature review and survey results. Royal College of Psychiatrists; 2015. Available from: https://www.rcpsych.ac.uk/docs/default-source/members/faculties/intellectual-disability/id-fr-id-06.pdf?sfvrsn=5a230b9c_2

39. **Valentim A, Valentim JP.** What I think of school: perceptions of school by people with intellectual disabilities. Disability & Society 2020;**35**(10):1618–40.

40. **Trollor JN, Ruffell B, Tracy J, Torr JJ, Durvasula S, Iacono T**, et al. Intellectual disability health content within medical curriculum: an audit of what our future doctors are taught. BMC Medical Education 2016;**16**:105.

41. **Trollor JN, Eagleson C, Turner B, Tracy J, Torr JJ, Durvasula S**, et al. Intellectual disability content within tertiary medical curriculum: how is it taught and by whom? BMC Medical Education 2018;**18**(1):182.

42. **Katsui H, Kumpuvuori J.** Human rights based approach to disability in development in Uganda: a way to fill the gap between political and social spaces? Scandinavian Journal of Disability Research 2008;**10**(4):227–36.

Chapter 9

Sexuality, marriage, and parenthood across cultures

Priyanka Tharian, Lucretia Thomas,
Ratnaraj Vaidya, and Chaya Kapugama

Introduction

Sexuality and relationships are a core element of the human condition, as en-shrined in Article 8 of the United Nations Declaration of Human Rights, giving all human beings the right to a private and family life (1). This is elucidated further in Article 23 of the United Nations Convention on the Rights of Persons with Disabilities, which states that 'parties shall take effective and appropriate measures to eliminate discrimination against persons with disabilities in all matters relating to marriage, family, parenthood, and relationships, on an equal basis with others' (2).

One of the challenges faced by clinicians is the ability to balance the rights of individuals with intellectual disability (ID) with their professional responsibil-ities of ensuring that these individuals are safe and protected from exploitation (3). Evidence and clinical practice show that people with ID desire intimate relationships much like the majority of the rest of the population, so clinicians must take this into account when providing holistic care (3).

However, in practice, people with ID can still face challenges with regard to forming and maintaining relationships, sometimes being unable to experience relationships as couples, unlike adults in the general population (4). Due to im-paired cognition, some may lack the knowledge and skills necessary to maintain a relationship, despite the motivation to do so (4,5). This is exacerbated by the lack of opportunities for people with ID to have interpersonal interactions out-side of family, carers, and peers based within their residential placements (4).

Historical context

Historically, the sexual and relationship rights of individuals with ID have been overlooked and, in some cases, actively targeted. People with ID have been vic-tims of non-consensual sterilization by the state throughout the nineteenth and twentieth centuries, being perceived to be unfit for relationships and parenthood (6). This is due in part to the ideology of 'negative eugenics', which discourages procreation among certain demographic groups deemed to be unsuitable for society (7).

Physicians have had an active role in the forced sterilization of people with ID, with approximately 60,000 such operations having taken place in the US in the twentieth century, with most of these taking place in the late 1920s and late 1930s (8). This rose to above 400,000 in the case of Nazi Germany, indicating that cultural differences and ideological variance have a direct impact on the sex lives and relationships of people with ID (9).

From this historical context, it is evident that people with ID have been discriminated against in sexual and relationship settings. However, from the latter half of the twentieth century onwards, the sexual rights of people with ID have been viewed more in line with the rest of the population (10). Though there is variability in each country's laws around extremes such as forced sterilization, case law acts as a useful precedent (11). One such landmark case was *Secretary, Department of Health and Community Services vs JWB and SMB*, also known as 'Marion's Case', which took place in 1992. This case focused on the reproductive rights of a 14-year-old girl with 'mental retardation' and 'behavioural problems', who was described as being unable to 'care for herself' (12: p 218). Marion's parents applied to the Family Court of Australia for a court order to authorize the performance of a hysterectomy and an oophorectomy on Marion in order to prevent pregnancy, menstruation, and the fluctuation of reproductive hormones; this request was overturned by the High Court of Australia due to her parents being unable to make a non-therapeutic decision of this nature (11,12). In post-reunification Germany, people with disabilities are legally entitled to a carer who is also a legal representative; this carer must take the views and wishes of the disabled person into account in legal decisions (13). These examples show the positive trajectory of a rights-focused legal attitude towards people with ID.

Perceptions of parents regarding sexuality

The role of the family is valuable in ensuring people with ID have a broad range of exposure to interpersonal interactions and social situations (5,14). Families provide support with regard to other aspects of individuals' lives (such as education, development, and advocacy), but less emphasis is placed on building social and interpersonal skills in the context of romantic relationships (15). A greater value being placed on promoting interpersonal interaction can help to build the confidence of people with ID in this aspect of life.

In addition, people with ID can also experience discrimination and harmful stereotypes with regard to how they are perceived in aspects of sex, sexuality, and relationships (16). Due to potentially increased risks of vulnerability and exploitation, the views of the general public can result in discriminatory attitudes towards those with ID, infantilizing them and holding negative views around their sexual rights (16).

In the Western world, parents of those with ID are not exempt from such discriminatory attitudes. Evidence suggests that parents of those with ID have fears around several themes: forming successful relationships, choosing appropriate partners, and managing sexual desire (5,17). As a result of this, parents can restrict the freedoms of those with ID and reduce their social exposure (5).

A contributory reason for these actions may be due to parental stressors themselves; parents of people with ID experience additional responsibilities, including (but not limited to) physical (directly assisting in personal care while ageing), emotional (facing uncertainty and worry), and financial responsibilities (having an additional dependant) (18). These can themselves make parents resistant to adding new complex social factors involving the care of people with ID.

Furthermore, some parental perceptions of relationships in people with ID are that they are primarily based on physical intimacy (5). However, people with ID do not view relationships as a purely sexual endeavour; warmth and affection are also key factors in interactions with others (19). The misconception that people with ID place more value on sexual intimacy than other aspects of a relationship, including companionship, compared to the general population, may negatively impact people with ID, since this may lead parents and carers to be less supportive of them entering into a relationship, as well as contributing to societal stigma regarding ID (5).

Parental perceptions of the challenges faced by people with ID in relationships also include issues around conduct and misinterpreting situations. Some parents believe that those with ID can be childish in their behaviours, resulting in them being inappropriate in certain settings. Parents can feel that people with ID are not able to stand up for themselves when navigating romantic relationships. Compounded with co-occurring neurodevelopmental conditions such as autism spectrum disorder, some parents fear that people with ID may misunderstand the social situations that comprise interpersonal relationships (5).

These attitudes have an impact on sex and relationship education for people with ID. Parents report feeling discomfort when discussing information about relationships to their children with ID (5). Concerns and worries include that their child may not be able to understand or comprehend it, and that instead of learning from parents, can fixate on sexual thoughts and ideas. Other parental perceptions can include fears around unplanned pregnancy and sexually trans-mitted infections (5). This emphasizes the value of tailored sex education for those with ID, such as around barrier contraceptives and sexually transmitted infection prevention, as a means to address such concerns.

Consequently, this has an impact on people with ID and their core rights to meaningful relationships, as parents tend to retain a greater degree of authority and information control over their children with ID relative to their non-ID peers (20). Parents of people with ID tend to refrain from discussing sexual and relationship matters altogether, opposing marriage and parenthood for people with ID. In a cross-sectional study including 40 parents of children with mild to moderate ID, it was reported that 32.5% ($n = 40$) of parents had not had a con-versation with their child regarding sexuality, whereas, 37.5% ($n = 40$) reported that their child with ID had asked them about sexuality (21).

From a cross-cultural perspective, these trends are amplified in the British South Asian population when compared to their White British counterparts. Evidence shows that some people from South Asian backgrounds have a signifi-cantly negative view towards the sexual rights of people with ID, with a greater emphasis on parental control (22).

However, a different dynamic is also present in South Asian populations as to the roles of marriage and parenthood as support mechanisms; key themes showed that some South Asians can view marriage as a way to 'overcome cog-nitive problems, secure good standing in their community and access a carer's support within marriage' (22). Consequently, perceptions towards marriage re-flect less on individualistic culture and more on collectivist culture, as reflected in South Asian ethnic heritage (22).

Such findings present a potential conflict of interest between the rights of the individual and the concerns of the parent. Clinicians should be aware of these potential clashes and act accordingly, preserving the dignity and human rights of people with ID while also ensuring that they are safe and happy.

Parental attitudes towards adolescents

The aforementioned parental attitudes are present before people with ID be-come adults. Caregivers may be less permissive of sexual activity among young people with ID (23). Similar parental control is echoed in the adult population, where parents maintain control over the pace at which their adult offspring with ID become involved romantically with others (21).

In addition, parents often form the relationship archetype for people with ID, with the majority of them learning about relationships from their parents. This sets the template for the rest of the lives of people with ID. As a result, parental influence within the formative years can have a lasting influence on individuals with ID (24).

Parents may be more protective, and thus limit social opportunities for adolescents with ID (17). For adolescents with autism spectrum disorder (and ID) who have social and communication difficulties, this may have multiplicative detrimental effects on forming relationships (17). The initial opportunities for socializing would be fewer due to parental restrictions, and subsequently they may struggle with those interactions when presented with others in a social context (17).

This can result in adolescents with ID having limited romantic conceptualizations, including understanding the distinction between friendships and romantic relationships. Evidence suggests that adolescents with ID have limited knowledge about sex, thus leaving them more vulnerable in their interactions with others (17).

Research findings exemplify this, with people who have ID having a greater risk of pregnancy and sexually transmitted infections compared to their peers without ID (24). This may at least be partially attributed to the impact of parental unwillingness to discuss and disclose sexual and relationship information on the health of young people with ID (21).

Attitudes of carers towards sexuality

In residential and day care settings, people with ID interact less with parents and more with carers and support workers. Consequently, the attitudes of these carers are also important regarding how people with ID are able to express their desire for sexuality and relationships. Attitudes from care workers can be variable depending on their age, experience of care, and their own cultural background. For instance, in Ireland, with a strong Catholic influence, cultural and religious attitudes towards sexual topics such as contraception and abortion influence the opinions of carers (26). As many services for people with ID have a religious ethos, this can result in additional implications for the people with ID who use and access such services (26).

Evidence shows that some carers can be hesitant to discuss and explore issues relating to sexuality (26). Some carers can have perceptions that discussing sexual themes can evoke sexual impulses in people with ID, or mark an infringement of service user privacy. This in turn results in fewer people with ID receiving adequate attention or access to sexual needs and desires, or access to relevant information (27).

In addition, beyond the direct impact on sexual health, the views of carers can be reflected in their clients with ID (28). Several older studies show that some people with ID have a low tolerance towards homosexual activity and pre-marital sexual intercourse, suggesting the conservative views of carers can affect the people they look after (29). This may lead people with ID to feel conflicted about their sexuality and urges. However, there is a strong likelihood that the liberalization of sexual attitudes has transferred to current care staff over time.

These issues tie into broader questions about the training which staff who care for people with ID receive in the fields of sex, sexuality, and relationships. A lack of policies and guidelines within care organizations is an issue identified by care workers, creating ambiguity around the expectations of service users and organizations themselves. Consequently, to ensure that policy frameworks are embedded in routine practice, information on how best to support people with ID in sex and relationships needs to be included in induction and education programmes (26).

Lesbian, gay, bisexual, and transgender individuals with intellectual disability

Alongside liberalization in sexual attitudes, there are an increasing number of individuals with ID identifying as lesbian, gay, bisexual, or transgender (LGBT). These LGBT individuals with ID have their own unique set of challenges with regard to sexual identity and sexual expression. However, there is a paucity of evidence around this topic, which requires further research.

From the data available, LGBT people with ID often express positive attitudes about their sexuality, actively using labels to define themselves and had 'come out' to one or more people (30). Those confided in were often support staff in residential settings, further cementing the need for good-quality training for such staff in matters of sex, sexuality, and relationships.

However, LGBT people with ID also report feelings of anxiety before coming out, and fear of rejection upon disclosing of their sexual identity. This is mitigated somewhat by LGBT role models in the media, who aim to raise awareness and can provide a valuable template to sharing their sexuality. Despite this, bullying is a common theme among young LGBT people with ID; much of this was centred around their sexuality (30).

The experiences of those with ID are different to the LGBT demographic as a whole; people with ID report that potential partners are rejected on the basis of moral judgements about their own rights to have relationships. This is exemplified by a quote from 'Kenneth', saying 'when you've got a disability they don't want to know you because they think it's wrong' (30).

With regard to service provision, LGBT people with ID reported that services only offer partial support; they either care only for sexuality needs, or ID needs. For LGBT people with ID, opinions were expressed that there is a need for more integrated service support which is inclusive of both the ID and LGBT aspects (30).

Forced marriage

Data collected by the UK Government Forced Marriage Unit indicate that people with ID are five times more likely to become a victim of forced marriage, compared to their peers without ID. These statistics also indicate that in contrast to the general population, where women are more likely to be the victim of forced marriage, this trend is not observed among individuals with ID, where men and woman are equally at risk (31–34). Epidemiological data also indicate that forced marriage is more prevalent among cultural and ethnic groups where arranged marriages are traditionally practised, including South Asian communities and religious groups including Orthodox Jewish communities; in the UK, forced marriage is most common among South Asian communities (32,35). However, it is important to note that forced marriage occurs across all ethnic groups within the UK and the particular ethnic and cultural groups in which forced marriage is most prevalent is likely to change as the demographic composition of the UK changes over time (31).

It is important to highlight the distinction between an arranged marriage and a forced marriage, since the understanding of this is critical in safeguarding individuals with ID against the risk of forced marriage while maintaining cultural sensitivity (31,36). In an arranged marriage, although the potential spouse is identified by parents or family members, both parties are able to freely decide whether they wish to proceed with the marriage and have the capacity to do so (31,35,36). In contrast, a forced marriage (as defined by the UK Government Forced Marriage Unit), takes place where one or both individuals involved either do not choose to freely give consent to be married, or do not have the capacity to make this decision (31,32,35). Forced marriage has also been defined as including an element of duress, which can include emotional, sexual, or financial pressure (36,37). However, it is important to note that where an individual does not have the capacity to consent to marriage, forced marriage may not always take place under duress; this is because an individual may be willing to marry without having sufficient understanding of what marriage means, including the roles and responsibilities it involves (31,35,36).

Forced marriage can result in significant harm for the individual who has been forced, including the risk of domestic violence, sexual assault, and rape

(36,38). Individuals with ID who are victims of forced marriage may also experience significant psychological distress resulting from entering into a complex relationship which they do not fully understand (35). They may be reluctant to seek help and support if they are dependent on their spouse, for example, for financial reasons or for support with activities of daily living (35). Furthermore, individuals with ID may also be unable to seek support if they are a victim of abuse or are experiencing psychological distress, for example, due to communication difficulties (31,35). The majority of reported cases of forced marriage are identified and reported by social services and other professionals who have safeguarding responsibilities, such as individuals working for the police or in educational settings, with a small percentage of cases being reported by victims themselves or their family or friends (31).

The arrangement of marriages between families in different countries, via the internet or through other relatives, may increase the risk of forced marriage, since less information may be available regarding the individuals involved (35).

While forced marriage cannot be excused or condoned, it is important to understand the circumstances within which it may occur, including the motivations of parents or family members who are involved in arranging the forced marriage. This understanding may enable health and social care professionals to better recognize forced marriage, and to work closely with family members to prevent it from occurring (32,35).

There are several factors which may underlie the occurrence of forced marriage, which largely stem from cultural beliefs and expectations regarding marriage and ID (31–33,39). These include concerns regarding securing long-term care and support for people with ID, but may also stem from a lack of understanding of the law relating to mental capacity and marriage (31–33,39).

The parents of an adult with ID may see marriage as a means of gaining acceptance of their child within their community and extended family; since marriage is often seen as a rite of passage, allowing their child to conform with this societal expectation may alleviate stigma (32,35). It has also been reported that, particularly within South Asian communities, a belief is sometimes held that getting married can reduce the severity of an individual's ID, and may alleviate this entirely (32,35,40). Marriage may also be seen as a means of securing long-term care for an individual with ID, relieving parents of this caring responsibility as they age; this belief may be compounded by mistrust of or lack of knowledge regarding community social care provision for individuals with ID, which is also thought to be particularly prevalent among South Asian communities (31–33,39,41–43).

Lack of awareness or understanding regarding mental capacity law may result in some parents and family members allowing a loved with ID to enter into a forced marriage, believing that this is in their best interests, without having insight into the fact that the marriage is forced due to their loved one lacking the capacity to make this particular decision (32,35). There have also been reports of the practice of individuals with ID who reside in the UK being forced to marry someone without ID who lives abroad for the purposes of immigration although it is unclear how frequently this practice occurs (32,44). However, protective factors have been identified which may reduce the risk of forced marriage, including concerns regarding abuse, particularly in the context of an individual with an ID marrying someone who does not have an ID. In addition, there may be concerns regarding increasing the burden of care on the parents and family of a person with ID if they marry another person with ID (32).

Parenthood

Supporting parents with ID to take an active role in parenting, while safeguarding their child or children from unintentional neglect, is an area of practice which professionals involved in the care and support of people with ID frequently find challenging and complex to navigate (45).

Much of the literature which is available regarding the experiences of parenthood among people with ID has focused on the barriers and inequities that individuals with ID may face during child protection processes (45–49).

Being a child of a parent with ID has been associated with an increased risk of various adverse experiences and outcomes, particularly when the parent does not receive adequate support. Such experiences and outcomes for the child include neglect, developmental delay, behavioural problems, and poor social–emotional well-being (46,51,52). However, it is important to emphasize that a wide range of social factors may influence the ability of an individual with ID to provide good-quality parental care, aside from their degree of ID (46,51,52).

Such psychosocial factors include financial hardship and having limited social networks, which have been reported to be disproportionately more common among individuals with ID compared to the general population (51).

It is important to note that many negative psychosocial factors including financial difficulties, lack of social support, having been a victim of abuse or neglect, or having a history of mental illness or substance abuse have been reported to be disproportionately more prevalent among people with ID, compared to the general population (51–53). Child protection systems have been criticized for overlooking these psychosocial factors when assessing the ability of parents with ID to provide adequate care to their offspring, and instead relying on an individual's IQ too heavily as a measure of assessing their parenting ability (52,53). This is reflected by evidence which has found that people with ID are over-represented at all stages of the legal child protection process, compared to individuals with other types of disability and those who do not have a disability (44,53,54).

It is becoming increasingly clear that, with appropriate and high-quality long-term support that is tailored to a parent's individual needs and their child's developmental stage, parents with ID are often able to provide adequate care which meets the physical, psychosocial, and developmental needs of their children (45,53,55,56). In countries where there are specialist ID services available, multidisciplinary teams are likely to play a crucial role in supporting parents with ID to develop their parenting skills and to provide parental support as independently as possible, while safeguarding the rights of the child (45).

It is also important to emphasize that family members often play a key role in supporting parents with ID to care for their children (54). This is thought to be particularly important in countries where there is a paucity of specialist ID services (54). Furthermore, an individual's cultural or ethnic group may have a strong influence on the extent to which they receive parental support from their extended family (44). A qualitative exploration of the attitudes and experiences of parents with ID and their families in a Bangladeshi community in the UK, conducted by Durling and colleagues, indicated that parenting is often seen as a shared responsibility of families belonging to this particular minority group (44). This type of family support may allow parents with ID to actively participate in parenting and develop a bond with their child. This is supported by evidence which indicates that increased social support may reduce parenting stress experienced by parents with ID and increase their satisfaction with the overall parental support they receive (51). However, it could also potentially hinder the ability of the parent with ID to develop their parenting skills and acquire more independence in their parenting responsibilities (54).

It is important to note that the majority of studies which have investigated the experiences of people with ID with regard to sexuality, marriage, and parenthood appear to have been conducted in the UK or US; there may therefore be a paucity of evidence regarding global attitudes to these topics.

References

1. European Court of Human Rights. Guide on Article 8 of the European Convention on Human Rights: right to respect for private and family life, home and correspondence. 2022. Available from: https://www.echr.coe.int/documents/guide_art_8_eng.pdf
2. Department of Economic and Social Affairs. Article 23—respect for home and the family. United Nations; n.d. Available from: https://www.un.org/development/desa/disabilities/convention-on-the-rights-of-persons-with-disabilities/article-23-respect-for-home-and-the-family.html

3. Kelly G, Crowley H, Hamilton C. Rights, sexuality and relationships in Ireland: 'It'd be nice to be kind of trusted.' British Journal of Learning Disabilities 2009;37(4):308–15.

4. Burgen B, Bigby C. The importance of friendship for young adults with intellectual disabilities. In: Bigby C, Ozanne E, Fyffe C, editors. Planning and Support for Adults with Intellectual Disabilities. London: Jessica Kingsley Publishers; 2007: 208–14.

5. Neuman R. Parents' perceptions regarding couple relationships of their adult children with intellectual disabilities. Journal of Applied Research in Intellectual Disabilities 2020;33(2):310–20.

6. Park DC, Radford JP. From the case files: reconstructing a history of involuntary sterilisation. Disability and Society 1998;13(3):317–42.

7. Rowlands S, Amy JJ. Sterilization of those with intellectual disability: evolution from non-consensual interventions to strict safeguards. Journal of Intellectual Disabilities 2019;23:233–49.

8. Kaelber L. Eugenics: Compulsory Sterilization in 50 American States. University of Vermont; 2012. Available from: https://www.uvm.edu/~lkaelber/eugenics/

9. Racial Hygiene: Medicine Under the Nazis, Robert N. Proctor. 1987. Harvard University Press, Cambridge, MA. 496 pages. ISBN: 0-674-74580-9. $34.95. Bulletin of Science, Technology & Society 1988;8(4):464.

10. Shandra CL, Hogan DP, Short SE. Planning for motherhood: fertility attitudes, desires and intentions among women with disabilities. Perspectives on Sexual and Reproductive Health 2014;46(4):203–10.

11. Parker M. 'Forced sterilisation': clarifying and challenging intuitions and models. Journal of Law and Medicine 2013;20(3):512–27.

12. Secretary, Department of Health and Community Services v JWB and SMB (1992) 175 CLR 218 (Marion's Case).

13. Dimopoulos A. Issues in Human Rights Protection of Intellectually Disabled Persons. London: Routledge; 2016.

14. Pownall JD, Jahoda A, Hastings R, Kerr L. Sexual understanding and development of young people with intellectual disabilities: mothers' perspectives of within-family context. American Journal on Intellectual and Developmental Disabilities 2011;116(3):205–19.

15. Pownall J, Wilson S, Jahoda A. Health knowledge and the impact of social exclusion on young people with intellectual disabilities. Journal of Applied Research in Intellectual Disabilities 2020;33(1):29–38.

16. Swango-Wilson A. Caregiver perception of sexual behaviors of individuals with intellectual disabilities. Sexuality and Disability 2008;26(2):75–81.

17. Heifetz M, Lake J, Weiss J, Isaacs B, Connolly J. Dating and romantic relationships of adolescents with intellectual and developmental disabilities. Journal of Adolescence 2020;79:39–48.

18. Dervishaliaj E. Parental stress in families of children with disabilities: a literature review. Journal of Educational and Social Research 2013;3(7):579–84.

19. Lafferty A, McConkey R, Taggart L. Beyond friendship: the nature and meaning of close personal relationships as perceived by people with learning disabilities. Disability and Society 2013;28(8):1074–88.

20. Evans DS, McGuire BE, Healy E, Carley SN. Sexuality and personal relationships for people with an intellectual disability. Part II: staff and family carer perspectives. Journal of Intellectual Disability Research 2009;53(11):913–21.

21. Isler A, Beytut D, Tas F, Conk Z. A study on sexuality with the parents of adolescents with intellectual disability. Sexuality and Disability 2009;27(4):229–37.

22. Sankhla D, Theodore K. British attitudes towards sexuality in men and women with intellectual disabilities: a comparison between white Westerners and South Asians. Sexuality and Disability 2015;33(4):429–45.

23. Shepperdson B. The control of sexuality in young people with Down's syndrome. Child: Care, Health and Development 1995;21(5):333–49.

24. Pownall JD, Jahoda A, Hastings RP. Sexuality and sex education of adolescents with intellectual disability: mothers' attitudes, experiences, and support needs. Intellectual and Developmental Disabilities 2012;50(2):140–54.

25. Cheng MM, Udry JR. Sexual experiences of adolescents with low cognitive abilities in the U.S. Journal of Developmental and Physical Disabilities 2005;17(2):155–72.

26. Healy E, McGuire BE, Evans DS, Carley SN. Sexuality and personal relationships for people with an intellectual disability. Part I: service-user perspectives. Journal of Intellectual Disability Research 2009;53(11):905–12.

27. Konstantareas MM, Lunsky YJ. Sociosexual knowledge, experience, attitudes, and interests of individuals with autistic disorder and developmental delay. Journal of Autism and Developmental Disorders 1997;27(4):397–413.

28. Murphy GH, O'Callaghan A. Capacity of adults with intellectual disabilities to consent to sexual relationships. Psychological Medicine 2004;34(7):1347–57.

29. Cuskelly M, Bryde R. Attitudes towards the sexuality of adults with an intellectual disability: parents, support staff, and a community sample. Journal of Intellectual and Developmental Disability 2004;29(3):255–64.

30. Dinwoodie R, Greenhill B, Cookson A. 'Them two things are what collide together': understanding the sexual identity experiences of lesbian, gay, bisexual and trans people labelled with intellectual disability. Journal of Applied Research in Intellectual Disabilities 2020;33(1):3–16.

31. Clawson R, Patterson A, Fyson R, McCarthy M. The demographics of forced marriage of people with learning disabilities: findings from a national database. Journal of Adult Protection. 2020;22(2):59–74.

32. McCarthy M, Clawson R, Patterson A, Fyson R, Khan L. Risk of forced marriage amongst people with learning disabilities in the UK: Perspectives of South Asian carers. Journal of Applied Research in Intellectual Disabilities 2021;34(1):200–10.

33. Patterson A, Clawson R, McCarthy M, Fyson R, Kitson D. My marriage my choice. Summary of findings. Project report. University of Nottingham; 2018. Available from: https://kar.kent.ac.uk/70153/

34. Forced Marriage Unit. Forced marriage unit statistics. Home Office and Foreign and Commonwealth Office; 2016. Available from: https://www gov uk/government/uploads/system/uploads/attachment_data/file/505827/Forced_Marriage_Unit_statistics_2015 pdf. 2016;

35. Groce N, Gazizova D, Hassiotis A. Forced marriage among persons with intellectual disabilities: discussion paper. Leonard Cheshire Disability and Inclusive Development Centre; 2014. Available from: https://discovery.ucl.ac.uk/id/eprint/10128025/

36. Rauf B, Saleem N, Clawson R, Sanghera M, Marston G. Forced marriage: implications for mental health and intellectual disability services. Advances in Psychiatric Treatment 2013;19(2):135–43.
37. Stobart E. Multi-Agency Practice Guidelines: Handling Cases of Forced Marriage. London: HM Government; 2009.
38. Chantler K, Gangoli G, Hester M. Forced marriage in the UK: religious, cultural, economic or state violence? Critical Social Policy 2009;29(4):587–612.
39. Clawson R, Fyson R. Forced marriage of people with learning disabilities: a human rights issue. Disability & Society 2017;32(6):810–30.
40. Manor-Binyamini I. Reasons for marriage of educated Bedouin women to Bedouin men with intellectual disability from the point of view of the women. Journal of Intellectual and Developmental Disability 2018;43(3):285–94.
41. Devapriam J, Thorp C, Tyrer F, Gangadharan S, Raju L, Bhaumik S. A comparative study of stress and unmet needs in carers of South Asian and white adults with learning disabilities. Ethnicity and Inequalities in Health and Social Care 2008;1(2):35–43.
42. Pryce L, Tweed A, Hilton A, Priest HM. Tolerating uncertainty: perceptions of the future for ageing parent carers and their adult children with intellectual disabilities. Journal of Applied Research in Intellectual Disabilities 2017;30(1):84–96.
43. Raghavan R, Waseem F. Services for young people with learning disabilities and mental health needs from South Asian communities. Advances in Mental Health and Learning Disabilities 2007;1(3):27–31.
44. Durling E, Chinn D, Scior K. Family and community in the lives of UK Bangladeshi parents with intellectual disabilities. Journal of Applied Research in Intellectual Disabilities 2018;31(6):1133–43.
45. Tarleton B, Turney D. Understanding 'successful practice/s' with parents with learning difficulties when there are concerns about child neglect: the contribution of social practice theory. Child Indicators Research 2020;13(2):387–409.
46. Aunos M, Feldman MA. Attitudes towards sexuality, sterilization and parenting rights of persons with intellectual disabilities. Journal of Applied Research in Intellectual Disabilities. 2002;15(4):285–96.
47. McConnell D, Llewellyn G, Ferronato L. Context-contingent decision-making in child protection practice. International Journal of Social Welfare 2006;15(3):230–9.
48. McConnell D, Llewellyn G. Stereotypes, parents with intellectual disability and child protection. Journal of Social Welfare and Family Law 2002;24(3):297–317.
49. Sigurjónsdóttir HB, Rice JG. Evidence of neglect as a form of structural violence: parents with intellectual disabilities and custody deprivation. Social Inclusion 2018;6(2):66–73.
50. Hindmarsh G, Llewellyn G, Emerson E. The social-emotional well-being of children of mothers with intellectual impairment: a population-based analysis. Journal of Applied Research in Intellectual Disabilities 2017;30(3):469–81.
51. Meppelder M, Hodes M, Kef S, Schuengel C. Parenting stress and child behaviour problems among parents with intellectual disabilities: the buffering role of resources. Journal of Intellectual Disability Research 2015;59(7):664–77.
52. Callow E, Tahir M, Feldman M. Judicial reliance on parental IQ in appellate-level child welfare cases involving parents with intellectual and developmental disabilities. Journal of Applied Research in Intellectual Disabilities 2017;30(3):553–62.

53. LaLiberte T, Piescher K, Mickelson N, Lee MH. Child protection services and parents with intellectual and developmental disabilities. Journal of Applied Research in Intellectual Disabilities 2017;30(3):521–32.

54. Chandra PS, Ragesh G, Kishore T, Ganjekar S, Sutar R, Desai G. Breaking stereotypes: helping mothers with intellectual disability to care for their infants. Journal of Psychosocial Rehabilitation and Mental Health 2017;4(1):111–16.

55. Azar ST, Maggi MC, Proctor SN. Practices changes in the child protection system to address the needs of parents with cognitive disabilities. Journal of Public Child Welfare 2013;7(5):610–32.

56. Macintyre G, Stewart A. For the record: the lived experience of parents with a learning disability—a pilot study examining the Scottish perspective. British Journal of Learning Disabilities 2012;40(1):5–14.

Part 3

Care of People with Intellectual Disability in cultural context

Chapter 10

Models of healthcare provision

Ashok Roy, Amala Jesu, Jayan Mendis,
Aisha M. Bakhiet, and Meera Roy

Factors influencing the development of models

Changing terminology used to describe intellectual disability (ID) over time
has meant that identification levels in general populations can be variable. The
recognition of ID in low- and middle-income (LAMI) countries is influenced
by other characteristics including educational levels and cultural aspects that
could influence the current measures of intellectual functioning as well as by
socioenvironmental factors impacting the person's adaptive capacity. This
makes the identification of mild and moderate ID particularly challenging (1).

The prevalence and incidence of ID is examined in greater detail in Chapter 1.
ID occurs in all cultures and Maulik et al. (2) found the global prevalence to be
10.37/1000 population, a rate of 1%. The rate was higher in males. Prevalence
was higher in LAMI countries with a rate that can be almost double that in
high-income countries. Maulik and Darmstadt (3) examined child disability in
LAMI countries which are spread across Asia, Africa, Eastern Europe, and Latin
America, and found the prevalence rate of ID ranging from 0.09% to 18.3%.
Usually, the prevalence of ID is extrapolated from Western studies. Lakhan et al.
(4) examined age-adjusted prevalence of ID in rural and urban populations and
its correlation with age in children and adults. They found an overall prevalence
of 10.5/1000 in ID with higher rates in urban areas. McKenzie et al. (5) extended a systematic review further to studies on prevalence between 2010 and
2015 and found considerable heterogeneity in study settings, methodologies,
age groups, and case definitions and reported a prevalence range of 0.05–1.55%.
In a systematic review, Fischer et al. (6) found locally developed screening tools
which were felt to be feasible for early identification of developmental disabilities in LAMI countries. These tools were acceptable in terms of sensitivity and
specificity, cost, access, low training time, and the need for health worker time
in day-to-day use.

In the majority of cases, the cause of ID was unknown. In those where the cause was identifiable, antenatal, perinatal, and postnatal factors were responsible in almost equal proportions. Birth injury, birth asphyxia, and intrauterine birth retardation were common perinatal causes and infections and developmental disorders were common postnatal causes. The cause of ID and the social context can drive the shape of the services that people receive.

Estimates from Africa suggest that asphyxia during birth, often resulting from the absence of a skilled attendant, leaves an estimated 1 million children with impairments such as cerebral palsy and learning difficulties while maternal iodine deficiency leads to 18 million babies being born each year with mental disabilities (7,8). Studies suggest that the prevalence of ID in South Africa is higher than in high-income countries with a high burden of preventable causes including nutritional causes and growth stunting, cognitive impairment due to HIV/AIDS, tuberculosis meningitis, trauma, and foetal alcohol syndrome. The challenge for African countries is that when childhood mortality comes down, the burden of neurocognitive impairment may increase (9).

In the developed world, the social model was developed to understand that barriers to activities in life were caused to a large extent by an environment that does not acknowledge the rights, abilities, and opportunities of people with ID. To take into account the variety of norms in society, a cultural–social model has been put forward to promote a culturally determined identity and community which embraces disability and does not reject it due to stigma, helping promote a person-centred approach based on strengths.

The World Health Organization's International Classification of Functioning, Disability and Health (2018) developed the biopsychosocial model by synthesizing elements of the medical and social models, without compromising the complex notion of disability. Models of disability which have been used in the developed world need to be modified to meet the social and cultural contexts in LAMI countries. In their analysis of policy development, Memari and Hafizi (10) note that the medical model of disability, while successful in dispelling unscientific and supernatural explanations of ID, has on its own been perceived to be a barrier to a better life for people with ID. Causes of ID and medical interventions contribute to the biological model while stigma will impinge on the social aspects.

Tilahun et al. (11) found that stigma was widespread in families with children with developmental delay with a significant number being attributed to both biomedical and supernatural causes accompanied with expectation of full recovery. Stigma did not vary with the nature of the disorder, age, or sex of the child or the educational level of the caregiver. This suggests that support for families must consider their existing beliefs and support systems including religious and traditional values. While South Africa is the only country with a constitution that makes special recognition of persons with a disability, Njenga (9) makes a strong plea on behalf of people with ID in Africa, saying that a negative attitude towards them is pervasive. It is particularly so towards mothers of those with ID with many medical practitioners and traditional healers who feel the mothers may be possessed by evil spirits.

In a Chinese study, He et al. (12) pointed out that the prevalence of psychiatric disorders in adults with ID is higher than the prevalence in the general population. A similar pattern can be observed in other developed and developing countries, and it is accompanied by the suboptimal use of psychiatric services by people with ID. Important risk factors for psychiatric disorders in adults with ID include greater age (due in part to a high prevalence of dementia), more severe ID, and urban residency.

In the UK, while people with an ID make up 2% of the population, only one in ten receive input from specialist ID services, and therefore many have unmet health and social care needs. The ongoing reduction of services means many people with a mild learning disability are becoming a hidden population. Qualitative research projects concerning the lives of people with a mild learning disability who live independently show that the participants' lives are shaped by poverty, limited social capital, and skills deficits relating to having a learning disability. The challenges experienced related to difficulties with literacy and numeracy skills, digital exclusion, tenancy issues, and lack of purposeful occupation. This group also experience health inequalities and fail to engage with available health screening and services. This group should be recognized as having a learning disability and receive proactive and preventative support for their health and independent living needs, accessible information, crisis support, and advocacy. This will enable them to enjoy fulfilled and safe lives, and full citizenship in accordance with the United Nations Convention on the Rights of Persons with Disabilities (13).

At the age of 21, the trajectory of services offered to youth with profound ID change significantly since access to specialized services is more limited. Despite the desire of parents to avoid any impact on their child, several factors can influence the course of this transition. However, there is little research on facilitators and obstacles to the transition to adulthood, and impacts on people with a profound ID. It is therefore difficult to provide solutions that meet their specific needs. In a descriptive qualitative study aimed to document the needs of parents and young adults with profound ID during and after the transition to adulthood, Gauthier-Boudreault et al. (14) found that many material, informative, cognitive, and emotional needs of young adults and their parents are not met. Obstacles, mainly organizational, persist and result in a particularly difficult transition to adulthood experience. By knowing the specific needs of these families, it is possible to develop and implement solutions tailored to their reality. The transition to adulthood is a critical period for families with young adults with an ID, a reality observed internationally.

Access to mainstream healthcare

In Sweden, where Bengt Nirje formulated the normalization principle, disability is seen in relation to the environment or a social situation which needs adapting, so no disability is evident (15). This is a mainstream issue and social insurance to fund financial security, personal assistance, and employment with people with severe disabilities including ID operates nationally. The regional authorities lead on health and municipal authorities on education and social support. Schooling is inclusive and can range from children with ID having classes in ordinary schools with support to special classes in special schools on the same sites as ordinary schools. Adults with ID are supported to live in their own homes with support or in group homes, usually individually equipped apartments with access to shared rooms and shared support.

In the US, reversing of institutional care began with President John. F. Kennedy initiating the President's Panel on Mental Retardation which led to the influential Community Mental Health Act of 1963, enabling states to build research facilities to focus on ID issues, build community-based mental health facilities, and train educators in effective methods in working with people with ID (16). The next important event involved how state services for people with ID were provided. In 1981, the Medicaid Home and Community-Based Services Waiver programme was authorized and Intermediate Care Facilities for the Mentally Retarded (now named Intermediate Care Facilities for Individuals with Intellectual Disability) provided the first Medicaid long-term services for people with ID. As a result, a vast majority of people with ID now receive their care from non-governmental organizations (NGOs). Traditionally, health, mental health, and behavioural services for people with ID are housed separately, funded and regulated by different government agencies, and this can be a challenge to people with ID and their parents and carers (17).

The situation in Greece is that although the rights of people with ID are protected with all state policies including them, there is no official record of them as a percentage of the total population (18). Greece is part of all major human rights conventions pertaining to people with ID and participated in developing standardized criteria for mental health Assessments in adults with Mental Retardation and European Intellectual Disability Research Network. There is access to education either in special schools or inclusion into mainstream schools, and diagnostic services through Child Guidance Clinics of the National Health System. Psychiatric care is provided through the Greek National Health System; there are no specialized services for people with ID. NGOs have been charged via the 'Psychargos' National Action Plan to provide residential care and possibly mental health services. It is likely that a large number of people with ID are under the care of the Ministry of Health and Social Solidarity in residential institutions. There have been developments in recent years of community care with social support, education, and training with meaningful day activities. People with ID have a right to a regular monthly benefit from the state with reduced taxation, subsidies on electricity and phone bills, and an interest-free loan to buy a home. There is also support to train people with ID for sheltered employment; however, opportunities for employment are limited.

Serbia has changed education policies to be inclusive and to provide additional support to children with ID, as they were traditionally segregated (19). There was also a strategy to reduce discrimination experienced by people with disabilities. In Bulgaria, there were similar moves on integration and providing equal opportunities for people with disabilities. Both in Serbia and Bulgaria, general practitioners and paediatricians tend to look after the health needs of adults and children with ID. Outpatient mental healthcare is not well developed; those requiring inpatient care have to be admitted to units in district general hospitals or specialist psychiatric units located in in university centres. Both countries have a large residential population of children who need packages of care including day centres and supported homes.

Within high-income countries, people from minority ethnic communities face inequalities in health and healthcare. A systematic review considered the question of what we know about the health and healthcare of children and adults with ID from ethnic minority communities in the UK. Twenty-three studies were identified, most commonly focusing on South Asian communities. Very little information was identified on physical health or physical healthcare, with the identified evidence tending to focus on mental healthcare, and access to specialist ID and inpatient services. Little is known about the health status of people with ID from minority ethnic groups in the UK. They are likely to experience barriers in accessing specialist ID services and other forms of healthcare (20).

ID is more common in LAMI countries than in high-income countries. Stigma and discrimination have contributed to barriers to people with ID accessing healthcare. As part of a larger study on caregiving for children with ID in urban Cape Town, South Africa, a subgroup of families who had never used the ID services available to them, or who had stopped using them, were interviewed using a qualitative research design and semi-structured interviews.

Results revealed that caregivers and parents of children with ID did not use the service due to financial difficulties, fragile care networks and opportunity costs, community stigma and lack of safety, lack of faith in services, and powerlessness at effecting changes and self-stigmatization. This highlights a need for increased intervention at community level and collaboration with community-based projects to facilitate access to services, and engagement with broader issues of social exclusion (21). Epilepsy is often a common comorbidity in children with ID (9) which should be better monitored as older, more sedative medications continue to be used which affect the children's potential to learn—many African children with ID and epilepsy spend time at school asleep.

In some LAMI countries, people with disabilities are more likely to have inequitable access to healthcare services than their counterparts without disabilities. A quantitative study explored the predictors and determents of access to healthcare for this population in Iran and showed that the mean level of access to healthcare among people with ID was significantly lower than their counterparts with physical disabilities. In the affordability dimension, type of disability, marital status, and supplemental health insurance could predict access to health services. In the availability dimension, only location predicted the outcome variable significantly. Also, the location and type of disability were predictors of access to health services in the acceptability dimension. The results indicate that various factors can limit access to health services. To achieve universal health coverage, vulnerable groups and their needs should be identified to increase equitable access to healthcare services. Also, the healthcare system should pay more attention to demographic differences when planning and providing affordable and acceptable healthcare for people with disabilities. Finally, the role of the government as the health stewardship was vital to promote healthcare access for people with disabilities in Iran (22).

China, home to 1.3 billion people of different ethnic groups, languages, and traditions, was estimated to have a prevalence of ID of 0.75% based on the national survey on disability carried out in 2006 (23). The prevalence in urban areas was lower at 0.4% compared to rural areas which was 1.02%. The constitution of the People's Republic of China states that people with disabilities have the right to receive assistance from the state and society and the Compulsory Education Law provides 9 years of compulsory education to all children reaching the age of 6 without tuition fees. China is also a signatory to the law of Protection of persons with Disabilities. Every third Sunday in May is set aside as the National Day for Helping the Disabled. In the National Development Programme for 2006 to 2010, the plan was to set up at least one special education school for children with ID in counties and cities with a population of 300,000 to provide the 9-year compulsory education. Education campaigns were launched about iodine deficiency, consanguineous marriage, infections, and poisoning. The government also supported services for adults including re-habilitation programmes and sheltered employment for people with ID. There are government targets for poverty alleviation and support for families looking after people with ID. The services are to be provided for children and adults by the government and NGOs. Despite the will to provide the services, there are difficulties in finding premises, securing funding, and recruiting staff to run services. After the Special Olympics in Shanghai and Paralympics in Beijing in 2008, cities were more open to the idea of community rehabilitation services. Kwok et al. (23) conclude by saying that access to services is patchy, less so in rural areas, and mental health needs are a neglected area.

Specialist services or support for people with intellectual disability to access timely and effective healthcare

He et al. (12) noted that the prevalence of psychiatric disorders in this popula-tion is higher than in the general population both in developed and developing countries and this is accompanied by suboptimal use of services. Important contributory factors were age, degree of disability, and urban residency.

Mercadante et al. (24) evaluated the services available to people with ID in Latin American countries and conclude that this is an emerging field. There was an epidemiological study from Chile which correlated an increasing inci-dence of children with Down syndrome with the mother's age and another two studies from Jamaica where the Ten Questionnaire (TQ) was standardized and a cross-sectional, door-to-door study carried out to establish the prevalence of ID, using the TQ. The authors suggest that these studies could lead to evidence-based service development.

Katz et al. (25) conclude that the prevalence of ID in Mexico has not been established and hospitals which provide care underestimate the presence of ID in adults and in children. They suggest that people with ID could be considered 'invisible' citizens as they do not have access to medical services and there are no programmes to foster their independence. Any service is provided by phil-anthropic and charitable organizations, usually set up by parents, for a local area and for people up to the age of 18 and often without any regard to scientific evidence. Education policies are oriented towards integrating children with ID into primary education and do not foster independent living. They conclude that one of the problems is that Mexico's National Institute of Psychiatry's policy has not included people with ID who are older than 18 years.

Jeevanandam (26) summarized the policy and services available to people with ID in South Asian countries including China, Hong Kong, India, Indonesia, Japan, South Korea, Malaysia, Mongolia, Nepal, Pakistan, Philippines, Singapore, Sri Lanka, Taiwan, and Thailand and found that all the states had at least one law or policy that promotes the well-being of persons with disabilities although Japan specifically has one for people with ID. These are to provide disability pensions, payment for courses, health security, and social security. The data from the World Health Organization appear to suggest primary care services are provided in all the countries for children with ID and specialist services in 80% of the countries; adults have primary healthcare and rehabilitation in 80% of the countries and specialist inpatient care falls to 50% of the countries.

Lin and Lin (27), in their review of services in Taiwan have indicated that in 2007, the number of institutions increased from 223 to 254 compared to 2002 and the beds increased from 16,664 to 20,707. Men were more likely to be admitted than women. They have also indicated that the health of staff looking after people with ID in institutions was poorer than that of the general population. Children with ID are entitled to full National Insurance coverage and access to regular care providers but often, caregivers are unaware of their entitlements and the children miss out on their entitlements. The health of people with ID in institutions can only improve by the creation of a supportive environment where they participate in the decision-making process. General practitioners did not feel they had the expertise in treating patients with ID and needed further training on the job.

In the Soviet Union, there were large institutions where children were cared for as the philosophy was one of 'defectology' where children with any deficiencies were to be separated from their families, so that the society could exist as if there were no disabled people. Since the breakup of the Soviet Union in 1991, Russia passed a significant amount of legislation intended to protect the rights of children to education (28). This has not fully translated into changing the old stereotypes of stigma and social exclusion. Mothers of children with disabilities including ID who choose to bring them up have been told by professionals to place them in institutions and try for another child without 'defects'. The concept of discriminatory language is new in Russia. As social work programmes in Russian universities prepare practitioners to develop programmes for children with disabilities, community resources may develop in time.

The philosophy of defectology has influenced what has happened to children and adults in Central and Eastern European countries. Vann and Siska (29) described the situation in the Czech Republic as a case in point where people with ID continued to be housed in large state-run institutions in rural areas.

There are NGOs providing alternatives to institutions, usually in the cities, but the supply exceeds demand. Some of the practices in the institutions amount to human rights violations but they continue to be built.

In a South African study, McKenzie and McConkey (30) found that family carers take on responsibility for long-term care without much support. Carers expressed concerns about a lack of day-to-day support as well as education, training, and life opportunities for their loved ones which constrained their lives and did not allow them to develop their full potential. Underfunding in residential services contributed to the priority of care becoming more protective and segregated and less focused on vocational and life skill development (31).

Immigrant and refugee populations and people with developmental disabilities are known to have inequitable access to a range of health services (32). Very little study has been undertaken, however, on immigrants who have disabilities and their experience of the American healthcare system. A qualitative study by Bogenschutz sought to discover the particular challenges that immigrants with disabilities face when accessing healthcare, and the facilitating factors that assist them in this process. Findings from this study suggest strong resilience among immigrant families with a member with a disability, as they continue to seek help despite experiencing confusion in navigating a complex healthcare system. Factors challenging access included difficulty finding accurate information on insurance and service providers, trouble with coordinating multiple specialist services, and a lack of cultural competence at all levels of health service provision. Access to healthcare services was facilitated by linguistically and culturally sensitive practitioners, favourable comparisons to the country of origin, and systems such as schools that helped to coordinate care. Much can be done to integrate and improve health services for immigrants with developmental disabilities. Emerging models such as 'medical home' may assist with coordination, and improvements in communication patterns could help to improve service access and outcomes.

Whittle et al. (33) examined multiple barriers that prevent people with ID from accessing appropriate services. They carried out a qualitative study designed to explore the lived experience of barriers and enablers to access to mental health services among people with ID in Australia. Barriers and enablers were identified across four key dimensions of access, including financial barriers, lack of services and distance, poor understanding of mental illnesses, behaviour problems and trauma, discriminatory eligibility criteria, and being of indigenous origin.

Wieland et al. (34) reviewed access to mental healthcare in the Netherlands and Flanders for people with borderline intellectual functioning or an ID. They found that insufficient knowledge about mental disorders in long-term ID care and insufficient knowledge of, and experience with, borderline intellectual functioning and ID among mental healthcare providers play a role in the limited access to good mental healthcare. They recommend exchange of knowledge and sharing of experience between mental health and ID services.

Bakhiet (35) describes factors such as poverty, consanguinity, iodine deficiency, and poor medical care in Sudan which contribute to increased rates of ID. Several challenges are faced in provision of specialized care for Sudanese children with ID. The Sudanese community can be quite reserved and has a very close social fabric and strong religious beliefs. Stigma against people with disabilities and mental illness constitutes a great obstacle for accessing services. Sudanese patients prefer seeking traditional healing as it is more accepted culturally than going to see a psychiatrist. However, in some Sudanese communities a disabled child can be regarded as a blessing. This can also expose them to exploitation, as they can be used as a source of income, when people come to them seeking blessings or healing of their ill. Families refrain from seeking healthcare or education for disabled children as they get used to their disability as a source of income for the family. Other obstacles in establishing specialized service for people with ID include the lack of accurate statistics, low priority given to this group, and insufficient resources. There are some specialized schools for children with ID owned and run by parents of disabled children. These centres offer lifespan service for children and adults with learning disabilities. There is no governmental supervisory body to govern these schools and there are no protocols or guidelines to guide practice in these centres. Training for staff is patchy and does not follow evidence-based practice. Most of these centres are too expensive for poor families to afford. Furthermore, often the staff is poorly paid as well as poorly trained. In most areas there is no clear referral pathway and no multidisciplinary teams. Services are clustered around the capital making them inaccessible to other parts of the country.

Culture-specific innovations in healthcare for people with ID

Countries like UK have specialist multidisciplinary teams within the health service to manage the mental health needs of individuals with ID. These teams work jointly with social services to offer holistic support to people with ID and their families. There is an emphasis on strengthening primary care services, led by general medical practitioners, and other mainstream services including acute hospital services, so they are equipped in the recognition and management of health needs in ID populations (36).

In many LAMI countries, mental health problems in individuals with ID are managed by generic mental health services or primary care depending on the place of residence and availability of services. There is significant variation in the provision of service for people with ID between high-income and LAMI countries. There is often a lack of health services particularly in the rural areas of LAMI countries and this, along with a lack of awareness of health needs in ID, can lead to poorer health outcomes. NGOs play a crucial role in the support and rehabilitation of individuals with ID in LAMI countries. Many of these NGOs promoting care in the community have been founded by the parents of people with ID. There is evidence to suggest that this model can be helpful in meeting the needs of individuals with ID in a culturally sensitive manner (37). Parents can take a lead in providing health interventions when there is lack of access to professionals (38). Some of these innovative community mental health models in LAMI countries for people with mental health problems have been successful (39,40). A sustainable model of care should therefore focus on empowering the families/carers with advice and support from healthcare professionals while ensuring that the model of care is appropriate to the needs and sociocultural context. This is particularly important in countries that do not have a welfare state as a safety net.

In a systematic review of research evidence, Cantrell et al. (41) suggested that regular health checks could help to identify the health needs of people with a learning disability, and that these were useful for improving care for people who had additional long-term conditions. Factors that helped access for people with a learning disability were consistency of care and support, staff training, good staff communication, sufficient time during appointments, joined-up working, and accurate record-keeping.

Heer et al. (42) explored the cultural context of caregiving among South Asian communities caring for a child with ID in the UK. They conducted focus groups with parents from Sikh and Muslim support groups who were all accessing ID services for their children. Emerging themes were making sense of the disability, feeling let down by services, and looking to the future, which explained difficulties when making sense of the disabilities and difficult interactions with services. The study makes recommendations for service delivery to ethnic minority groups including being aware of intragroup variations in the interpretations and responses of South Asian parents. It makes recommendations for developing culturally sensitive support and interventions for ethnic minority groups which is important given the increase in multi-ethnic populations in the UK.

Girimaji and Srinath (43) summarize the prevalence studies carried out in India and suggest that prevalence may cluster around 10–30/1000 including all degrees of ID. India is a signatory to a number of international conventions and declarations on the rights of people with disabilities. There are several Acts formulated relating to ID: Persons with Disabilities Act, 1995, National Trust for Welfare of Persons with Autism, Cerebral palsy, Mental Retardation and Multiple Disabilities Act, 1999; and the Rehabilitation Council Act of India, 1992. In India, families are a major source of support and it has long been the tradition to involve families in the management of individuals with ID by training them in behaviour modification techniques and use of self-help skills. An approach that relies on the strength of parent–professional partnerships has gradually grown though there may be variations in goals and methods of delivery (44–46) both in India and other countries like Singapore (47). In larger cities, there are child guidance and specialist clinics for children with ID. Identifying people with ID using population-based screening tools can be expensive and time-consuming. An alternative approach was described by Lakhan and Mawson (48) showing high correlation in cases identified through focus group interviews within the communities where the young people lived compared to a standardized survey. They suggest that early engagement of communities tends to accelerate acceptance of subsequent support. In another study, carer reports of delayed acquisition of motor skills such as sitting alone, standing alone, and walking alone proved to be effective in screening for autism, thus providing a low-cost screening at a younger age to enable early help to be provided (49).

Masulane-Mwale et al. (50) from Malawi describe a step-by-step approach wherein they reviewed literature to arrive at two models from which they derived interventions likely to be effective in the local setting. They carried out a qualitative study to gain insights into the lived experience of parents of children and young people with ID. Expert panels reviewed the final package and this was then piloted in the local community for acceptability and feasibility. The authors demonstrated that culturally sensitive and effective interventions can be developed and used in LAMI countries.

In his overview of service delivery models for people with ID in LAMI countries, Kishore (51) emphasized the need for services for an ID population that is 'marginalised and excluded, often facing misconceptions, stigma, discrimination and severe human rights violations among all groups of people with disabilities'. He cited an example in Laos of difficulties in identification of people with ID seen in some developing countries, a problem exacerbated by familial fear of stigma. Service delivery models need to understand the local culture notions of disability. In this study, parent groups and advocates were raising awareness and demonstrating the effectiveness of specialized services. In Bolivia where a shortage of expertise and the high costs of specialist therapists were highlighted, abandonment of the medical model is recommended with the adoption of a new model based on shared practical and expert knowledge among families. Some post-Soviet republics tended to stigmatize and exclude people with disabilities in large institutions. Urgent restructuring of the service provider–client relationship and changing the professional culture of educational, social, and health organizations was needed. In a bottom-up approach, local volunteers were trained as Community Resource Persons in rural South India. They were well received by families caring for people with ID and led to the development of neighbourhood centres as local activity and information sharing hubs.

Menon et al. (52) describe a national framework in India which is developing group homes, respite, health insurance, and care training, as well as promoting community awareness and interaction. It is based on a socioecological framework and works holistically to meet social and health needs and is supported by a legal guardianship programme managed by local level committees who are legally empowered to act in the best interests of the person with ID. The authors recommend the framework for use in other LAMI countries as well as ongoing evaluation and development.

Conclusion

Models of healthcare provision vary widely across the world and are often influenced by local culture, resources both professional and societal, levels of stigma, and the level of support available for investment and development of services.

References

1. **Odiyoor MM, Jaydeokar S.** Intellectual disability in rural backgrounds: challenges and solutions. In: **Chaturvedi S,** editor. Mental Health and Illness in Rural World. Mental Health and Illness Worldwide. Singapore: Springer; 2019.

2. **Maulik PK, Mascarenhas MN, Mathers CD, Dua T, Saxena S.** Prevalence of intellectual disability: a meta-analysis of population-based studies. Research in Developmental Disabilities 2011;**32**(2):419–36.

3. **Maulik PK, Darmstadt GL.** Childhood disability in low- and middle-income countries: overview of screening, prevention, services, legislation, and epidemiology. Pediatrics 2007;**120**:182–5.

4. **Lakhan R, Ekúndayò OT, Shahbazi M.** An estimation of the prevalence of intellectual disabilities and its association with age in rural and urban populations in India. Journal of Neurosciences in Rural Practice 2015;**6**(4):523–8.

5. **McKenzie K, Milton M, Smith G, Ouellette-Kuntz H.** Systematic review of the prevalence and incidence of intellectual disabilities: current trends and issues. Current Developmental Disorders Report 2016;**3**:104–15.

6. **Fischer VJ, Morris J, Martines J.** Developmental screening tools: feasibility of use at primary healthcare level in low and middle-income settings. Journal of Health, Population and Nutrition 2014;**32**(2):314–26.

7. **Tesemma ST.** Educating Children with Disabilities in Africa: Towards a Policy of Inclusion. Addis Ababa: The African Child Policy Forum; 2011.

8. **Adnams CM.** Perspectives of intellectual disability in South Africa: epidemiology, policy, services for children and adults. Current Opinion in Psychiatry 2010;**23**(5):436–40.

9. **Njenga F.** Perspectives of intellectual disability in Africa: epidemiology and policy services for children and adults. Current Opinion in Psychiatry 2009;**22**(5):457–61.

10. **Memari AH, Hafizi S.** People with intellectual disability and socio-political life participation: a commitment to inclusive policy in less developed countries. Journal of Policy and Practice in Intellectual Disabilities 2015;**12**(1):37–41.

11. **Tilahun D, Hanlon C, Fekadu A, Tekola B, Baheretibeb Y, Hoekstra R.** Stigma, explanatory models and unmet needs of caregivers of children with developmental disorders in a low-income African country: a cross-sectional facility-based survey. BMC Health Services Research 2016;**16**(152):1–12.

12. **He P, Chen G, Wang Z, Guo C, Li N, Yun C,** et al. Adults with intellectual disabilities in China: comorbid psychiatric disorder and its association with health service utilisation. Journal of Intellectual Disability Research 2018;**62**(2):106–14.

13. **Tilly L.** Challenges to a full life for people with mild learning disability living without support. Journal of Intellectual Disability Research 2019;**63**(7):846.

14. **Gauthier-Boudreault C, Gallagher F, Couture M.** Specific needs of families of young adults with profound intellectual disability during and after transition to adulthood: what are we missing? Research in Developmental Disabilities 2017;**66**:16–26.

15. **Tideman M.** Education and support for people with intellectual disabilities in Sweden: policy and practice. Research and Practice in Intellectual and Developmental Disabilities 2015;**2**(2):116–25.

16. **Conrad JA.** On intellectual and developmental disabilities in the United States: a historical perspective. Journal of Intellectual Disabilities 2020;**24**(1):85–101.

17. **Ervin DA, Williams A, Merrick J.** Primary care: mental and behavioural health and persons with intellectual and developmental disabilities. Frontiers in Health 2014;**2**:76.

18. **Anagnostopoulos DC, Soumaki E.** Perspectives of intellectual disability in Greece: epidemiology, policy, services for children and adults. Current Opinion in Psychiatry 2011;**24**(5):425–30.

19. **Ispanovic-Radojkovic V, Stancheva-Popkostadinova V.** Perspectives of intellectual disability in Serbia and Bulgaria: epidemiology, policy and services for children and adults. Current Opinion in Psychiatry 2011;**24**(5):419–24.

20. **Robertson J, Raghavan R, Emerson E, Baines S, Hatton C.** What do we know about the health and health care of people with intellectual disabilities from minority ethnic groups in the United Kingdom? A systematic review. Journal of Applied Research in Intellectual Disabilities 2019;**32**(6):1310–34.

21. **Mkabile S, Swartz L.** 'I waited for it until forever': community barriers to accessing intellectual disability services for children and their families in Cape Town, South Africa. International Journal of Environmental Research and Public Health 2020;**17**(22):8504.

22. **Matin BK, Kamali M, Williamson HJ, Moradi F.** The predictors of access to health services for people with disabilities: a cross sectional study in Iranian context. Journal of Medical Council of Islamic Republic of Iran 2019;**33**(1):1–7.

23. **Kwok HWM, Cui Y, Li J.** Perspectives of intellectual disability in People's Republic of China: epidemiology, policy, services for children and adults. Current Opinion in Psychiatry 2011;**24**(5):408–12.

24. **Mercadante, MT, Evans-Lacko S, Paula CS.** Perspectives of intellectual disability in Latin American countries: epidemiology, policy, and services for children and adults. Current Opinion in Psychiatry 2009;**22**(5):469–74.

25. **Katz G, Marquez-Caraveo ME, Lazcano-Ponce E.** Perspectives of intellectual disability in Mexico: epidemiology, policy and services for children and adults. Current Opinion in Psychiatry 2010;**23**(5):432–5.

26. **Jeevanandam L.** Perspectives of intellectual disability in Asia: epidemiology, policy, and services for children and adults. Current Opinions in Psychiatry 2009;**22**(5):462–8.

27. **Lin LP, Lin JD.** Perspectives on intellectual disability in Taiwan: epidemiology, policy and services for children and adults. Current Opinions in Psychiatry 2011;**24**(5):413–18.

28. **Iarskaia-Smirnova E.** What the future will bring I do not know: mothering children with disabilities in Russia and the politics of exclusion. Frontiers: A Journal of Womens Studies 1999;**20**(2):68–86.

29. **Vann BH, Siska J.** From 'cage beds' to inclusion: the long road for individuals with intellectual disability in the Czech Republic. Disability & Society 2006;**21**(5):425–39.

30. **Mckenzie J, McConkey R.** Caring for adults with intellectual disability: the perspectives of family carers in South Africa. Journal of Applied Research in Intellectual Disabilities 2015;**29**:531–41.

31. **McKenzie J, MacConkey R, Adnams C.** Residential facilities for adults with intellectual disability in a developing country: a case study from South Africa. Journal of Intellectual and Developmental Disability 2014;**39**(1):45–54.

32. **Bogenschutz M.** 'We find a way': challenges and facilitators for health care access among immigrants and refugees with intellectual and developmental disabilities. Medical Care 2014;**52**(10 Suppl 3):S64–70.

33. **Whittle EL, Fisher KR, Reppermund S, Trollor J.** Access to mental health services: the experiences of people with intellectual disabilities. Journal of Applied Research in Intellectual Disabilities 2019;**32**(2):368–79.

34. **Wieland J, Denayer A, van Amelsvoort TAMJ.** Mental health care for people with borderline intellectual functioning or intellectual disabilities. Tijdschift voor Psychiatrie 2019;**61**(11):819–24.

35. **Bakhiet A.** Challenges of practicing learning disability psychiatry in Sudan. Sudanese Journal of Paediatrics 2015;**15**(1):96–7.

36. **Bhaumik S, Kiani R, Michael DM, Gangavati S, Kahn S, Torales J**, et al. World Psychiatric Association (WPA) report on mental health issues in people with intellectual disability. International Journal of Culture and Mental Health 2016;**9**(4):417–44.

37. **Aldersey HM.** Family perceptions of intellectual disability: understanding and support in Dar es Salaam. African Journal of Disability 2012;**1**(1):32.

38. **Einfeld SL, Stancliffe RJ, Gray KM, Sofronoff K, Rice L, Emerson E**, et al. Interventions provided by parents for children with intellectual disabilities in low and middle income countries. Journal of Applied Research in Intellectual Disabilities 2012;**25**(2):135–42.

39. **Manoj Kumar T.** Community psychiatry—transcontinental lessons of the last quarter century. Indian Journal of Social Psychiatry 2018;**34**(4):292–5.

40. **Samarasekara N, Davies M, Siribaddana S.** The stigma of mental illness in Sri Lanka: the perspectives of community mental health workers. Stigma Research and Action 2012;**2**(2):93–9.

41. **Cantrell A, Croot E, Johnson M, Wong R, Chambers D, Baxter SK**, et al. Access to primary and community health-care services for people 16 years and over with intellectual disabilities: a mapping and targeted systematic review. Health Services and Delivery Research 2020;**8**(5):1–142.

42. **Heer K, Larkin L, Burchess I.** Culture specific innovations in health care for people with ID. Advances in Mental Health and Intellectual Disabilities 2012;**6**(4):179–91.

43. **Girimaji SC, Srinath S.** Perspectives of intellectual disability in India: epidemiology, policy, services for children and adults. Current Opinion in Psychiatry 2010;**23**:441–6.

44. **Russell PSS, John JK, Jayaseelan L.** Family intervention for intellectually disabled children—randomised controlled trial. British Journal of Psychiatry 1999;**174**(3):254–8.

45. **Girimaji SR.** Family focused intervention in mental retardation—Indian models. In: **Bhatti RS, Varghese M, Raguram A**, editors. Changing Marital and Family Systems: Challenges to Conventional Models in Mental Health. Bengaluru: National Institute of Mental Health and Neuro Science; 2003: 192–9.

46. **Girimaji SC.** Intellectual disability in India: the evolving patterns of care. International Journal of Psychiatry 2011;**8**(2):28–31.

47. **Rainbow Centre.** Training. n.d. Available from: https://rainbowcentre.org.sg/training/

48. **Lakhan R, Mawson R.** Identifying children with intellectual disabilities in the tribal population of Barwani district in the estate of Madhya Pradesh, India. Journal of Applied Research in Intellectual Disabilities 2013;**29**:211–19.

49. **Arabameri E, Sotoodeh MS.** Early developmental delay in children with autism: a study from a developing country. Infant Behaviour and Development 2015;**39**:118–23.

50. **Masulani-Mwale C, Kauye F, Gladstone M, Mathanga D.** Development of a psycho-social intervention for reducing psychological distress among parents of children with intellectual disabilities in Malawi. PLoS One 2019;**14**(2):e0210855.

51. **Kishore MT.** Service delivery models for people with intellectual disabilities in low and middle income countries: strategies and solutions can emerge from within. Journal of Intellectual Disabilities 2017;**21**(3):201–2.

52. **Menon DK, Kishore MT, Sivakumar T, Maulik PK, Kumar D, Lakhan R**, et al. The National Trust: a viable model of care for adults with intellectual disabilities in India. Journal of Intellectual Disabilities 2017;**21**(3):259–69.

Chapter 11

Culture and therapies

Alison Drewett, Louis Busch, Jessica Cremasco, Pauline Ndigirwa, and Natalie Yiu

Introduction

Using the perspectives from three allied healthcare professional groups, namely speech and language therapists (SLTs), behaviour analysts, and occupational therapists (OTs), this chapter illustrates culturally sensitive practices, evidenced by the frontline experiences of clinicians from both the UK and Canada, and reference is made to cultural competency frameworks to explore real-world issues in implementation (1). A systematic review identified nine such frameworks across the world, and established four core themes: awareness of diversity, ability to care, non-judgemental openness, and competency as a lifelong development (2). A specialist model developed for SLT practice in the US called VISION is applied to the practice examples provided by the SLTs and OTs in this chapter (3). VISION stands for (V) values and beliefs, (I) interpretation of experiences, (S) structure of the professional and family relationship, (I) interaction styles, (O) operational strategies to achieve expectations and goals, and (N) family and professional needs. The VISION model is relevant to the family-centred approach in working with individuals with intellectual disability (ID) and applicable across disciplines. The behaviour analysts have utilized a framework from Mushquash (4) that describes culturally sensitive practices with the indigenous population.

Speech and language therapy approach

SLTs in the UK work with people with ID focusing on their speech, language, and communication needs, as well as eating and drinking difficulties (dysphagia) (5). It is estimated that almost 58% of people with ID have communication difficulties, nearly a quarter have severe difficulties, and half have problems communicating with professionals (6). These include difficulties in expressive, receptive, and social communication skills. People with ID are also more likely to have speech difficulties such as dysarthria (a motor speech disorder), as well as memory issues, and processing and literacy difficulties. Communication is also negatively impacted because of the additional risk of people with ID having visual and hearing impairments. There may be additional communication challenges for people with ID with Black and minority ethnic backgrounds whose first language is not English, as well as multilingual speakers in UK and non-UK countries (7). These difficulties widen health inequalities that people with ID face (8), compounded by ethnicity (9).

The professional approach of SLTs in the UK is governed by the Royal College of Speech and Language Therapists, the Health and Care Professions Council, and the National Health Service. Critically, the approach is guided by a biopsychosocial framework which means practice needs to give equal respect to all languages (whether spoken, signed, or written), and consideration given to the cultural contexts in which communication takes place (10). The Royal College of Speech and Language Therapists has promoted the need for therapists to be culturally competent. Despite this, scholars argue that *how* SLTs develop cultural intelligence is still under-researched (11). This section examining SLT practice highlights three key professional approaches to illustrate how SLTs (can) routinely demonstrate cultural competency: indirect working or working with others (12,13), inclusive communication (10), and the Means, Reasons, and Opportunities (MRO) framework (14).

Due to the nature of the cognitive disability, families of people with ID often support the person over a lifetime, which means that they need to be central to therapeutic input. In English-speaking countries, it is widely considered to be a sign of independence for the person with ID to leave the family home and move into supported care in the community, but this is not the same for all cultures. Additionally, conceptualizations about the causes of disability are inherently culturally derived so that spiritual, religious, and social understandings are central to how SLTs navigate therapeutic engagement. This relates very clearly to the 'V' part of the VISION model.

An example of this is that there are often issues arising that need to be discussed concerning family-held beliefs about the aetiology of the ID, as well as ideas about independence and adult identity that reflect different cultural norms and expectations. The chapter authors have experience of both African and Asian-born parents who believed that their son or daughter's ID was caused by a curse placed on them deliberately by someone who had a grudge against them or was a punishment for something that they or their ancestors had done. These beliefs may leave some families feeling helpless as they believe that their situations could not improve, while for others it offered the possibility that, if the curse could be lifted, the intellectual impairment would expire. In contrast, some families conceptualized their family member's ID as a special gift and that they had been specifically chosen to care for them. The downside of this positive framing was that for one family this resulted in the parents passively accepting all of their son's behaviour and not placing boundaries which subsequently led to an escalation of challenging behaviours.

There were also beliefs regarding personal responsibility for causing the ID. People stated that the ID was due to the mother's behaviour in pregnancy, for example, because of the items she had eaten or drunk. Subsequently, mothers felt guilty and were even blamed by other family members. Alongside these attributions, intellectual impairment was often linked to a specific event in the early life of the person such as falling into a ditch, being frightened by a dog, or a specific childhood illness. These are examples of cultural differences in interpretation when applied to the VISION model.

These commonly held cultural ideas about disability also extend to perceptions of challenging behaviour. Commonly, SLTs offer support around ways to manage and reduce challenging behaviour viewing it as a (mal)adaptive way of communicating, and as socially and culturally constructed (15). In cultures where respect for elders is very important, behaviour that is seen to disrespect parents or other parental figures within the community is viewed negatively and can lead to serious consequences for the individual and their family. In short, the challenging behaviour is not viewed as related to the person's ID and their communication difficulties but individualized and constructed as bad behaviour.

Policy and practice guidance highlight that family and client involvement in SLT assessment is essential, and that therapists need to demonstrate respect towards diversity. This means therapists need to address carers' understanding of ID and the perceived role of the therapist because it has a direct bearing on carers' expectation of the professional ('S' and 'O' in VISION). Families may expect the therapist will *cure* the ID, or even have a medicine or treatment that would return the person to normal cognitive functioning. These views can significantly impact their engagement with and acceptance of interventions. Sometimes, their expectation could be that the professional would *do something to* the person with ID and work directly with them one to one. This individualized approach, more suited to a biomedical model whereby treatment is directed to the person, does not sit easily with the more *indirect* approach of SLTs.

The rationale for an indirect approach is the principle that better communication is the responsibility of both the client and the communication partner and that given the developmental nature of the disability, significant change is unlikely to occur by focusing on the adult with the ID alone. Thus, working collaboratively with the person's communication partners is beneficial to identify communication opportunities, address ways to promote independence, and model good communication skills. However, this social approach would not always be received well by families expecting a more didactic 'expert knows best approach'. This difference may severely hamper goal setting and the therapeutic relationship. In contrast, for SLTs, the MRO model underlines how important it is to consider not only how the person communicates (means), but also to ensure that they have reasons to interact with others (to be able to ask for things, share ideas, and so on) and that they have opportunities to communicate (to see others in a variety of settings) (14). The SLT will work with families to address how the person is able to do this in a meaningful and culturally sensitive way for them.

Practice that adapts an inclusive communication approach is also central to SLT therapeutic input. This is an approach that recognizes the right of individuals to personal choice and values any *means* of communication. In the Western world, there is a greater value placed on literacy and being able to read, write, and converse using spoken language. An inclusive communication approach uses any other form of communication (e.g., visual information such as pictures, symbols, drawings, and photos, signing and gestural systems, alternative and augmentative communication, using objects of reference) are alongside the more traditional approaches.

As therapists, we would want the assessment materials we use to reflect culturally familiar vocabulary, grammatical structures, and language concepts. However, what was challenging, particularly in one of the therapist's experiences of working in Tanzania, was the lack of familiarity with pictures or visual aids as a form of material. The pictures typically found in SLT assessments and visual support materials were incomprehensible to those with ID and even to family members without ID. The therapist needed to use real objects (objects of reference), act out scenarios, or sometimes utilize photos in therapy. In this way, it is clear that cultural competency is critical to operational goal setting, and to work effectively with diverse backgrounds.

Cultural competency is also relevant in relation to providing professional guidance to families following assessment and intervention. It is easy to assume that the carer(s) accompanying the person with ID to an appointment are the primary caregivers, and therefore the most relevant recipients of recommendations. However, this assumption is not always true for people from ethnic minorities, and it is important to identify who is the best person to liaise with from the outset. In addition, there may be a younger family member or paid member of the household providing the care, so it is also important to ensure that they are involved in discussions. Within these relationships, it is important to explain that interaction and communication is bi-directional as this is often not the expectation ('S' in the model). Therapists also need to be mindful of the etiquette surrounding the rules of social interaction before they embark on *social skills training* for the client. For example, greetings are not permitted to be initiated by a younger person in the company of an older person in some cultures. Given the roles that people with ID may have in the family home and community, it is important to provide recommendations that are functional and related to everyday household tasks. This considers the needs of both the family and professionals in the VISION model ('N').

Finally, a note about community acceptance as a way of thinking about cultural diversity and the environmental context in which therapy happens. We have had some experience of communities where the person with ID was kept separate. However, in the majority of cases, the opposite has been found and people with ID are treated as integrated and valued members of their community. This acceptance has a significant impact on the development of self-esteem and well-being and lessens the impact of the ID, for example, on participation and activity (16). This also has a helpful impact on communication skills as individuals are interacting with a range of different people for a variety of reasons and with many opportunities—the MRO model in action.

An example of this was Nelson, an individual with ID who had no verbal communication. After assessment, it was decided that teaching signing to him and his mother would give him a way to communicate with others. His mother was taught a small vocabulary of signs and booked in for another session in 3 weeks. After speaking to his mother about how she had approached the signing, it was discovered that she had gone back to her community and taught everyone the signs: her family, neighbours, local shopkeepers, and the bus drivers. She was delighted to share that Nelson could now go to the shop independently to buy selected items. When she was praised for her approach, she replied, 'Well how will he learn to communicate if others don't know what he's saying?'

Behaviour analytic approach

Applied behaviour analysis is a subdiscipline of operant-behavioural psychology which uses the principles of learning to address behavioural health challenges and other issues of social importance. For people with ID, behavioural health challenges may range from skill deficits which make social interaction or tasks of daily living difficult, to responsive behaviours that put them and others at a risk of harm (e.g. severe self-injury, physical aggression, and environmental destruction) (17). Behaviour analysts use functional behavioural assessments to understand the function of harmful behaviour within each individual's unique context. After identifying variables which may be maintaining challenges, such as an individual being removed from a group activity after screaming loudly, skills are taught, and adaptations are made to the environment. For example, the individual is taught to raise their hand to ask for a break, while staff are trained to identify and respond to that request quickly and consistently. Interventions based on functional behavioural assessments focus on building replacement skills and are more effective than default strategies (18). A behaviour analytic approach is highly individualized for each person in their unique context, and seeks to promote safety, independence, and improved quality of life (19).

Behaviour analysts are often involved in the support of individuals with ID and behavioural health issues in diverse community settings. Although most behaviour analysts receive graduate-level training in assessment, treatment, and skill-building methods specific to individuals with ID, many behaviour analysts do not receive training in cultural safety, competency, or humility (20). The assessment and treatment of behavioural health challenges require careful attention to cultural consideration, when working with diverse and marginalized groups. Mushquash (an Indigenous clinical-academic) provides guidelines for culturally sensitive psychological assessment with Indigenous people living with ID (4). This section extends the 'Mushquash' framework to behaviour analytic work in Indigenous communities as an example of cultural considerations and adaptations to improve the safety of healthcare and social services for marginalized groups.

Mushquash (4) suggests beginning with a self-assessment of potential biases and prejudices while learning as much as possible about a culture to approach the relationship with humility and to address existing stereotypes. Self-assessment tools exist that are specific to behaviour analysts (21) and specific to work with Indigenous peoples (22) which could be useful in this endeavour. Mushquash cautions clinicians to acknowledge the diversity of Indigenous language and culture and to avoid a pan-Indigenous approach in this process (4). Each Indigenous nation, and even communities within similar nations in close geographical regions, can be extremely distinct in their cultural practices, languages, histories, and experiences with settler populations, and care should be taken to appreciate these differences.

The framework underscores the importance of understanding variables in the broader context which may impact clinical work and to acknowledge potential barriers of distrust which may exist within Indigenous communities. The historical and present-day impacts of colonization contribute to significant disparities in the availability, accessibility, and acceptability of health and social care for Indigenous populations across the world (23). In Canada, for example, many clinicians are likely to be unaware of (i) the existence of segregated 'Indian Hospitals' which operated from the 1920s to the 1980s, and contributed to the deaths of thousands of Indigenous peoples in extremely inhumane conditions (24); (ii) lethal and non-consensual starvation experiments conducted on Indigenous children by the Government of Canada in partnership with paediatricians at the country's leading children's hospital (25); (iii) deceptive research practices such as those examining the effect of radioactive isotopes on the human thyroid, which were provided to Alaska Natives and Inuk peoples, including children and pregnant women, under the false pretence of medical treatment (26); or, (iv) the alarmingly high number of coerced sterilizations conducted on Indigenous women across the Canada within the last decade alone (27).

Similarly, many therapists will not be aware of the destructive impact that social services have had in the lives of Indigenous peoples. The residential school system which operated for 165 years across Canada, saw forced familial separation and institutionalization of approximately 150,000 Indigenous children, as young as 4 years of age. Moreover, an excess of 6000 children died from malnutrition, disease, and child homicide in these state- and church-run facilities. Many others who survived were left with enduring trauma from severe emotional, physical, and sexual abuses which were reported at facilities across the country up until the last facility closed in 1996 (28). The child welfare system has also done, and continues to do, considerable harm in Canada, with forced displacement and adoption of thousands of Indigenous children away from their communities and cultures beginning in the 1960s and continuing to the present day. Indigenous children are 15 times more likely to be in care than non-Indigenous children in Canada (29).

These are just a few examples of the experiences of Indigenous people in contact with the health and social care system in Canada, but they are relevant to effective intercultural practice. An intimate knowledge of historical and ongoing acts of oppression and discrimination, and, importantly, the experiences of Indigenous peoples from the perspective of Indigenous peoples, is a necessary prerequisite to safe and effective behavioural health support for Indigenous people living with ID. Due to this history, a well-earned mistrust of external practitioners, and their clinical and research methods, must be anticipated and acknowledged by practitioners when it occurs.

An understanding of the differences between worldviews grounded within Western social science and medical models and those of Indigenous peoples is important. While each Indigenous nation is unique in its cultural, educational, medical, governance, and spiritual practices, many groups share a holistic perspective of wellness that emphasizes relationality and balance rather than compartmentalization across physical, mental, emotional, and spiritual health domains that is often found in Western service models. In an examination of Navajo perspectives on autism, for example, Kapp (30) suggests that an understanding of 'intercultural commonalities and differences' could foster inclusion and have a positive impact on attitudes towards disability. For example, prioritizing efforts at 'raising autistic people's adaptive skills and quality of life, but also to change the social environment for intercultural survivance' (30: p 18). Assessments designed by Indigenous researchers and health practitioners which evaluate wellness and cultural connectedness from an Indigenous perspective should be considered when working with Indigenous peoples (31,32).

Although many psychosocial assessment procedures include assessments of physical environments, family or caregiver dynamics, community resources, and broader socioeconomic supports and risks, few assessment methods explore important cultural variables which are relevant to the lives of diverse groups. The Mushquash framework focuses on assessment procedures that are culturally safe and relevant, and provides several recommendations for safe and effective clinical engagement with Indigenous peoples (4). It advocates that clinical assessments are implemented and interpreted in the individual's preferred language; immediate and extended family members and relevant community members (e.g. elders) are included when appropriate; a multi-method assessment approach is applied; and there is a period of prior relationship building with the individual and their caregivers. For behaviour analysts, this may mean applying functional assessment measures with multiple respondents, assessing in a variety of contexts (home, school, community centre, extended family's home), identifying culturally appropriate activities and replacement skills, and spending significant time in the community building relationships prior to engaging in clinical work.

Cultural translation, integration, and indigenization of clinical procedures may also be an effective way to promote cultural safety and trusting relationships while providing behavioural health supports. Many modern psychosocial approaches applied to teach skills and address challenges have been applied by Indigenous peoples in some way over many generations. As an example, in translating a cognitive behavioural therapy-based parent–child intervention for Alaskan Native families, Bigfoot and Funderbunk drew connections to positive reinforcement procedures used to teach new skills to the traditional practices of recognizing youth traditions such as honorary dinners, giveaways, or naming ceremonies (33). By connecting the tradition of recognizing an individual following some personal success or pro-social behaviour to the use of reinforcement-based shaping procedures described in many behavioural procedures, the approach may be viewed as more familiar and acceptable. This translation and integration work is necessarily done by Indigenous people, for Indigenous people, rather than in a performative, superficial, or tokenistic way.

When conducting research or delivering behavioural health interventions, acknowledging the importance of self-determination, data sovereignty, and sustainability of supports in Indigenous communities is paramount (34). As a result of systemic racism and neo-colonial structures, many communities face barriers to the availability, accessibility, and acceptability of services (35). The tiered-service mediator models often applied in the support of individuals with developmental disabilities, may not be appropriate or suitable for all communities. It is not uncommon for an expert-level consultant to train frontline staff to apply teaching and support strategies and monitor effectiveness of procedures in many resource-rich urban settings, but this may not be successful in some remote communities. Adaptations which include involvement of natural change agents (caregivers, community members), train-the-trainer procedures, or the use of ongoing support via telehealth may be necessary for successful outcomes. Investing the time to engage and form relationships in the community is vital, as is relinquishing control of the decision-making process to stakeholders.

When working with Indigenous communities, behaviour analysts must attend to the individual and micro-level ecological contexts that are frequently the target of functional assessment and function-based behavioural interventions, but also to the more complex macro-, exo-, and chrono-system dynamics involved in the Indigenous determinants of health. Integrating behaviour analytic approaches with Indigenous perspectives on wellness and building reciprocal and respecting relationships is vital to successful outcomes for Indigenous peoples with ID. In examining behavioural interventions in diverse school populations, Wilson (36) suggests recognition of sociocultural differences, inclusion of community in determining goals and expectations, incorporation of the voices of cultural leaders and knowledge keepers throughout the clinical process, and acceptance and mindful judgement when approaching behavioural health challenges; these are tenants which could be effectively applied to work with Indigenous peoples. Although these suggestions are presented in the context of clinical partnerships with Indigenous populations in Canada, they could be extended to marginalized groups across the world, with a careful effort to understand and safely respond to each unique context.

Occupational therapy approach

OTs help people to 'engage in everyday activities or occupations that they want and need to do in a manner that supports health and participation' (37). OTs champion occupational justice, or everyone's right to have access to occupations that are meaningful and valued to them (38). Individuals with ID may experience occupational injustice in the form of reduced community participation, social relationships, employment, and leisure opportunities (39). OTs engage with clients and families to identify their occupational needs, interests, strengths, and future goals, as well as any concerns with adaptive functioning. These may include barriers such as motor, emotional regulation, or sensory processing challenges prevalent among this population. In Canada and the US, OTs play a crucial role in teaching and training people with ID in life and vocational skills, supporting caregivers, and advocating for inclusion, participation, and community integration (40).

Occupational therapy theory was developed with a Eurocentric perspective, and this theological basis perpetuates Westernized assumptions, values, and worldviews (41). What results is an underlying assumption that the subsequent theories and models developed in a Western context are universally applicable and relevant to others. Thus, there is a strong case for cultural humility as an approach to therapy; as therapists we must take the time as part of the assessment to learn about the client's life, their experiences, priorities, and occupational choices. We must ask and listen to the client, to consider how their ID and perceived physical, cognitive, and/or sensory difference(s) may interact with environmental and sociocultural contexts. We must also learn how this interaction may facilitate or impede adaptive functioning (42), and ultimately, how the cultural status of ID can affect opportunities for, and barriers to, occupation.

The Canadian Occupational Performance Measure is conducted as a semistructured interview, so OTs can adapt the assessment to address cultural considerations within the measure (38). However, the authors do recognize that the Canadian Occupational Performance Measure may be more difficult to use with clients of non-Westernized cultures; an example being where the client may be uncomfortable with expressing needs, setting goals, and accepting help from someone outside their family. For other cultures, occupations are difficult to conceptualize into the conventional Western categories of self-care, productivity, and leisure, or to consider occupations across these categories as equally influential on one's health and well-being. Hammell gives the example of leisure (e.g. recreational activities and play) sometimes being considered as irrelevant by certain populations facing socioeconomic constraints, such as poverty (43). Alternatively, the American Occupational Therapy Association's Occupational Profile Template offers a more direct approach to discussing what aspect(s) of the client's cultural context the client/family sees as a support or a barrier to occupational engagement (37). Furthermore, therapists need to skilfully broaden the inquiry to include activities that may not be captured by the traditional self-care, productivity, and leisure categories such as caring for and connecting with others, and culturally specific occupations such as ceremonies.

Constructed norms of societal roles influence participation in occupation; being classified outside of these norms, as an individual with ID might be, can negatively impact occupational opportunities. Established within a culture is the inherent assignment of differing values to activities. Imposing meaningful occupations on individuals based on Western cultural norms and evaluating 'success' based on the accomplishment of occupational roles (e.g. paid worker, spouse, parent) can be detrimental. An example of this is a woman with ID who does not have the ability, or desire, to manage a household and raise children independently. Her family may have to modify what they view as valuable or successful and find fresh meanings for the person's role within the family. This corresponds to the 'V' in the VISION model; the focus on developing an awareness and understanding of the values and beliefs of the family, and of your own as the professional (3).

Respectful communication between clinician and client is important throughout the therapeutic process and requires special consideration when sharing occupational therapy assessment findings and intervention. Often the care team may present to the client and caregivers as a panel of 'professionals', with multiple disciplines present at one time. The meeting may take place in the clinic rather than the client's own environment, further highlighting the power differential between client and clinician. The interaction style of verbal and non-verbal communication of family and professional (second 'I' in VISION) should strive for 'respectful, reciprocal and responsive interactions' (44). As OTs our focus is on identifying and promoting the assets and resilience of clients with ID and their families; our language is centred on functions rather than impairments, and we provide examples that they can relate to in their everyday life.

Therapists need to consider how occupations are practised within a family, the family's views on independence, their priorities, and goals for therapy (45). A case study example helps to shed light on the therapy process, and what these elements mean in practice. Shara, a client in her forties, was referred to occupational therapy for the first time to facilitate future housing and support planning. Occupational therapy assessment determined that her mother would like for Shara to continue receiving assistance for certain self-care activities, such as bathing. Therefore, the therapist aligned with the family's goal, which was to find support to continue providing the same level of care for Shara as her parents aged. Therapist also made recommendations to facilitate Shara's collaboration and co-participation in these activities as opposed to achieving independence with life skills. This case study illustrates the 'N' in VISION (3).

Therapists are encouraged to present clients and families with options regarding assessments and interventions with special consideration for the activities of daily living (such as bathing or dressing), that warrant privacy to respect the client. OTs commonly employ observation-based assessments, which allow them to personalize assessments according to the activity needs as well as cultural values and unique environments of clients and their families. However, the traditional model of observing activities does not always work well with culturally diverse families. OTs should ask directly about any concerns with modesty and privacy. Alternative methods to assessment and intervention may be explored, such as interviews with clients or caregivers, sitting outside the door while clients or caregivers narrate their actions, using visual supports, and coaching caregivers in implementing the intervention programmes. The client or caregiver may appreciate being directly asked about any plan for intervention, 'Does this go against your culture?' This demonstrates the 'O' in the VISION model (3).

It is also evident that many widely used standardized assessment tools are based on Western and predominantly White populations as the norm, such as the Adolescent/Adult Sensory Profile (46). The original English version makes assumptions around how individuals experience sensory events based on Western customs (e.g. adding spices to food or touching others when talking), and environments (e.g. assuming easy access to big shopping centres). Some translated versions have been developed, for instance, an Arabic version is validated for use with Arabic speakers and contains adjusted cut-off scores for this population (47). At the same time, specific translations might not be easily accessible in a Western clinic for use with diverse populations. Therapists need to highlight the limitations of the assessment, use scores only to present general patterns of sensory behaviour, and supplement the analysis with real-life examples and observations. Therapists must critically analyse the Eurocentric evidence used in practice and exercise clinical judgement about the application and interpretation of standardized tools with persons of colour and diverse cultures.

Therapists, clients, and their families need to establish trust and mutual respect before they can engage in therapy readily and provide information on the most intimate parts of their lives. By adopting a longer engagement and assessment process, OTs working with families with language barriers or cultural diversity strive to create a meaningful alliance. It can be very useful for therapists to spend some time with clients at school, day centre, or home at the start to observe clients in different settings and get to know the various caregivers and community members involved in clients' lives. Therapists also seek to collaborate with families and community members beyond the Western norm of nuclear families. Many immigrant families reside in multigenerational households. For example, a young man with autism received more involved care from his grandparents as his parents worked long hours outside of the home. The therapist was acutely aware of a distinct cultural and generational difference in their view of disability and realized a need for diverse communication strategies even within one family. Structuring the relationship between the professional and family (the 'S' in VISION) involves determining who should be included in the clinical process and the degree of family participation (3).

Many individuals with an ID and autism are visual learners. However, their learning might be hindered when their culture is not portrayed in the social stories, visual schedules, or videos provided during intervention. Visual support software offers some customization, but therapists may find clients prefer photos of themselves in their actual environment, with translations in their native language.

Finally, therapists need to critically reflect on the impact their own cultural identities, values, beliefs, and assumptions have on their professional practice, and acknowledge the power imbalance between therapists and clients (39). In the midst of the Black Lives Matter movement, interdisciplinary clinicians from Surrey Place in Toronto, Canada, created an ongoing space during team meetings for knowledge sharing, group discussion, guidance for personal reflection, and exploring plans for change within their own practice. Dedicating the time to learn and grow as a culturally sensitive clinician with the ID population is as important as any professional development.

Conclusion

When applied cross-culturally in the support of individuals living with ID, therapeutic approaches need to be carefully adapted to be safe, relevant, and effective. Understanding the inherent biases in the frameworks, assessment methods, and teaching tools that we use is an important first step. The use of cultural competency frameworks should likewise be flexible, interdisciplinary, and pragmatic in their application. Building cultural competency and promoting cultural safety are important initial goals which should be followed by a vision of cultural humility in which clinicians make, 'a lifelong commitment to self-evaluation and critique, to redressing power imbalances and to developing mutually beneficial and non-paternalistic partnerships with communities on behalf of individuals and defined populations' (48). ID occurs across all cultures and is impacted by complex sociocultural variables. To be effective in the important work of supporting individuals with ID to live their best possible lives, clinicians from all cultures must be responsive to the values, norms, and practices, of our clients' unique cultures.

References

1. **Purnell L.** The Purnell model for cultural competence. Journal of Multicultural Nursing & Health 2005;**11**(2):7–15.

2. Jirwe M, Gerrish K, Emami A. The theoretical framework of cultural competence. Journal of Multicultural Nursing & Health 2006;**12**(3):6–16.

3. Bellon-Harn ML, Garrett MT. VISION: a model of cultural responsiveness for speech-language pathologists working in family partnerships. Communication Disorders Quarterly 2008;**29**(3):141–8.

4. Mushquash CJ, Bova DL. Cross-cultural assessment and measurement issues. Journal on Developmental Disabilities 2007;**13**(1):53–65.

5. Baker V, Oldnall L, Birkett E, McCluskey G, Morris J. Adults with Learning Disabilities (ALD). Royal College of Speech and Language Therapists Position Paper. London: Royal College of Speech and Language Therapists; 2010.

6. Smith M, Manduchi B, Burke É, Carroll R, McCallion P, McCarron M. Communication difficulties in adults with intellectual disability: results from a national cross-sectional study. Research in Developmental Disabilities 2020;**97**:103557.

7. Royal College of Speech and Language Therapists. Good Practice for Speech and Language Therapists Working with Clients from Linguistic Minority Communities. London: Royal College of Speech and Language Therapists; 2007.

8. Chinn D. Review of interventions to enhance the health communication of people with intellectual disabilities: a communicative health literacy perspective. Journal of Applied Research in Intellectual Disabilities 2017;**30**(2):345–59.

9. Ali A, Scior K, Ratti V, Strydom A, King M, Hassiotis A. Discrimination and other barriers to accessing health care: perspectives of patients with mild and moderate intellectual disability and their carers. PLoS One 2013;**8**(8):e70855.

10. Money D. Inclusive Communication and the Role of Speech and Language Therapy. Royal College of Speech and Language Therapists Position Paper. London: Royal College of Speech and Language Therapists; 2016.

11. Leadbeater C, Litosseliti L. The importance of cultural competence for speech and language therapists. Journal of Interactional Research in Communication Disorders 2014;**5**(1):1–26.

12. Royal College of Speech and Language Therapists. Five Good Communication Standards: Reasonable Adjustments to Communication that Individuals with Learning Disability and/or Autism Should Expect in Specialist Hospital and Residential Settings. London: Royal College of Speech and Language Therapists; 2013.

13. Money D. A comparison of three approaches to delivering a speech and language therapy service to people with learning disabilities. European Journal of Disorders of Communication 1997;**32**(4):449–66.

14. Money D, Thurman S. Towards a Model of Inclusive Communication: Speech and Language Therapy in Practice. London: Royal College of Speech and Language Therapists; 2002.

15. Barclay JE. Challenging Behaviour: A Unified Approach. College Report CR144. London: Royal College of Psychiatrists; 2007.

16. World Health Organization. International Classification of Functioning, Disability, and Health: Children & Youth Version: ICF-CY. Geneva: World Health Organization; 2007.

17. Emerson E, Kiernan C, Alborz A, Reeves D, Mason H, Swarbrick R, et al. The prevalence of challenging behaviors: a total population study. Research in Developmental Disabilities 2001;**22**(1):77–93.

18. **Heyvaert M, Saenen L, Campbell JM, Maes B, Onghena P.** Efficacy of behavioral interventions for reducing problem behavior in persons with autism: an updated quantitative synthesis of single-subject research. Research in Developmental Disabilities 2014;**35**(10):2463–76.

19. **Hassiotis A, Robotham D, Canagasabey A, Romeo R, Langridge D, Blizard R,** et al. Randomized, single-blind, controlled trial of a specialist behavior therapy team for challenging behavior in adults with intellectual disabilities. American Journal of Psychiatry 2009;**166**(11):1278–85.

20. **Fong EH, Ficklin S, Lee HY.** Increasing cultural understanding and diversity in applied behavior analysis. Behavior Analysis: Research and Practice 2017;**17**(2):103–13.

21. **Beaulieu L, Addington J, Almeida D.** Behavior analysts' training and practices regarding cultural diversity: the case for culturally competent care. Behavior Analysis in Practice 2019;**12**(3):557–75.

22. **Indigenous Corporate Trainings Inc.** Indigenous cultural competency self-assessment checklist. 2016. Available from: https://www.ictinc.ca/blog/indigenous-cultural-com petency-self-assessment-checklist

23. **Talaga T.** All Our Relations: Finding the Path Forward. Toronto: House of Anansi; 2018.

24. **Lux MK.** Separate Beds: A History of Indian Hospitals in Canada, 1920s–1980s. Toronto: University of Toronto Press; 2016.

25. **Mosby I.** Administering colonial science: nutrition research and human biomedical experimentation in Aboriginal communities and residential schools, 1942–1952. Histoire Sociale/Social History 2013;**46**(1):145–72.

26. **Hodge FS.** No meaningful apology for American Indian unethical research abuses. Ethics & Behavior 2012;**22**(6):431–44.

27. **Dhaliwal RK.** Settler colonialism and the contemporary coerced sterilizations of Indigenous women. Political Science Undergraduate Review 2019;**4**(1):29–39.

28. **Miller JR.** Final report of the Truth and Reconciliation Commission of Canada. Volume one: summary 'Honouring the Truth, Reconciling for the Future'. BC Studies 2016;**191**:167.

29. **Blackstock C.** The complainant: the Canadian human rights case on First Nations child welfare. McGill Law Journal/Revue de droit de McGill 2016;**62**(2):285–328.

30. **Kapp SK.** Navajo and autism: the beauty of harmony. Disability & Society 2011;**26**(5):583–95.

31. **Fiedeldey-Van Dijk C, Rowan M, Dell C, Mushquash C, Hopkins C, Fornssler B,** et al. Honoring Indigenous culture-as-intervention: development and validity of the Native Wellness Assessment™. Journal of Ethnicity in Substance Abuse 2017;**16**(2):181–218.

32. **Snowshoe A, Crooks CV, Tremblay PF, Hinson RE.** Cultural connectedness and its relation to mental wellness for First Nations youth. Journal of Primary Prevention 2017;**38**(1–2):67–86.

33. **BigFoot DS, Funderburk BW.** Honoring children, making relatives: the cultural translation of parent-child interaction therapy for American Indian and Alaska Native families. Journal of Psychoactive Drugs 2011;**43**(4):309–18.

34. **Mecredy G, Sutherland R, Jones C.** First Nations Data Governance, Privacy, and the Importance of the OCAP® principles. International Journal of Population Data Science 2018;**3**(4).

35. **Ward AF, Smylie D, Firestone M.** Evidence Brief: Wise Practices for Indigenous-specific Cultural Safety Training. Toronto: Southwest Ontario Aboriginal Health Access Centre and the Well Living House; 2017.

36. **Wilson AN.** A critique of sociocultural values in PBIS. Behavior Analysis in Practice 2015;**8**:92–4.

37. **American Occupational Therapy Association**. Occupational therapy practice framework: domain and process (2nd ed.). American Journal of Occupational Therapy 2008;**62**:625–83.

38. **Canadian Association of Occupational Therapists**. The Canadian Occupational Performance Measure. Cross-cultural applications of the COPM. n.d. Available from: https://www.thecopm.ca/advanced/cross-cultural-applications-of-the-copm/

39. **Verdonschot MM, De Witte LP, Reichrath E, Buntinx WH, Curfs LM.** Community participation of people with an intellectual disability: a review of empirical findings. Journal of Intellectual Disability Research 2009;**53**(4):303–18.

40. **Johnson KR, Blaskowitz M, Mahoney WJ.** Occupational therapy practice with adults with intellectual disability: what more can we do? Open Journal of Occupational Therapy 2019;**7**(2):12.

41. **Hammell KRW.** Occupation, well-being, and culture: theory and cultural humility/ Occupation, bien-être et culture: la théorie et l'humilité culturelle. Canadian Journal of Occupational Therapy 2013;**80**(4):224–34.

42. **Mona LR, Cameron RP, Clemency Cordes C.** Disability culturally competent sexual healthcare. American Psychology 2017;**72**(9):1000–10.

43. **Hammell KW.** Sacred texts: a sceptical exploration of the assumptions underpinning theories of occupation. Canadian Journal of Occupational Therapy 2009;**76**(1):6–13.

44. **Barrera I, Corso RM.** Cultural competency as skilled dialogue. Topics in Early Childhood Special Education 2002;**22**(2):103–13.

45. **Lindsay S, Tétrault S, Desmaris C, King GA, Piérart G.** The cultural brokerage work of occupational therapists in providing culturally sensitive care: Le travail de médiation culturelle effectué par des ergothérapeutes offrant des soins adaptés à la culture. Canadian Journal of Occupational Therapy 2014;**81**(2):114–23.

46. **Brown C, Dunn W.** Adolescent/Adult Sensory Profile. San Antonio, TX: Pearson; 2002.

47. **Al-Momani F, Alghadir AH, Al-Momani MO, Alharethy S, Al-Sharman A, Al-Dibii R**, et al. Performance of the Arabic population on the adolescent-adult sensory profile: an observational study. Neuropsychiatric Disease and Treatment 2020;**16**:35–42.

48. **Tervalon M, Murray-Garcia J.** Cultural humility versus cultural competence: a critical distinction in defining physician training outcomes in multicultural education. Journal of Health Care for the Poor and Underserved 1998;**9**(2):117–25.

Chapter 12

Family networks and voluntary sector participation in the care of people with intellectual disability

Raghu Raghavan and Keir Jones

Introduction

Intellectual disability (ID) affects 2.6% of the world's population; however, some estimates suggest that over 80% of people with ID live in the Global South (1). Due to the lack of relevant and reliable epidemiological data in India and across Africa, it is hard to precisely estimate the prevalence of ID, but estimates suggest that 1–3% of the African population have ID and 2.6% of the Indian population have ID (1). IDs have been defined by the World Health Organization (WHO) as:

> a significantly reduced ability to understand new or complex information and to learn and apply new skills (impaired intelligence) (2). This results in a reduced ability to cope independently (impaired social functioning), and begins before adulthood, with a lasting effect on development. Disability depends not only on a child's health conditions or impairments but also and crucially on the extent to which environmental factors support the child's full participation and inclusion in society.

People with ID are among the most marginalized groups globally. They are subjected to far more social exclusion than their non-disabled counterparts and this experience is exacerbated within contexts of poverty such as those seen on the African continent as well as South Asian countries, including India. Due to the lack of resources and services available to people with ID, there can be an increased reliance on family members to provide care and support throughout the person's life, compared to the Global North. While this can cause notably added stress for the family, there is little evidence that examines the importance of family networks to people with ID from a global perspective. The situation for people with ID in Africa and low- and middle-income countries (LMICs) is starkly different to that of the countries in the

Global North, which will be elaborated upon in this chapter. These differences remain little understood or researched in the global research literature.

International context

Global North perspectives of people with intellectual disability

Research into people with ID has been predominantly conducted in Global North countries or high-income countries. Internationally, the inclusion of people with disabilities into mainstream society has been promoted through social policy aiming to improve acceptance and integration (e.g. International Association for the Scientific Study of Intellectual Disabilities, 2001) The aim of social policy should be to create a community in which people with disabilities are 'able and allowed to be themselves among others' (3). Attitudes and perspectives of people with ID have been assessed across several Global North countries, including Australia (4), the UK, Austria, Germany (5), the US (6), and Japan (7), across various population groups, including children, students, health professionals, and older adults (8).

Attitudes and perspectives towards people with ID involve multidimensional evaluation of people, which can be either positive or negative, or a combination of both (9). Several studies have investigated the effects of various attitudes, such as how positive social attitudes can help with inclusion and acceptance by family, friends, and employers (10); nonetheless, negative attitudes can lead to low expectations, discrimination, and marginalization. More specifically, evidence indicated that negative attitudes of healthcare professionals act as a barrier for the participation of individuals with disabilities in several domains such as physical activity, fitness, and education settings (11). Given the global situation and the importance of attitude, the public must be urged to rethink and promote their attitudes towards people with disabilities, to build a more inclusive society.

Evidence shows that a focus on social inclusion, community participation, and empowerment of people with disabilities drives more inclusive policies and services to provide better care for people with ID (12). Public attitudes towards people with ID not only affect their integration into the community and access to public services (13) but also affect their daily lives and social participation (10), such as employment (14). A systematic review by Wang et al. of 27 studies examined the different aspects of factors that influence public attitudes towards people with a disability in Global North countries, including the US, China, and Netherlands (15). The main finding was that familiarity and contact with people with disabilities were the factors that more powerfully influenced positive opinions towards people with ID. Other studies support the finding that having contact with people with ID leads to more positive attitudes (12,16). Having regular contact with people with ID reduces fear and anxiety and creates a more balanced and realistic perspective about people with a disability regarding their functional capacity and ability (17).

Indeed, there was a greater perception of improvements to views of certain rights and capabilities of people with ID in some countries more than others. For example, in a study by McConkey et al. (18) examining the perceptions of 26,876 people towards the rights and capabilities of people with ID in the US, there was a greater perception that they were more capable of having friends, holding down a job, and graduating from high school than concerning other tasks such as managing a business. It was noted that a large minority of participants gave low ratings to both capability and rights of people with ID, suggesting that the public could be more likely to support the rights of those they perceive to be more capable and like themselves, rather than people with more severe disabilities. In comparison, Horner-Johnson et al. 2015 (6) investigated attitudes of healthcare staff towards people with ID in Japan and the US. The major findings were that Japanese staff exhibited a greater tendency towards sheltering and exclusion of people with ID and a lower endorsement of empowerment of people with ID than staff in the US. This was significantly affected by the age and education of the staff, indicating that attitudes shift as newer generations of staff enter the workplace. There is a need to explore public attitudes and perspectives for the rights of people with ID and their acceptance in local communities. This has rarely been studied internationally, comparing the perspectives of Global North countries and Global South countries.

Global South perspectives of people with intellectual disability

There are very few studies examining the perspectives of people with ID living in the Global South. Unlike their Global North counterparts, people with ID in Global South countries are more likely to face several additional barriers in their everyday lives due to poor resource allocation. These lead to additional challenges as culturally appropriate diagnostic and support services are extremely limited (19). These challenges are exacerbated especially in African countries due to HIV, wars, and internal displacement (20). Therefore, it is unsurprising that the level of stigma and prejudice against people with ID is still significantly higher in Global South countries (21).

Stigma and prejudice can have a devastating effect on the well-being of people with ID as seen in several studies comparing disabled and non-disabled people in Global South countries. It has been found that people with ID are more likely to have their fundamental rights and freedoms denied (21). Many people with ID experience higher levels of inequality in several basic areas including health, social, and financial (22). For example, children with ID in African countries have been found to have high mortality rates and only 2 out of 100 children with disabilities go to school in developing countries (23). Scior et al. found that people with ID, particularly children, are also more suspectable to sexual, emotional, and physical abuse and still widely viewed as unable to live independently or contribute to society (24).

Over the years, there has been a mixture of data examining attitudes of different cultures and countries towards people with ID. For example, in an anthropological study in South Africa, children who lived in rural communities were found to be more accepted among their peers due to the integral role they played in the household and the community. Whereas, it has been found in other studies, especially in India (25) and Nigeria (26), that traditional beliefs and misconceptions about the causes of ID can lead to the people affected, and often their families, being viewed with suspicion and ostracized from their communities (27). McKenzie et al. (22) have explained that this contradiction across countries and cultures can be due to several factors, including the severity of ID, the competence of the person, degree of ID, and so on. For example, someone who is more socially competent and contributes to both the household and community will be more accepted among their peers. However, if a person is highly dependent on their family members for financial aid and care time, there could be less acceptance especially if family resources are already limited. This pattern was seen recently in a study by Scior et al. (24) who examined ID stigma across 88 countries. The main finding was that respondents in African and Asian countries, and former states of the Soviet Union still expressed their desire to segregate people with IDs from society due to deep-rooted prejudice. It was seen in many African countries that people still had misconceptions and stigmatizing beliefs about the causes of ID. It was concluded that in many LMICs, equal rights for people with ID appear to be a 'distant vision'. Therefore, there is urgent importance in the need for family support and advocacy as well as community interventions to improve the stigma surrounding people with ID in the Global South.

In comparing and contrasting the role of the family in the Global North compared to the Global South in broad terms, four key themes emerge that we shall explore further.

Theme 1: the primacy of the family in terms of support

The importance of the family in providing support for people with ID is highlighted by researchers in the Global South. Particularly in LMICs, the duty of care for individuals with an ID often falls to family members (22). This can lead to an increased burden of caregiving, as well as negative emotional consequences of providing support. Despite this, research in South Africa found that family caregivers show a strong commitment to care (28). Family members often viewed themselves as protectors of their relatives, with the burden of care increasing a sense of responsibility. For example, caregivers would express concerns about who would look after their relative if they were unable to do so (28–30). These concerns led to family caregivers becoming increasingly protective of their relative with an ID. Research in India has shown a similar theme of families accepting the responsibility of care. Parents of children with an ID recognized the help of other close relatives, including the child's sibling(s) who would assist in caregiving duties (30). This provided parents with hope that the sibling would assume responsibility for care in the future. Hence, research in the Global South shows the emphasis placed on the family as the main source of support for individuals with an ID.

The burden of caregiving is largely placed on the mother, and this theme is observed by researchers in rural South Africa and Nigeria (28,29,31), as well as India (30,32). Mothers have additional responsibilities of looking after the rest of the family and were more bound by traditional male–female roles. Additional stressors of caregiving include traditional gender roles, financial issues, reduced leisure, social lives of caregivers, and lack of healthcare resources (25). Mothers experienced greater responsibility for the child's healthcare needs (28) and struggled to meet physical care needs such as feeding and mobility (31). This was particularly challenging in situations where the father may reject the family, possibly due to stigma or fear of financial consequences (29,31). In comparison, mothers who had the support of their spouse were able to cope and manage the needs of the child better, demonstrating the importance of family cohesion. The mother's role in providing emotional security is also emphasized, as this can influence whether the child develops a secure attachment style (32). The development of a secure attachment style for children with ID is important as this may improve social interaction skills (33). Compared to average attachment scores in the Global North, the mean security scores among children with an ID in India are significantly lower (32). Perhaps this reflects the increased burden of care placed on mothers in the Global South, limiting their ability to meet the physical and/or emotional needs of their children.

There is not simply the emotional and physical burden of caregiving but the stigma and prejudice associated with caring for someone with ID. There have been suggestions that many family members feel incredibly isolated and judged because they look after someone with ID in many Global South countries. In a study by McKenzie and McConkey, many of their South African participants who were carers of people with ID felt embarrassed by behavioural difficulties when going out in public or if people came to the house (34). This would often lead to both the carers and the family member with ID being isolated. One respondent even wanted the wider community to be educated about ID, as they heard their children being called a 'deformed child'. Some children with ID do see the harm that it has on family members, especially those who feel as if they cannot socialize with other people. They can internalize the stigma and live with a sense of failure in themselves, which can lead to feelings of depression and suicide (34). As the family members are key to people with ID, there is a need for an intervention to target the stigmatizing beliefs the community members have about people with ID.

Given the importance of family caregivers, services designed to support families looking after their relatives with an ID may improve their quality of life (35,36). For example, the completion of an 'interactive group psychoeducation' programme led to significant clinical improvements in child-rearing skills and improved knowledge of ID (37). This programme also assessed parental attitudes towards ID in southern India. It was found that participation in group psychoeducation was effective in changing negative parental attitudes. These family-based interventions are useful in areas where resources are limited. Information programmes involving the wider community may also address the stigma associated with ID (38).

Theme 2: models of understanding the diagnosis and the impact of this on families

The way families conceptualize ID in their relative varies across the Global South. This may include medical models, similar to those used in Global North, as well as social and spiritual explanations. The concepts used to understand ID have an important influence on the caregiving approaches used by families. In terms of the medical model, it was common for parents to search for the right treatment, and importance was placed on finding the 'best doctors' (30). However, disappointment with the doctors' ability to provide answers led to caregivers seeking alternative explanations and treatments. A lack of information available about ID may also motivate caregivers to move away from mainstream medicine (25,30). This is important to consider within services for ID as information about the diagnosis may provide families with problem-focused coping strategies (32).

There is a need to further explore and understand how different people conceptualize ID, especially to re-examine the dominant Western constructions of knowledge and practice and to endeavour to gain a deeper understanding of how different cultures understand ID. The most common model is the biomedical model, which attempts to allow for cultural variation, but is based on a universal and 'Westernized' approach to explain disability, with almost no attention to local variation (39). The other model of explaining diagnosis is the sociocultural model, which focuses on impairment not being pathological but due to environmental or spiritual factors. In different countries and cultures, there is a combination of both models being used to explain and understand the diagnosis of ID. This was seen in a study by Mkabile and Swartz (40), which examined the explanatory models of ID from the perspective of parents and caregivers in South Africa. Caregivers and parents employed a wide range of explanatory models to explain the causes of ID in their children. These included biomedical and sociocultural explanations where they believed that witchcraft, bad spirits, and bewitchment may have caused the ID. Many participants admitted using both Western-trained doctors as well as traditional healers to understand and treat their children. This shows there is a different understanding around the diagnosis of ID based on their private belief system.

In a similar review by McKenzie et al. in South Africa, they were more rooted in negative feelings, such as bewitchment and fear of curses from their ancestors (22). This would lead to parents/caregivers taking their child with ID to traditional healers to seek a 'cure' and appease the ancestors. However, this was not seen in African countries such as Tanzania, where some beliefs encouraged positive behaviour towards those diagnosed with ID. This was due to the belief that it was a 'test' for the family members from God (39). This led to more positive views around understanding the ID and encouraged better coping strategies for both the child with ID and the caregivers.

A reliance on traditional beliefs such as bewitchment as a cause of ID was also common across many countries in Africa (22,41–43). While some beliefs, especially those that suggest that disability is a blessing from God, can lead to positive appraisals (41), some may promote stigmatization and marginalize individuals with disabilities (41). However, it is suggested by researchers that these beliefs varies with age and education, with younger, Western-educated individuals being less likely to hold these beliefs (40). Therefore, spiritual leaders and religion can influence the approach used by families to support their relatives. This is also seen where many families use religion and prayer as coping mechanisms. When examining the support and coping mechanism of caregivers of people with ID, prayer and religious beliefs were often used as a source of comfort and hope. Edwardraj et al. found that the majority of participants in their study, specifically health workers, would recommend to caregivers to take medicines and have faith (25). It was expressed that individual faith was the best help rather than organized religious support. Therefore, seeking information and treatments from traditional healers and churches may provide families with coping strategies (22,41).

Another salient theme in literature was denial or minimization of diagnosis, used as a coping strategy by families of those with milder ID (44). While this may lead to them being more accepted in society and reduce stigmatization, the needs of the individual with an ID may be overlooked. For example, accessing services for support may be deemed unnecessary for families adopting denial as a coping mechanism. For some families who adopt the denial mechanism for coping with family members with ID, it can often lead to blaming other members of the family as the cause for ID. In some cases, this can be seen between a husband and wife, which in turn can affect their marriage and sometimes lead to separation. This also led to some caregivers from lower socioeconomic backgrounds in South Africa feeling as if their child was a burden and wishing that the child would die (25). Many people, especially those with a low socioeconomic background, do not have the resources to care for the child and would not consider treatment unless there is a prospect of the child becoming completely normal. This highlights the fact that people with limited resources would not be able to pay for any treatment, and simply would ignore the issue. Despite this, this coping strategy was successful in terms of integrating individuals into wider society (44), an aspect that may be hindered using medical labels.

Theme 3: barriers to accessing services and the impact on the family

Stigma towards people with an ID is a key factor contributing to the barriers in accessing healthcare (20,42,45). Although the issue of stigma is also prominent across the Global North, the lack of wider support services and economic resources may exacerbate its effect in the Global South. Even when ID services are available in close proximity, community stigma can lead parents to stop taking their child to these services (40), which can lead to poor health outcomes. In some cases, parents self-prescribed medication and waited for symptoms to persist before accessing services, to avoid negative public attitudes (25). This can be particularly damaging for individuals with a severe ID, who require healthcare the most, and yet are more likely to be shielded by caregivers.

A prominent barrier perceived in accessing services was the difficulty in accessing services and the quality of the services. In South Africa, specifically very rural areas of South Africa, being able to get to the different hospitals or specialized treatment services can be very difficult. It is not only the problem of affording the travel costs to get there but also travelling with a child who could be physically disabled or has outbursts in reactions to different sounds, smells, or sights. This is partially related to the stigma of caring for someone with an ID, as some people feel embarrassed if their child has an episode or the fear that people will mock and judge them. Even if caregivers manage to gain access to specialized services, many people especially in South Africa (40), Nigeria (45), and India (46) felt as if the care and services provided were neither sufficient nor effective. McKenzie and McConkey (34) found that carers in South Africa had been let down by services, from the State, social workers, and paid helpers. This was due to misunderstandings around the person's disorder and not knowing what help to offer people. A predominant issue highlighted by one carer is that paid caregivers or residential homes could not be trusted, as people with ID would be left on their own for hours or would often be victims of theft and abuse. Due to the dearth of services for people with ID in LMICs, it is not surprising that many people feel let down.

Primary caregivers of children with ID were often left without knowing what ID is, how to deal with behavioural outbursts, violence, and what a life of a child with ID entailed. A barrier that was perceived by caregivers in South Africa was that there was no information released to them about the management of a child with ID or services (25). A few people have recommended the need for information booklets or guidelines on managing a child with ID. Hashemi et al.'s (2020) meta-analysis of 41 studies from LMICs looked at families' perceptions of why they could not access services revealed many people only received a diagnosis, without any information on how to manage it or what their rights were (47). This highlights the need for better information to be given to caregivers and family members surrounding caring for a person with ID.

Researchers found that language can be a significant barrier affecting access to healthcare (48). In South Africa, many ID services are offered in either English or Afrikaans. However, with 11 official languages spoken across the country, challenges in communication can significantly limit access for individuals with an ID. Families living in poorer areas of the country are more likely to encounter these language barriers, due to differing local dialects. This shows that in addition to the scarcity of services available, language barriers need to be addressed in order to make these services useful for the wider community.

Living in extreme poverty can pose significant economic barriers in accessing not only healthcare, but also education, community support centres, and transport to these services (20,40,48). In many communities, services may only be accessible by economically advantaged families. For example, the shift from regular schools to 'special schools' in India may not be attainable for families living in poverty (25,49). This can limit social and educational outcomes for the child with an ID, and they may feel excluded in regular schools. The cost of public transport is another significant financial barrier, affecting individuals' access to healthcare (40). Some caregivers' financial challenges are exacerbated by a lack of support from extended family, leading them to give up employment to fulfil caregiving duties. This shows that simply providing services may be insufficient without considering other financial barriers affecting families' ability to make use of these services. Given the financial challenges experienced by many families, accessibility including transport facilities to ID services may need to be considered (50).

Aside from stigma and financial barriers, families express further concerns for the safety of their relative with an ID (40,48). Some caregivers reported incidences of physical and sexual abuse towards their child (48), which may lead to families becoming protective and shielding the child from public view. High violence within the community also prevented participation in community activities that were otherwise enjoyable for families (50). Caregivers emphasized the need for safety measures and increased security within the community to feel safer in public. It was also suggested that support from other caregivers of children with ID would be useful in enhancing social inclusion (50).

Theme 4: community-based rehabilitation, special schools, and family interventions

Initiatives that involve the wider community may overcome issues related to the stigma and social exclusion of individuals with an ID, particularly in the Global South context. For example, community-based rehabilitation programmes have been implemented to reduce stigma by moving away from the 'medical model' (51). These programmes are supported by health professionals and involve people with disabilities, family members, and volunteers (52). However, there are barriers that limit the effectiveness of these programmes, such as a lack of local expertise. This led to 'task-shifting' in which volunteer family members can be trained by professionals to deliver evidence-based interventions. This attempts to address the gap between the needs of carers and the available healthcare services in LMICs (52). Families are also able to collaborate and work towards reducing the stigma associated with ID. However, many caregivers stated that time constraints and domestic responsibilities would prevent them from volunteering in such a programme (52). Additionally, the quality of evidence for the efficacy of community-based rehabilitation programmes is 'very low' (51). Some children accessing programmes show progress, while others show very few beneficial outcomes. However, this may be due to an insufficient evidence base, rather than the inefficacy of community rehabilitation programmes (51).

Community-based interventions may be good at reducing stigma, but due to the insufficient number of specialist therapies and the difficulty of travelling to specialist centres, it may not be the best way forward. Family-based interventions can be delivered by non-specialist community workers or parents of the child with ID. Parents are commonly the caregivers of the child with ID, due to the lack of services and care provided in LMICs. Therefore, parents have frequent and consistent contact with their child across a range of settings so would be effective in implementing these interventions. A systematic review by Einfeld et al. (53) recommended a 'Stepping Stones Triple P' parenting programme be implemented in LMICs due to the extensive evidence base. This intervention involves training parent coaches or other volunteers to deliver Triple P to families (54). Triple P would be delivered in various formats with increasingly intensive interventions from 'level 1 (universal communication strategy) to level 5 (intensive support for families with complex needs)'. An advisory group would recommend what programmes suited the community best and would be tailored to their needs. This intervention was also recommended by Turner et al. (55) as an exemplar of evidence-based parent support programmes due to its versatility in being adapted across 39 different countries. As mentioned previously as a disadvantage of community-based rehabilitation programmes, some parents, especially mothers, did not have time to take part in these programmes and thus would drop out. However, these programmes are fully flexible, adapted into different languages, and suitable for the community (56).

As well as using community interventions and parent-based interventions to help improve child behaviour, knowledge around the disorder improves the mental and physical health of both parent and child. One suggestion made in the literature after examining personal perspectives of family carers in South Africa was for community-based education, training, and leisure options that help make the person with ID more independent (34). This can help relieve parental stress and can allow people with ID to be more integrated into society (57). This intervention would work well in conjunction with an anti-stigma community-based intervention so the community can understand the needs of people with ID. This sort of intervention has been noted to be used in rural communities in South Africa (25), as many members with ID are very well integrated into the community.

A major issue raised frequently in the literature is the lack of access to inclusive schools in the Global South countries including the Republic of the Congo, India, Liberia, Nepal, Nigeria, and Uganda (58). A study by Scior et al. (58) found that most often children with ID did not attend school at all in countries such as Bangladesh, Iran, and Kenya. This was due to several reasons including affordability of travel, distance, or affordability of the school fee. Tackling resource limitation has been suggested as a possible way to ensure that children and adults with ID have access to inclusive schools as well as special schools (58). However, Scior et al. suggested 'developing resources go hand in hand with educating the public about ID and tackling the intense stigma associated with them' (58). If stigma interventions are put forward, people may feel more comfortable with sending their children to schools, as to not shield them so much from the outside world.

In Global North countries, possibly in the context of a culture of multigenerational homes being less common, there is often a well-developed network of residential homes and supported living settings for adults with an ID. This move to an external setting can result in some relatives feeling 'shut out' from the care of their loved ones, perhaps in a way that would be unlikely to happen in the Global South, where many people with ID remain within a family setting. In the UK, for example, one response to this has been to develop a network of national voluntary organizations specifically for relatives of people with ID, such as Contact (www.contact.org.uk) or Sibs (www.sibs.org.uk). This is in addition to high-profile charities working in the field with a wider remit such as Mencap and SCOPE, who in addition to lobbying government and providing support to individuals with ID, also provide a range of services for families.

Conclusion

There are many different challenges faced by the families of people with an ID depending on where they are in the world and we have aimed to present some of the broad themes in the literature when contrasting the Global North and Global South perspectives. For example, there is clear evidence that stigma and prejudice still exist around intellectual disorders in Global South countries, including South Africa and India, and this clearly presents families with many additional challenges. Alongside stigma, several other barriers make it difficult for parents and caregivers to access services for their family member with ID, including lack of information about the disorder, insufficient services, language barriers, and financial poverty. Therefore, it is the recommendation of this chapter to put forward a community-based anti-stigma campaign which promotes active communication between people with ID and people without ID as well as a parent-based intervention to improve knowledge about ID.

References

1. **Girimaji SC, Srinath S.** Perspectives of intellectual disability in India: epidemiology, policy, services for children and adults. Current Opinion in Psychiatry 2010;**23**(5):441–6. https://doi.org/10.1097/yco.0b013e32833ad95c

2. **World Health Organization.** Definition: intellectual disability. n.d. Available from: https://www.euro.who.int/en/health-topics/noncommunicable-diseases/men tal-health/news/news/2010/15/childrens-right-to-family-life/definition-intellectual-dis ability

3. **Nirje B.** The basis and logic of the normalization principle. Australia and New Zealand Journal of Developmental Disabilities 1985;**11**(2):65–8. https://doi.org/10.3109/136682 58509008747

4. **Yazbeck M, McVilly K, Parmenter TR.** Attitudes toward people with intellectual disabilities. Journal of Disability Policy Studies 2004;**15**(2):97–111. https://doi.org/10.1177/10442073040150020401

5. **Zeilinger EL, Stiehl KAM, Bagnall H, Scior K.** Intellectual disability literacy and its connection to stigma: a multinational comparison study in three European countries. PLoS One 2020;**15**(10):e0239936. https://doi.org/10.1371/journal.pone.0239936

6. **Horner-Johnson W, Keys CB, Henry D, Yamaki K, Watanabe K, Oi F,** et al. Staff attitudes towards people with intellectual disabilities in Japan and the United States. Journal of Intellectual Disability Research 2015;**59**(10):942–7. https://doi.org/10.1111/jir.12179

7. **Tachibana T, Watanabe K.** Schemata and attitudes toward persons with intellectual disability in Japan. Psychological Reports 2003;**93**(3 Suppl):1161–72. https://doi.org/10.2466/pr0.2003.93.3f.1161

8. **Pelleboer-Gunnink HA, van Oorsouw WMWJ, van Weeghel J, Embregts PJCM.** Mainstream health professionals' stigmatising attitudes towards people with intellectual disabilities: a systematic review. Journal of Intellectual Disability Research 2017;**61**(5):411–34. https://doi.org/10.1111/jir.12353

9. **Dunn DS, Andrews EE.** Person-first and identity-first language: developing psychologists' cultural competence using disability language. American Psychologist 2015;**70**(3):255–64. https://doi.org/10.1037/a0038636

10. **Findler, L, Vilchinsky, N, Werner, S.** Multidimensional Attitudes Scale toward Persons with Disabilities. PsycTESTS Dataset; 2007. https://doi.org/10.1037/t48910-000

11. **Rimmer JH, Riley B, Wang E, Rauworth A, Jurkowski J.** Physical activity participation among persons with disabilities. American Journal of Preventive Medicine 2004;**26**(5):419–25. https://doi.org/10.1016/j.amepre.2004.02.002

12. **Morin D, Rivard M, Crocker AG, Boursier CP, Caron J.** Public attitudes towards intellectual disability: a multidimensional perspective. Journal of Intellectual Disability Research 2012;**57**(3):279–92. https://doi.org/10.1111/jir.12008

13. **Verdonschot MML, de Witte LP, Reichrath E, Buntinx WHE, Curfs LMG.** Community participation of people with an intellectual disability: a review of empirical findings. Journal of Intellectual Disability Research 2009;**53**(4):303–18. https://doi.org/10.1111/j.1365-2788.2008.01144.x

14. **Burge P, Ouellette-Kuntz H, Lysaght R.** Public views on employment of people with intellectual disability. Journal of Vocational Rehabilitation 2007;**26**(1):29–37.

15. **Wang Z, Xu X, Han Q, Chen Y, Jiang J, Ni GX.** Factors associated with public attitudes towards persons with disabilities: a systematic review. BMC Public Health 2021;**21**:1058. https://doi.org/10.1186/s12889-021-11139-3

16. **ten Klooster PM, Dannenberg JW, Taal E, Burger G, Rasker JJ.** Attitudes towards people with physical or intellectual disabilities: nursing students and non-nursing peers. Journal of Advanced Nursing 2009;**65**(12):2562–73. https://doi.org/10.1111/j.1365-2648.2009.05146.x

17. **Alnahdi GH, Schwab S.** Special education major or attitudes to predict teachers' self-efficacy for teaching in inclusive education. Frontiers in Psychology 2021;**12**:680909. https://doi.org/10.3389/fpsyg.2021.680909

18. **McConkey R, Slater P, Smith A, Dubois L, Shellard A.** Perceptions of the rights and capabilities of people with intellectual disability in the United States. Journal of Applied Research in Intellectual Disabilities 2020;**34**(2):537–45. https://doi.org/10.1111/jar.12819

19. **Scherzer AL, Chhagan M, Kauchali S, Susser E.** Global perspective on early diagnosis and intervention for children with developmental delays and disabilities. Developmental Medicine & Child Neurology 2012;**54**(12):1079–84. https://doi.org/10.1111/j.1469-8749.2012.04348.x

20. **Njenga F.** Perspectives of intellectual disability in Africa: epidemiology and policy services for children and adults. Current Opinion in Psychiatry 2009;**22**(5):457–61. https://doi.org/10.1097/yco.0b013e32832e63a1

21. **Scior K, Werner S.** Changing attitudes to learning disability: a review of the evidence. Mencap; 2015. Available from: https://www.mencap.org.uk/sites/default/files/2016-08/Attitudes_Changing_Report.pdf

22. **Mckenzie JA, McConkey R, Adnams C.** Intellectual disability in Africa: implications for research and service development. Disability and Rehabilitation 2013;**35**(20):1750–5. https://doi.org/10.3109/09638288.2012.751461

23. **Salvador-Carulla L, Garcia-Gutierrez C.** The WHO construct of health-related functioning (HrF) and its implications for health policy. BMC Public Health 2011;**11**(Suppl 4):S9. https://doi.org/10.1186/1471-2458-11-s4-s9

24. **Scior K, Hamid A, Hastings R, Werner S, Belton C, Laniyan A**, et al. Consigned to the margins: a call for global action to challenge intellectual disability stigma. Lancet Global Health 2016;**4**(5):e294–5. https://doi.org/10.1016/s2214-109x(16)00060-7

25. **Edwardraj S, Mumtaj K, Prasad JH, Kuruvilla A, Jacob KS.** Perceptions about intellectual disability: a qualitative study from Vellore, South India. Journal of Intellectual Disability Research 2010;**54**(8):736–48. https://doi.org/10.1111/j.1365-2788.2010.01301.x

26. **McKenzie J, Ohajunwa CO.** Understanding disability in Nigeria: a commentary on 'Country profile: intellectual and developmental disability in Nigeria'. Tizard Learning Disability Review 2017;**22**(2):94–8. https://doi.org/10.1108/tldr-02-2017-0008

27. **Mung'omba J.** Comparative policy brief: status of intellectual disabilities in the Republic of Zambia. Journal of Policy and Practice in Intellectual Disabilities 2008;**5**(2):142–4. https://doi.org/10.1111/j.1741-1130.2008.00163.x

28. **McKenzie J, McConkey R, Adnams C.** Residential facilities for adults with intellectual disability in a developing country: a case study from South Africa. Journal of Intellectual and Developmental Disability 2014;**39**(1):45–54.

29. **Aldersey HM.** Family perceptions of intellectual disability: understanding and support in Dar es Salaam. African Journal of Disability 2012;**1**(1):32.

30. **John A, Bailey LE, Jones JL.** Culture and context: exploring attributions and caregiving approaches of parents of children with an intellectual disability in urban India. Child & Family Social Work 2017;**22**(2):670–9.

31. **Ntswane AM, Van Rhyn L.** The life-world of mothers who care for mentally retarded children: the Katutura township experience. Curationis 2007;**30**(1):85–96.

32. **John A, Morris AS, Halliburton AL.** Looking beyond maternal sensitivity: mother-child correlates of attachment security among children with intellectual disabilities in urban India. Journal of Autism and Developmental Disorders 2012;**42**(11):2335–45.

33. **Willemsen-Swinkels SH, Bakermans-Kranenburg MJ, Buitelaar JK, IJzendoorn MHV, Engeland HV.** Insecure and disorganised attachment in children with a pervasive developmental disorder: relationship with social interaction and heart rate. Journal of Child Psychology and Psychiatry 2000;**41**(6):759–67.

34. **McKenzie J, McConkey R.** Caring for adults with intellectual disability: the perspectives of family carers in South Africa. Journal of Applied Research in Intellectual Disabilities 2015;**29**(6):531–41. https://doi.org/10.1111/jar.12209

35. **Aldersey HM, Turnbull HR III, Turnbull AP.** Intellectual and developmental disabilities in Kinshasa, Democratic Republic of the Congo: causality and implications for resilience and support. Intellectual and Developmental Disabilities 2014;**52**(3):220–33.

36. **Gona JK, Mung'ala-Odera V, Newton CR, Hartley S.** Caring for children with disabilities in Kilifi, Kenya: what is the caregiver's experience? Child: Care, Health and Development 2011;**37**(2):175–83.

37. **Russell PSS, John JK, Lakshmanan JL.** Family intervention for intellectually disabled children: randomised controlled trial. British Journal of Psychiatry 1999;**174**(3):254–8.

38. **Alnahdi GH, Schwab S.** Special education major or attitudes to predict teachers' self-efficacy for teaching in inclusive education. Frontiers in Psychology 2021;**12**:680909. https://doi.org/10.3389/fpsyg.2021.680909

39. **Kpobi L, Swartz L.** Indigenous and faith healing in Ghana: a brief examination of the formalising process and collaborative efforts with the biomedical health system. African Journal of Primary Health Care & Family Medicine 2019;**11**(1):e1–5. https://doi.org/10.4102/phcfm.v11i1.2035

40. **Mkabile S, Swartz L.** 'I waited for it until forever': community barriers to accessing intellectual disability services for children and their families in Cape Town, South Africa. International Journal of Environmental Research and Public Health 2020;**17**(22):8504. https://doi.org/10.3390/ijerph17228504

41. **Gona JK, Newton CR, Rimba K, Mapenzi R, Kihara M, Van de Vijver FJR,** et al. Parents' and professionals' perceptions on causes and treatment options for autism spectrum disorders (ASD) in a multicultural context on the Kenyan coast. PLoS One 2015;**10**(8):e0132729.

42. **Mkabile S, Garrun KL, Shelton M, Swartz L.** African families' and caregivers' experiences of raising a child with intellectual disability: a narrative synthesis of qualitative studies. African Journal of Disability 2021;**10**(0):a827.

43. **Ndlovu HL.** African beliefs concerning people with disabilities: Implications for theological education. Journal of Disability & Religion 2016;**20**(1–2):29–39.

44. **Chukwu NE, Okoye UO, Onyeneho NG, Okeibunor JC.** Coping strategies of families of persons with learning disability in Imo state of Nigeria. Journal of Health, Population and Nutrition 2019;**38**(1):1–9.

45. **Eseigbe EE, Nuhu FT, Sheikh TL, Eseigbe P, Sanni KA, Olisah VO.** Knowledge of childhood autism and challenges of management among medical doctors in Kaduna State, Northwest Nigeria. Autism Research and Treatment, 2015;**2015**:1–6. https://doi. org/10.1155/2015/892301

46. **Minhas A, Vajaratkar V, Divan G, Hamdani SU, Leadbitter K, Taylor C,** et al. Parents' perspectives on care of children with autistic spectrum disorder in South Asia—views from Pakistan and India. International Review of Psychiatry 2015;**27**(3):247–56. https:// doi.org/10.3109/09540261.2015.1049128

47. **Hashemi G, Wickenden M, Bright T, Kuper H.** Barriers to accessing primary healthcare services for people with disabilities in low and middle income countries, a meta-synthesis of qualitative studies. Disability and Rehabilitation 2022;**44**(8):1207–20. https://doi.org/10.1080/09638288.2020.1817984

48. **Mkabile S, Swartz L.** Caregivers' and parents' explanatory models of intellectual disability in Khayelitsha, Cape Town, South Africa. Journal of Applied Research in Intellectual Disabilities 2020;**33**(5):1026–37.

49. **Rao LG, Suryaprakasam B.** Effective teamwork in special schools for children with intellectual disabilities in India. Journal of Policy and Practice in Intellectual Disabilities 2004;**1**(2):79–87.

50. **McKenzie JA, Kahonde C, Mostert K, Aldersey HM.** Community participation of families of children with profound intellectual and multiple disabilities in South Africa. Journal of Applied Research in Intellectual Disabilities 2021;**34**(2):525–36.

51. **Robertson J, Emerson E, Hatton C, Yasamy MT.** Efficacy of community-based rehabilitation for children with or at significant risk of intellectual disabilities in low- and middle-income countries: a review. Journal of Applied Research in Intellectual Disabilities 2012;**25**(2):143–54.

52. **Hamdani SU, Atif N, Tariq M, Minhas FA, Iqbal Z, Rahman A.** Family networks to improve outcomes in children with intellectual and developmental disorders: a qualitative study. International Journal of Mental Health Systems 2014;**8**(1):1–8.

53. **Einfeld SL, Stancliffe RJ, Gray KM, Sofronoff K, Rice L, Emerson E,** et al. Interventions provided by parents for children with intellectual disabilities in low and middle income countries. Journal of Applied Research in Intellectual Disabilities 2012;**25**(2):135–42. https://doi.org/10.1111/j.1468-3148.2011.00678.x

54. **Tellegen CL, Sanders MR.** Stepping Stones Triple P—positive parenting program for children with disability: a systematic review and meta-analysis. Research in Developmental Disabilities 2013;**34**(5):1556–71. https://doi.org/10.1016/ j.ridd.2013.01.022

55. **Turner RR, Arden MA, Reale S, Sutton E, Taylor SJC, Bourke L,** et al. The development of a theory and evidence-based intervention to aid implementation of exercise into the prostate cancer care pathway with a focus on healthcare professional behaviour, the STAMINA trial. BMC Health Services Research 2021;**21**(1):273. https://doi.org/10.1186/s12913-021-06266-x

56. **Andersson E, McIlduff C, Turner K, Thomas S, Davies J, Elliott EJ,** et al. Jandu Yani U 'For All Families' Triple P—positive parenting program in remote Australian Aboriginal communities: a study protocol for a community intervention trial. BMJ Open 2019;**9**(10):e032559. https://doi.org/10.1136/bmjopen-2019-032559

57. **Cramm J, Nieboer A, Finkenflügel H, Lorenzo T.** Disabled youth in South Africa: barriers to education. International Journal on Disability and Human Development 2013;**12**(1):31–5. https://doi.org/10.1515/ijdhd-2012-0122

58. **Scior K, Hamid A, Hastings R, Werner S.** Intellectual disability stigma and initiatives to challenge it and promote inclusion around the globe. Journal of Policy and Practice in Intellectual Disabilities 2020;**17**(2):165–75. https://doi.org/10.1111/jppi.12330

Chapter 13

Intellectual disability, spirituality, religion, and social inclusion across cultures

Ayomipo J. Amiola, Nusra Khodabux,
Mohammad Farhad Peerally, Phil Temple,
Rosie Bunn, K.A.L.A. Kuruppuarachchi,
Meera Roy, Sheila Hollins, and
Regi T. Alexander

Introduction

Religion and spirituality play an important role in the lives of many people, in fact they are a central part of many cultures (1); although spirituality and religion have overlapping meanings and are often used interchangeably, they are not the same (2,3).

There are diverse definitions of spirituality in literature which vary according to context and authorship. The Royal College of Psychiatrists' position statement on spirituality and religion defines spirituality as:

> a distinctive, potentially creative, and universal dimension of human experience arising both within the inner subjective awareness of individuals and within communities, social groups and traditions. It may be experienced as a relationship with that which is intimately 'inner', immanent, and personal, within the self and others, and/or as a relationship with that which is wholly 'other', transcendent and beyond the self. It is experienced as being of fundamental or ultimate importance and is thus concerned with matters of meaning and purpose in life, truth, and values. (4,5)

There are significant difficulties involved in any attempt to define religion, difficulties stemming from both the diversity and complexity of the phenomena (6); while some authors emphasize the personal and others the social, some emphasize belief and others behaviour, some emphasize tradition and others function (2). While 'spirituality' is understood for instance by Swinton as that aspect of life that gives it its 'humanness' (7), religion as defined by Cook and Sims is that grounding of faith and basis of life to which one regards oneself as being bound for one's survival, a rope that ties one to God and to other believers (2). Religion therefore tends to be concerned with socially and traditionally shared beliefs and experience, including personal and subjective dimensions.

Historically, much of psychiatric care globally was provided within a religious context although not without egregious cases of abuse (2,8–15); however, it is only recently that scholarly research has identified the impact (largely positive) of spirituality/religion on mental health (16–20). Evidence suggests that spirituality plays important roles in the lives of many people with intellectual disability (21–24) and their families (25–27); however, participation in religious communities is often difficult for people with disabilities and their families (26, 28–30).

The Judeo-Christian religions

In this section, we aim to summarize the views of the Judeo-Christian culture and tradition on intellectual disability. These views will be informed by the writings of the Hebrew scriptures, the Christian Bible, and narrative accounts of how people in these traditions have engaged with the issues of intellectual disability over the years. Most of the scholarly work in this area comes from disability studies, rather than intellectual disability per se. Those insights, however, can be applied to intellectual disability and other neurodevelopmental conditions.

Judaism and Christianity are two religions that share a lot in common yet have significant differences (31). The Hebrew Bible of the Jews (*Tanakh*) is the Old Testament of the Christians, they share common beliefs in one transcendent God (monotheistic), all-powerful, all-Holy and all-good who made all people in His image. Both Christianity and Judaism view the world as a place of divine activity and human responsibility, yet both acknowledge the presence of evil and injustice in the world including human responsibility to live ethically before God. Both religions believe in the future redemption of mankind and the ushering in of an age of bliss.

Despite these similarities, there are major differences. Orthodox Christians have a Trinitarian view of one God who exists in three persons. Christians also believe in Jesus Christ, the Messiah, who is the second person of the Trinity; however, Judaism looks forward to a coming messiah (or in some circles, a messianic age). Perhaps more importantly, Christians believe that salvation is entirely a gift from God, made possible for everyone through the incarnation and sacrificial death of Jesus Christ whereas in Judaism, salvation has been primarily conceived in terms of the destiny of Israel as the chosen people of Yahweh, and offered through membership in the ethnic Jewish nation (32–34).

The concept of intellectual disability in Judaism and Christianity

The *Tanakh*, the *Talmud*, and indeed the New Testament do not particularly refer to intellectual disability or neurodevelopmental conditions as diagnosed in the present day (35,36) although the concept of mental disorders, their manifestations, and the larger reality of disability were known and understood (37–39). Throughout the *Tanakh* and the New Testament Scriptures, the word 'fool' repeatedly occurs; however, this rather than referring to someone's intelligence quotient is more an ethical description of a life lived in ignorance of God and his law. The *Halakhah* (40), a compendium of laws and ordinances that have evolved since biblical times to regulate religious observances and the daily life and conduct of the Jewish people, differentiates between people who have developed normally and those defined as simple-minded (*shoteh*; plural: *shotim*), that is, those ones whose 'mental capacity is disordered and whose thought processes or behavioural processes have been impaired' (36). Although descriptively like the label of intellectual disability, the causes of 'simple-mindedness' include mental illness, melancholy, brain injury, and diseases of old age, among other things (36). Others (41,42) have argued that the diagnostic category of the *shoteh* should be understood as defining a concept rather than as a fixed clinical entity and that another Hebrew word *peti* (loosely translated to English as fool), which describes someone of very low intelligence and impaired function is more appropriate in describing intellectual disability. Both approaches appear to acknowledge that the *shoteh* category can include those with very severe forms of intellectual disability.

In the Christian tradition, the history of engagement with disability in general, and intellectual disability in particular, is complex. Starting in the seventeenth century, the development of the present-day concept of intellectual disability saw theologians and philosophers attempting to solve a conundrum as to the essential nature of mankind (43). Although the Bible does not explicitly mention intellectual disability, it commonly refers to physical disabilities either as existential realities, divine punishments due to personal sin (38) or as metaphors for personal/social sin (44). In the Old Testament, priests with some forms of physical disabilities were excluded from some aspect of ministry (45,46); however, the Bible also includes several injunctions for God's covenant people to care for the disabled and uphold the rights of the vulnerable. It records stories of healings and cure of disabilities although these always seem to have a programmatic significance, portraying God's redemptive intervention and culminating in Christ, representative of his work of deliverance from sin (47–51).

Early Christian doctrine in the Patristic period (as seen in the writings of the North African Fathers Clement of Alexandria, Tertullian, and Lactantius) promoted the view that all people are created in the image of God and consequently are of equal worth and dignity. Early Christians had a countercultural attitude towards human life; hence they reacted against dominant attitudes such as exposure of defective babies and social exclusion of the lame, the blind, children, the poor, and other social outcasts (52). St Thomas Aquinas, an immensely influential philosopher-theologian in discussing *amentia* (a profound cognitive impairment similar to the present-day concept of intellectual disability) averred that the *amens* (the cognitively impaired individual) though suffering from an infirmity is not hindered in the active imaging of God nor are they prevented from participating in the supernatural life; hence, *amentia* cannot keep an individual from responding to God's grace nor able to prevent the *amens* from realizing their ultimate good (53).

However, in later periods, divergent views emerged: while some thought disability was a punishment from God, others believed that those with disabilities were more pious than non-disabled people; still, some with severe intellectual disability were seen as demon possessed and subjected to exorcisms and other inhumane acts. Many quote Luther's suggestion in *Table Talk*, No. 5207 that a 12-year-old boy, likely suffering from Prader–Willi syndrome, be suffocated. However, a more considered reflection is found in his written and spoken arguments across 30 years (1517–1546) concerned with childbirth and infancy, devils, superstitions, changelings, prodigies, folly, disablement, deafness, participation in Christian sacraments. These and his exegesis of Biblical texts on disabled people, give a more reliable, comprehensive, and interesting guide to his views (54–57).

In the present day, Christian theologians, many with a personal experience of intellectual disability or other neurodevelopmental conditions, have sought to formulate a coherent theology of disability that is faithful to the Scriptures but also celebrates diversity and disability, in the unity of all of God's children. Amos Yong (58), an evangelical theologian, suggests a summary of scriptural teaching about disability:

1. The existential truth that the disabled are to 'endure patiently the outworking of God's inscrutable plan, given the hope that God's ultimate intentions include their well-being and vindication'.

2. The theological insight that under God's sovereignty all 'disabilities are part of God's plan'.

3. The pastoral injunction to the church to meet the needs of people with disabilities.

Inclusion of people with intellectual disability in Judaism and Christianity

In Judaism, views concerning the place of people with disability are somewhat diverse; historically, there were rabbinic interpretations of the Torah that seem to perpetuate discriminatory attitudes towards those with disabilities yet there are other traditional interpretations that affirm the humanity, identity, and value of people with disabilities as being equal to that of others in the community. Jewish law explicitly expresses positive attitudes towards people with disabilities; the law, in principle, grants the individual with intellectual disability obligations and privileges equal to that of people with normal development in participating in religious life (36). Jewish law and scholars over time have stressed the need for education, acceptance, and obligations towards people with an intellectual disability (59). Nevertheless, inclusion of individuals and families where disability is present remains a challenge in the community, specifically regarding social life, synagogues, and education (39).

Despite reports of exclusion and rejection that people with intellectual disability and their families have experienced from members of the Christian community, throughout history there were also those who loved, supported, and cherished people with disabilities. For example, in the medieval period, a large section of the public saw the 'disabled' as possessing special gifts which were indicative of their privileged status as recipients of God's grace; also, since there was no state provision for people with disabilities, they were provided with humane care either at home or in monasteries cared for by monks and nuns based on the teachings of the Church (60,61). In the present day, L'arche communities (founded in 1964 by the Canadian Jean Vanier and two men with learning disabilities, Raphaël Simi and Philippe Seux) offer faith-centred, shared community living for individuals with and without intellectual disability. Today, L'Arche International is a Federation working in 38 countries worldwide, made up of 156 Communities and 26 community projects, with each community seeking to embody L'Arche's values, rooted in the Christian tradition, within the diversity of local customs and religious expressions.

For Christians with intellectual disability who want to read the Bible, 'Children's Bibles' are often offered; although this may assist comprehension, many consider this patronizing and there is a real risk that over time, this may leave people feeling embarrassed and excluded. To promote inclusion, many churches and Christian organizations have sought to remedy this inequity by encouraging an ecclesiology that acknowledges the reality of disability and thus regain the historical Christian vision of an inclusive and diverse body of Christ. To improve Bible literacy among those with intellectual disability, Scripture Union in association with Causeway PROSPECTS launched a project in 2006 where a set of 'Bible Prospects' books each containing 30 short Bible readings from the easy-to-read-version, simple notes to encourage understanding and response, and short prayers were published especially for people with learning disabilities. Similarly, Biblica (formerly the International Bible Society) started the Accessible Bible Project in 2016; this was about publishing a Bible edition that utilizes special fonts, illustrations, and layouts that make for easier reading and comprehension. The text is based on the New International Reader's version which makes the text easy to read and understand. The Accessible Edition includes audio and digital versions and has been developed specifically for those with intellectual disability, moderate sight loss, lower levels of literacy, and/or English as a second language.

Islam

In this section, we aim to summarize the rights of people with intellectual disability in Islam, based on Qur'anic principles and practices from the *Sunnah* (sayings and practices of the Prophet Muhammad).

Islam is a monotheistic, Abrahamic religion and is considered as the world's second largest religious group. Data from 2015 show that Islam has 1.8 billion followers, making up about 24.1% of the world's population (62). Currently, there are 1.5 million people with intellectual disability in the UK, with an estimate of 7% of children with intellectual disability being Muslim (63). Muslims believe that the Qur'an, their holy book, was revealed by Allah to the Prophet Muhammad, and they consider the Qur'an to be the primary source of information on religious, legal, moral, civic, and familial matters. The other source of such matters in Islam is the *Sunnah*, based on a collection of sayings from the prophet Muhammad, referred to as the *hadith*, and his way of life.

The concept of intellectual disability in Islam

Islamic principles promote the concept of egalitarianism and emphasize the importance of protection of the underprivileged, including both those who are ill and those who are disabled, physically or mentally (64). While neither the Qur'an nor the *Sunnah* use a generic term for 'intellectual disability' as is used in English, they have multiple descriptive references to specific disabilities, both physical and intellectual, such as *a'maa* (blind), *asamm* (deaf), *a'raj* (lame), *da'if* (weak), and *marid* (sick). Wentz clarifies that the use of such terms in the

Qur'an and in the *Sunnah* do not carry any negative meanings, being linguistically neutral (65). The Qur'an and the *Sunnah* consider disabilities as a normal and acceptable part of humanity, viewing any form of disability as morally neutral, that is, neither a blessing nor a punishment (66) and Islamic teaching provides both guiding principles and practical suggestions for caring for disabled people, ensuring the maintenance of their societal rights at all levels.

Social inclusion of Muslims with intellectual disability

From an Islamic perspective, the wider community is responsible for caring for those with any additional needs, including those with intellectual disability. Islamic teachings further highlight the rewards associated with ensuring the protection and inclusion of the weaker segments of society, including the disabled (67). This responsibility is facilitated through the mandatory practice of *Zakat* (charity based on a fixed percentage of a Muslim's savings beyond a certain limit) for those members of the Muslim community able to do so. Funds raised through *Zakat* can be used to ensure basic human rights ranging from food, shelter, access to education, and healthcare for the needy, including those with intellectual disability (68).

Research into societal inclusion of Muslims with intellectual disability is particularly scarce. Islamic principles and relevant examples from Islamic history give an account of the inalienable rights afforded to people with disabilities and the challenges they face in accessing these rights.

Right to basic care and protection from harm

It is the collective responsibility of the Muslim society to look after those with any additional needs (67), such actions are encouraged with the guarantee of divine rewards based on both Qur'anic writings and the *Sunnah*. For instance, Ibn Umar (an early follower of the prophet's teachings) reported that the prophet Muhammad said: 'The one who meets the needs of his brother, Allah will meet his needs. Whoever relieves a Muslim of distress, Allah will relieve him on the Day of Resurrection.' (69). Al-Aoufi (67) further highlights a Qur'anic verse illustrating the right to shelter, clothing and even kindness for those with disabilities: provide for them [*those with disabilities*] with it [*your property*] and clothe them and speak to them words of appropriate kindness (70).

Some sections of the early Islamic world also recognized the societal need for supported care for people with disabilities; for example, al Walid ibn Abd al Malik, a caliph in Damascus, Syria, set up the first care home for people with intellectual disability and allocated caregivers (71). Another caliph, Umar ibn Abdul Aziz facilitated the payment of carers for those with disabilities (72). Certain Islamic countries, such as Saudi Arabia, Jordan (67), Iran (73),

Indonesia (74), and Pakistan (75) have national policies outlining the responsibility of both government and the citizens to respect the human rights of people with special needs. Despite the presence of such policies and Islamic rulings promoting equality, there is often a lack of mechanism to ensure that they are implemented (73). Societal stigmas, economic difficulties, and traditional beliefs surrounding the cause of disability and potential 'treatments' fuel illegal, immoral, and religiously prohibited practices towards people with intellectual disability within certain sections of the Islamic world, such as in sub-Saharan Africa. Examples include occasional reports of infanticide, not registering disabled children at birth, abuse, violent 'cures', and ostracism (76).

Inclusion in healthcare

Evidence from both research and practice has highlighted the overall poorer physical health of people with intellectual disability (77–79). There is no reason to believe this to be different for Muslims. As discussed previously, Islamic principles guarantee equality for those with disabilities and promote their protection, which includes access to healthcare. Current societal barriers may, however, negatively influence healthcare accessibility and experience. Muslims in lower-income countries are often cared for in under-resourced mental health settings, where competing health priorities often take precedence. Perceived social stigma and lack of awareness surrounding the nature and cause of disabilities remain pervasive problems. These beliefs and lack of infrastructure fuel the drive for consultations with traditional healers (74,80).

In higher-income countries, Muslims are predominantly migrants, thus there may be a cross-cultural gap between Muslims with intellectual disability, their families, and healthcare professionals. Hasnain and colleagues highlight the importance of recognizing and addressing this gap to avoid poor engagement and treatment outcomes. This gap may exist because of numerous reasons: lack of awareness of available health and social care support services, language barriers, clinical assessment tools not validated in the Muslim population, and perceived social stigma, among others (80).

Inclusion in education

Islamic teaching highlights the importance of universal education and the obligation upon everyone, including the disabled, when possible, to seek education. Universal education is kept in such high regard that a Quranic verse describes how Allah reproached the prophet Muhammad for initially turning away a blind man who wished to increase his knowledge of Islam (70). The Prophet eventually called the man back and taught him to become one of the two callers to prayer in one of the holy cities (66,67). Numerous Muslim countries have developed educational policies promoting the inclusion of students with special educational needs, including those with intellectual disability (81,82). In practice, however, numerous challenges abound when providing quality education, as reported by Ibrahim and colleagues (72) including lack of specialist material (e.g. Braille documents for the visually impaired) or skills (e.g. lack of staff trained in sign language and speech and language therapists), poor staffing ratios, lack of schools offering inclusive education, and the perceived burden by certain teachers of the presence of students with special educational needs within mainstream education (81).

While access to inclusive education is more common in the West, disabled female Muslims in the West, including those with intellectual disability, are reportedly less motivated than males to access mainstream education, particularly among children of first-generation migrants. Hasnain et al. suggest a cultural reason engrained in traditional familial expectations for this difference: the belief that education is an investment for the future that is less likely to be profitable for females with intellectual disability (80).

Therefore, while Islamic principles promote the need for society to demonstrate care and compassion towards people with all forms of disabilities, and offer examples promoting their social inclusion, including through the mandatory practice of charity (*Zakat*), stigma, traditional practices in Muslim countries, and barriers faced by migrant Muslims in Western countries hamper true social inclusion of Muslims with intellectual disability. The scarcity of research specifically looking at the challenges of this segment of the population illustrates the amplitude of the task ahead. An international research agenda, driven by academic institutions, non-governmental organizations, and relevant governments should aim to explore the enablers and barriers to social inclusion by Muslims with intellectual disability within different settings.

Buddhism

Buddhism is regarded as a religion as well as a philosophy in many Eastern and Western countries. Prince Siddartha Gouthama, the founder of Buddhism, was born in North India about 2600 years ago during an era of spiritual awakening. According to Buddhism, the material world is impermanent and attachment to the world is seen as the cause of suffering among human beings (83). There is no place for the soul (Anatta doctrine) or God in Buddhism. Instead, it emphasizes human potential and the ability to change one's destiny if attempted (84,85). Influences of Buddhism may reasonably be claimed to have reached as many as 2 billion people currently alive, mostly within Asia who live in regions where there is a long history of Buddhist teaching and practice, which has some ongoing influence on the way most people think and behave (86). Zen

Buddhism, a 'stripped-down, determined, uncompromising, cut-to-the-chase, meditation-based Buddhism that takes no interest in doctrinal refinements or relying on scripture, doctrine or ritual' (87) is practised by many in Western nations.

Concept of intellectual disability in Buddhism

Seeing that there are many schools of thought within Buddhism, it is somewhat difficult to categorically state what Buddhism says or teaches about disability in general or intellectual disability. However, important sources of information that illuminate the topic of intellectual disability in Buddhist thought will include what the Buddha reportedly said about the matter (including scholarly and folk interpretations of his discourse); what modern Buddhist authorities have said, and, importantly, iconographic representations of disability; Buddhist medical, legal, ethical, or educational responses to disability; practical caring responses to children or adults with disabilities in areas with Buddhist influences; and disabled lives in Asia where Buddhist influence seems entirely absent (86).

Karma and rebirth are two central elements of Buddhist thought; based on these, some have said that to be born with a disability is very widely considered a negative condition, indicating 'bad karma'. Hence disability is not seen as a reward, or as promotion to a higher condition (although to be born human, even with disability, is seen as a better condition than being born as an animal or an insect) (86,88–89). Bejoian (90) argues that such a view is completely contradictory to Buddhist philosophy and practice since the law of karma (cause and effect) is not that simple to understand or explain. Hence implying that there is an obvious and linear causality between karma and disability is extremely insufficient and inadequate. Drawing on the *Jathaka* tales of the Buddha where he accommodated himself to the intellectual capacity of his audience thus aiding their understanding and learning including the story of *Pantaka*, who could be perceived as being 'mentally handicapped' yet was able to achieve enlightenment, Bejoian (90) shows that being disabled does not preclude the possibility of learning, gaining wisdom, or reaching the final goal of enlightenment.

Social inclusion of people with intellectual disability in Buddhism

Buddhism as a psychotherapy

There are '*Jathaka* stories' in Buddhism which are in very simple language and eventually give an important message to people, particularly the distressed. These stories are taught in schools as well as Sunday schools or Daham pasal conducted in Buddhist temples in Sri Lanka; these lessons are well attended by many young people including people with intellectual disability who find these stories easy to understand. There is a lesson to learn in every '*Jathaka*' story and they may be useful in psychotherapeutic interventions (91). The principles of Buddhism have been incorporated in many psychotherapeutic interventions such as cognitive behavioural therapy, dialectical behavioural therapy, and mindfulness training. In addition, meditation and relaxation techniques are practised all over the globe. These forms of therapy can be adapted for people with intellectual disability (92,93).

Rituals in Buddhism

Traditionally, most Buddhist extended families have worked together to support parents and children with disabilities in the home. Most Buddhist temples are in calm environments and there are Bo trees (*Ficus religiosa*), statues of the Lord Buddha, and various culturally important deities/gods in the temple precincts. Many people feel such an environment is calming and soothing and helps to relax and reduce distress and disturbance. Such environments are useful in caring for people with intellectual disability. Rituals like lighting oil lamps, pouring water to the Bo trees, worshiping statues of the Lord Buddha and other culturally important deities/gods, and so on are easy to follow for anyone and this form of religious practice is considered suitable for people with intellectual disability and other neurodevelopmental conditions.

Coping with anger and impulse control

In Buddhism it has been widely highlighted that people should not harm any living being in the world. Mindfulness training, importance of forgiveness, spreading and cultivating loving kindness towards people, and curbing anger are important concepts (94). Buddhism also teaches the importance of refraining from substances like alcohol and avoiding intoxication. These precepts or basic principles regarding 'Sila' (foremost of all good conditions) are refraining from taking one's life, stealing, immoral sexual conduct, telling lies and excessive drinking (84). They are expressed in simple language and are accessible to people with intellectual disability. Meditation techniques and relaxation training are also practised and encouraged. These practices help to overcome the anger and impulse control problems which are commonly encountered in some people with neurodevelopmental conditions and behaviours that challenge.

Astrology and intellectual disability

In Eastern countries like Sri Lanka, parents, family members, and friends seek advice from fortune tellers and astrologers regarding their disabled children. They also ask them to do various rituals and make offerings to various Gods, though Buddhist teachings do not encourage such activities. Many people believe in horoscopes or bad planetary influence as a cause of conditions such as intellectual disability and seek remedies from fortune tellers including wearing enchanted threads, various forms of gems, and talismans to ward off evil or seek solace from their misfortunes. Traditional healing practices such as exorcism are still practised for mental illnesses in countries like Sri Lanka (95). However, many have argued that traditional Buddhist religion discourages such attitudes and emphasizes the importance of believing in oneself and one's potential to have a change and positive outcome.

Protecting human rights

Lord Buddha gave equal rights to women and the disabled including the intellectual disabled who were very oppressed during those days. He condemned every form of discrimination including that based on the caste system which was widely prevalent in India in his time (84,85); as explained before, disabilities need not prevent one from achieving the goal of enlightenment.

Hinduism

Hinduism is known as the world's oldest surviving religion. Its origin dates back more than 4000 years. It is mainly practised in India but spread around the globe, internationally there are approximately 1.16 billion followers of Hinduism at present, representing about 15% of the world's population. Hinduism does not have a singular doctrinal focus and draws on the wisdom of innumerable writings compiled over thousands of years. 'Hinduism' is not the original name of an Indian religion but a nineteenth-century British invention; and those who followed the same tradition since the ancient times never gave it any name except for '*dharma*', which simply means 'the eternal law that supports and sustains those who practise it'. The term 'Hindu' was first used by the ancient Persians to refer to the people living near the river Indus, it then became convenient shorthand for the rulers of India and later it defined those who were not Muslims or Christians but followed the teachings of a large body of books called the 'Vedas' (96,97). There are multiple sources from which the teachings of Hinduism have been drawn. For example, some strands of Hindu thought are pluralistic and incorporate teachings from other religions, while orthodox Hinduism only accepts teachings from the Vedic tradition. Nevertheless, there are consistent themes that shape Hindu thought, such as the concept of the four *Purusharthas*, four goals of all mankind—*artha* (wealth), *kama* (desire), *dharma* (righteousness), and *moksha* (liberation), including the teaching of karma, which has important implications for people with disabilities (98).

Concept of intellectual disability in Hinduism

In Hinduism, there is no exact word, for the concept of intellectual disability (99). Gabel, in her 2004 ethnographic study, described a Hindi word, *mundh buddhi*, which literally translated applies to a person who has bad desires (*buddhi*) of the heart (*mundh*). There was no consensus as to its meaning in her research, several prominent meanings of this term surfaced in the data analysis, including the idea that a person with intellectual disability is as able as those without intellectual disability but only lazy (100,101).

According to Miles (102), in Hindu texts, disabilities are frequently understood as a retributive consequence for past actions. This sometimes is presented with a positive element, for example, people who were 'over-intellectual' or 'domineering' in a previous life might need the 'rehabilitative' experience of having an intellectual disability in the next life 'to overcome the arrogant tendency and thus enable the soul to progress towards enlightenment'.

Inclusion of people with intellectual disability in Hinduism

Historically, the teachings of Hinduism have profoundly affected the treatment of people with disabilities in India, often in unhelpful ways. The concept of disability was frequently explained in Hinduism as being 'sent by deity, fate [or] karma; often associated with parental or personal sin' (98). Yet, there are positive representations of disability as throughout Indian heritage, people with disabilities were seen as contributing members of the larger society as musicians, rulers, and philosophers (103).

In a study done among Hindu participants (predominantly first-generation immigrants), adult Hindus demonstrated fewer positive attitudes than Hindu adolescents, suggesting that age, or acculturation in a more inclusive society, could impact attitudes towards people with intellectual disability (101,104). In Indian society, some seem to hold views that are incompatible with the social inclusion of those with learning disabilities, especially in contemporary Indian communities where services for people with intellectual disability are lacking. In contrast, rural and agrarian communities demonstrate that inclusive and integrated practices can be supported (101).

Africa and social inclusion of people with intellectual disability

Africa is a heterogeneous and diverse continent. Although many cultures in sub-Saharan Africa share commonalities, the people and their views on disability in general and intellectual disability in particular are diverse, complex, and often contradictory. According to the most recent meta-analysis findings, the prevalence of intellectual disability ranges from 0.05% to 1.55% globally (105); however, the highest prevalence is found in low- and middle-income countries (106). Although intellectual disability is probably the largest impairment grouping on the African continent, few indigenous research and evaluation studies have been undertaken in the region.

The multinational study of attitudes towards individuals with intellectual disability (107) commissioned by the Special Olympics and the Attitudes of the Public in South Africa Toward People with Intellectual Disabilities study (108) included people from three African nations (Nigeria, Egypt, and South Africa). In the study, people in different cultures perceive individuals with intellectual disability very differently. In some countries, the public envisions a mildly challenged person, while in other countries the public sees a severely impaired person; generally speaking, in the African countries, the public's perceptions of capabilities are lower than that from the US and several European countries, particularly on the simple skills.

A substantial percentage of the public in Nigeria, South Africa, and Egypt believe that institutions are the best place for people with intellectual disability to live and most of the public in South Africa and Egypt believe that people with intellectual disability are best employed in special workshops and their Nigerian counterparts, unskilled jobs. Like participants in other parts of the world, many African people believe that children with intellectual disability should be educated in special schools, separately from other children. Compared with Western nations that are more accepting of inclusive practices, most people in Africa expect that including individuals with intellectual disability in the workplace and schools will create more accidents on the job, cause discipline problems in the classroom, lower productivity, and negatively affect the learning of other students.

The concept of intellectual disability in sub-Saharan Africa

As a vast continent with diverse cultural and religious values, there are a variety of perceptions of disability. While some communities believe that disabilities are caused by adultery, witchcraft, juju, or other supernatural forces thus negatively appraising those with disabilities, others consider people with disabilities to be special, even sacred (109). Disability studies have shown that in many African communities, perceptions of disability and people with disability include outright hostility, veneration, and tolerant views where those with disabilities are seen as hopeless, helpless, and harmless. In some communities, both positive and negative views can coexist (e.g. among the Igbos of South-eastern Nigeria, treatment of children with disabilities can range from total rejection to pampering) whereas in others, disability always carries the stigma of a divine curse; especially concerning intellectual disability, beliefs about supernatural causes of disability such as divine retribution or witchcraft are more common, and they have severe consequences for people with intellectual disability (110–113).

Among the Yorùbá of West Africa, disabilities always have some supernatural significance, for example, precolonial Yorùbá society saw albinos as incarnations of the gods and so treated them with deference. In a myth, Òrìṣà-ńlá, the Yorùbá sculptor divinity was depicted as a lover of palm wine who fashioned people with impairments and deformities while intoxicated, hence the Yorùbá language and oral tradition are replete with sayings that establish those with disabilities as Ẹni Òrìṣà (the votaries of the Òrìṣà), special and sacred to the deity; Adegbindin (114) has suggested that the hunchback, the cripple, the albino, and the dwarf are categorized as the major Ẹni Òrìṣà and others—the blind, the dumb, people with 'invisible disabilities', and so on—as the minor Ẹni Òrìṣà.

This myth apart from providing a cultural explanation of the origin of disabilities, as argued by Adegbindin (114), questions the assumptions associated with the recognition of the dichotomy between 'normality' and 'abnormality' but also teaches about the acceptance (perhaps even veneration) of those with disabilities (115).

Among the Ashanti in Ghana, people with disabilities were rejected, and children born with severe intellectual disability were seen as animal-like, somewhat like views held by Plato and Aristotle (116), and left to die; also, men with physical disabilities were precluded from chieftaincy positions. In contrast, the Chagga of East Africa perceived those with physical disabilities as pacifiers of evil spirits hence they were treated with respect and protection; in some communities in The Republic of Benin, children with disabilities have full acceptance in the community and are seen as harbingers of good luck and specially protected by benevolent spirits. Similarly, the Ga of Accra, Ghana, believed that those with intellectual disability were the reincarnation of a deity, hence they were perceived with awe and always treated with great kindness, gentleness, and patience (117).

Social inclusion of those with intellectual disability

Africans live in communities and relate within social groups; this understanding is captured in the Ubuntu ethic of Bantu-speaking regions of Africa expressed clearly in John Mbiti's 'I am, because we are; and since we are therefore I am'. This concept provides an African social ethic of inclusion, where people with intellectual disability have their dignity of personhood restored. Some have argued that industrialization and Westernization are responsible for the very concept of intellectual disability, in rural and agrarian communities, with less emphasis on formal/Western education, people with intellectual disability have greater opportunities for social competence and contributing to the community hence they do not pick up the label of intellectual disability (116,118).

Studies have shown that religion and spirituality are important to people with disabilities in many societies. Essentially, spiritual beliefs may greatly influence perceptions of people with disabilities, of themselves, others, and the world. In the present day, due to negative indigenous beliefs, the influence of European biomedical model of disability and what some have called 'disabling theology' (109,119,120), many hold negative attitudes and perpetrate discriminatory behaviour towards people with disabilities. In some cases, those with disabilities are seen as charity cases where those deemed 'normal' give handouts to them. Although this may offer much needed practical help, it may also perpetuate discriminatory attitudes (120,121).

Nevertheless, many people with disabilities and their families who belong to religious organizations report that religion and spirituality play both formal and informal functions in their lives ranging from a sense of belonging and fellowship with others to provision of practical help such as education and employment opportunities (120,122). In addition, indigenous African religious groups that appropriate positive elements of the African traditional worldview often practise a syncretistic African spirituality that provides people with disabilities (and their families) with resilience and the ability to cope with negative emotions that arise from their disability experiences. Unfortunately, many of these religious institutions propagate beliefs that people with intellectual disability are suffering from demon possession and spiritual attacks. The search for spiritual healing and deliverance often draws those with disabilities and their families to such places where many are exploited and they suffer abuses at the hands of their caregivers such as incarceration, molestation, and sexual harassment (120,123).

Conclusion

For most of human history, the major world religions have provided an all-encompassing social context which informed peoples' beliefs and attitudes (101). There is now a growing body of literature emerging from the health and social care professions, which suggests that spirituality is a basic human need and a necessary component of both mental and physical health. In spite of this, there is still a paucity of research on the impact of religious practices and beliefs on people with intellectual disability. In terms of the role religion plays in views towards people with intellectual disability, it is impossible to be reductionistic as religious beliefs can generate both positive and negative attitudes, they can promote understanding, foster resilience and support, but can also perpetuate discrimination and exploitation. Nevertheless, available research has confirmed the difficulties many people with disabilities and their families face in participating in their local faith communities (124) despite the high importance religious activities hold for those with intellectual disability and their families (23,24,26). Currently, many faith communities express the goal of embracing inclusivity (125), in line with the worldwide move towards physical integration of those with disabilities (126,127). However, the assumed benefits of increased physical integration without social integration have been questioned (128). The proponents of this approach argue that it is social integration and not simply physical integration that has a positive influence on the well-being of people with intellectual disability. Although this is arguably a very significant insight, practically, it may be difficult to delineate between physical and social integration. Beyond ideas of inclusion, there is a need to move to the practices of belonging and to reframe our practices from political rhetoric to activities motivated by love (129). In line with this, research has shown that more inclusive communities are those who feature faith leaders who were more committed to inclusion, who used educational resources to address disability-related issues, portrayed people with disabilities positively in their religious teachings, had stronger ties to disability organizations, and had a stronger orientation towards promoting social justice (125).

References

1. **Royal College of Psychiatrists**. Spirituality and mental health. Royal College of Psychiatrists; 2006 (updated 2020). Available from: https://www.rcpsych.ac.uk/mental-health/treatments-and-wellbeing/spirituality-and-mental-health

2. **Sims A, Cook CCH.** Spirituality in psychiatry. In: **Cook CCH, Powell A, Sims A,** editors. Spirituality and Psychiatry. London: Royal College of Psychiatrists; 2009: 1–15.

3. **Zinnbauer BJ, Pargament KI, Cole B, Rye MS, Butfer EM, Belavich TG,** et al. Religion and spirituality: unfuzzying the fuzzy. In: **Mirola W, Emerson M, Monahan S,** editors. Sociology of Religion: A Reader. New York: Routledge; 2015: 29–34.

4. **Cook CC.** Recommendations for Psychiatrists on Spirituality and Religion: Position Statement PS03/2013. London: Royal College of Psychiatrists; 2013.

5. **Cook CC.** Addiction and spirituality. Addiction 2004;**99**(5):539–51.

6. **Dawes G, Maclaurin J.** What is religion?: identifying the explanandum. In: **Maclaurin J, Dawes GW,** editors. A New Science of Religion. London: Routledge; 2013: 10–25.

7. **Fellinger J, Bertelli MO, Lassi S, Gaventa B.** Spiritual issues. In: **Bertelli MO, Deb S, Munir K, Hassiotis A, Salvador-Carulla L,** editors. Textbook of Psychiatry for Intellectual Disability and Autism Spectrum Disorder. Cham: Springer; 2022: 985–1001.

8. **Burns JK, Tomita A.** Traditional and religious healers in the pathway to care for people with mental disorders in Africa: a systematic review and meta-analysis. Social Psychiatry and Psychiatric Epidemiology 2015;**50**(6):867–77.

9. **Lambo TA.** A form of social Psychiatry in Africa (with special reference to general features of psychotherapy with Africans). World Mental Health 1961;**13**(4):190–203.

10. **Lambo TA.** Mental health in Nigeria—research and its technical problems. World Mental Health 1959;**11**:131–8.

11. **Lucas AO, Hendrickse RG.** Yoruba ideas of disease revealed by hospital patients. In: Proceedings of a Symposium on the Traditional Background to Medical Practice in Nigeria 20–23 April 1966. (Edited as occasional publication, University of Ibadan, 1971.)

12. **Odejide AO, Olatawura MO, Sanda AO, Oyeneye AO.** Traditional healers and mental illness in the city of Ibadan. Journal of Black Studies 1978;**9**(2):195–205.

13. **Orley JH.** Culture and Mental Illness: A Study from Uganda. Nairobi: East African Publishing House; 1970.

14. **Prince R.** Some Yoruba views on the causes and modes of treatment of antisocial behaviour. African Journal of Psychiatry 1975;**1**:133–7.

15. **Twumasi PA.** Ashanti traditional medicine. Transition 1972;**41**:50–63.

16. **Koenig HG.** Research on religion, spirituality, and mental health: a review. Canadian Journal of Psychiatry 2009;**54**(5):283–91.

17. **Koenig HG.** Religion, spirituality, and health: the research and clinical implications. International Scholarly Research Notices 2012;**2012**:278730.

18. **Koenig HG, Al Zaben F, Khalifa DA.** Religion, spirituality and mental health in the West and the Middle East. Asian Journal of Psychiatry 2012;**5**(2):180–2.

19. **Bertelli MO, Del Furia C, Bonadiman M, Rondini E, Banks R, Lassi S.** The relationship between spiritual life and quality of life in people with intellectual disability and/or low-functioning autism spectrum disorders. Journal of Religion and Health 2020;**59**(4):1996–2018.

20. **Weber SR, Pargament KI.** The role of religion and spirituality in mental health. Current Opinion in Psychiatry 2014;**27**(5):358–63.

21. **Swinton J.** Spirituality and the lives of people with learning disabilities. Tizard Learning Disability Review 2002;**7**(4):29–35.

22. **Turner S, Hatton C, Shah R, Stansfield J, Rahim N.** Religious expression amongst adults with intellectual disabilities. Journal of Applied Research in Intellectual Disabilities 2004;**17**(3):161–71.

23. **Shogren KA, Rye MS.** Religion and individuals with intellectual disabilities: an exploratory study of self-reported perspectives. Journal of Religion, Disability & Health 2005;**9**(1):29–53.

24. **Liu EX, Carter EW, Boehm TL, Annandale NH, Taylor CE.** In their own words: the place of faith in the lives of young people with autism and intellectual disability. Intellectual and Developmental Disabilities 2014;**52**(5):388–404.

25. **Weisner TS, Beizer L, Stolze L.** Religion and families of children with developmental delays. American Journal on Mental Retardation 1991;**95**(6):647–62.

26. **Gillibrand J.** Disabled Church—Disabled Society: The Implications of Autism for Philosophy, Theology and Politics. London: Jessica Kingsley Publishers; 2009.

27. **Lassi S, Mugnaini D, Fondelli E.** Research on spirituality, mental health and resilience in caregivers: a review. Psyche and spirit: connecting psychiatry and spirituality. WPA Newsletter of the Section on Religion, Spirituality and Psychiatry 2014;**3**(2):8–9.

28. **Gaventa W.** Faith and spirituality: supporting caregivers of individuals with disabilities. In: Multiple Dimensions of Caregiving and Disability. New York: Springer; 2012: 117–34.

29. **Ault MJ, Collins BC, Carter EW.** Factors associated with participation in faith communities for individuals with developmental disabilities and their families. Journal of Religion, Disability & Health 2013;**17**(2):184–211.

30. **Hendershot G.** A statistical note on the religiosity of persons with disabilities. Disability Studies Quarterly 2006;**26**(4).

31. **Spiro JD.** Judaism and Christianity: sources of convergence. Religious Education 1981;**76**(6):605–25.

32. **Brandon S.** Salvation: definition, nature, methods, varieties, & facts. Encyclopedia Britannica; 2022. Available from: https://www.britannica.com/topic/salvation-religion

33. **Cohen G, Greenberg M, Feldman L, Gaster T, Silberman L, Hertzberg A.** Judaism | Definition, origin, history, beliefs, & facts. Encyclopedia Britannica; 2022. Available from: https://www.britannica.com/topic/Judaism

34. **McGrath AE.** Christian Theology: An Introduction. Hoboken, NJ: John Wiley & Sons; 2016.

35. **Macaskill G.** Autism and biblical studies: establishing and extending the field beyond preliminary reflection. Journal of Disability & Religion 2021;**25**(4):388–411.

36. **Lifshitz H, Glaubman R.** Religious and secular students' sense of self-efficacy and attitudes towards inclusion of pupils with intellectual disability and other types of needs. Journal of Intellectual Disability Research 2002;**46**(5):405–18.

37. **Sims A.** Feigned insanity. British Journal of Psychiatry 2014;**204**(1):35.

38. **Otieno PA.** Biblical and theological perspectives on disability: implications on the rights of persons with disability in Kenya. Disability Studies Quarterly 2009;**29**(4).

39. **Fogelman F.** Disability matters within Judaism. Jewishideas.org; 2022. Available from: https://www.jewishideas.org/article/disability-matters-within-judaism

40. **Editors of Encyclopedia Britannica.** Halakhah: definition, history, & facts. Encyclopedia Britannica; 2022. Available from: https://www.britannica.com/topic/Halakhah

41. **Strous R.** The Shoteh and psychosis in Halakhah with contemporary clinical application. The Torah u-Madda Journal 2004;**12**:158–78.

42. **Lau B.** The Status of People with Disabilities in the Jewish Tradition. Israel: The Israel Democracy Institute; 2016.

43. **Goodey CF, Stainton T.** Intellectual disability and the myth of the changeling myth. Journal of the History of the Behavioral Sciences 2001;**37**(3):223–40.

44. **Jacobs NL.** The Upside-down Kingdom of God: A Disability Studies Perspective on Disabled People's Experiences in Churches and Theologies of Disability. Doctoral dissertation, SOAS University of London; 2019.

45. **Bible Gateway.** Leviticus 21. New International Version. 2022. Available from: https://www.biblegateway.com/passage/?search=Leviticus%2021&version=NIV

46. **Bible Gateway.** Leviticus 23. New International Version. 2022. Available from: https://www.biblegateway.com/passage/?search=Leviticus%2023&version=NIV

47. **Strawn BA.** The Old Testament: A Concise Introduction. London: Routledge; 2019.

48. **Bible Gateway.** Leviticus 19:14. New International Version. 2022. Available from: https://www.biblegateway.com/passage/?search=Leviticus%2019%3A14&version=NIV

49. **Walton JH, Matthews VH, Chavalas MW.** The IVP Bible Background Commentary: Old Testament. Westmont, IL: InterVarsity Press; 2012.

50. **Bible Gateway.** Acts 10:38. New International Version. 2022. Available from: https://www.biblegateway.com/passage/?search=Acts%2010%3A38&version=NIV

51. **Bible Gateway.** Isaiah 53. New International Version. 2022. Available from: https://www.biblegateway.com/passage/?search=Isaiah+53&version=NIV

52. **Caspary A.** The patristic era: early Christian attitudes toward the disfigured outcast. In: **Brock B, Swinton J,** editors. Disability in the Christian Tradition: A Reader. Grand Rapids, MI: WB Eerdmans; 2012: 24–64.

53. **Romero MI.** Aquinas on the corporis infirmitas: broken flesh and the grammar of grace. In: **Brock B, Swinton J,** editors. Disability in the Christian Tradition: A Reader. Grand Rapids, MI: WB Eerdmans; 2012: 101–51.

54. **Munyi CW.** Past and present perceptions towards disability: a historical perspective. Disability Studies Quarterly 2012;**32**(2).

55. **Miles M.** Martin Luther and Childhood Disability in 16th Century Germany: What Did He Write? What Did He Say? Farsta, Sweden: Independent Living Institute; 2005.

56. **Heuser S.** The human condition as seen from the cross: Luther and disability. In: **Brock B, Swinton J,** editors. Disability in the Christian Tradition: A Reader. Grand Rapids, MI: WB Eerdmans; 2012: 184–215.

57. **Wilder C.** Luther, the catechisms, and intellectual disability. Intersections 2018;**2018**(47):10.

58. **Yong A.** Theology and Down Syndrome: Reimagining Disability in Late Modernity. Waco, TX: Baylor University Press; 2007.

59. **Merrick J, Gabbay Y, Lifshitz H.** Judaism and the person with intellectual disability. Journal of Religion, Disability & Health 2001;**5**(2–3):49–63.

60. **Cusack CM.** Graciosi: medieval Christian attitudes to disability. Disability and Rehabilitation 1997;**19**(10):414–19.

61. **Kundu CL,** editor. Status of Disability in India—2000. New Delhi: Rehabilitation Council of India; 2000.

62. **Lipka M, Hackett C.** Why Muslims are the world's fastest-growing religious group. Pew Research Center; 2022. Available from: https://www.pewresearch.org/fact-tank/2017/04/06/why-muslims-are-the-worlds-fastest-growing-religious-group/

63. **Emerson E, Hatton C.** Future trends in the ethnic composition of British society and among British citizens with learning disabilities. Tizard Learning Disability Review 1999;**4**(4):28–32.

64. **Marlow L.** Hierarchy and Egalitarianism in Islamic Thought. Cambridge: Cambridge University Press; 2002.

65. **Wentz A.** Disability in Islamic law: historical applications and today's challenges. 2018. Available from: http://repozytorium.uni.wroc.pl/Content/93971/027_Wentz_A_Disability_in_Islamic_Law_historical_applications_and_today%E2%80%99s_challenges.pdf

66. **Bazna MS, Hatab TA.** Disability in the Qur'an: the Islamic alternative to defining, viewing, and relating to disability. Journal of Religion, Disability & Health 2005;**9**(1):5–27.

67. **Al-Aoufi H, Al-Zyoud N, Shahminan N.** Islam and the cultural conceptualisation of disability. International Journal of Adolescence and Youth 2012;**17**(4):205–19.

68. **Senturk OF.** Charity in Islam: A Comprehensive Guide to Zakat. Clifton, NJ: Tughra Books; 2007.

69. **Siddiqui AH.** Sahih Muslim. Karachi: Peace Vision; 1976.

70. **Ali AY.** The Holy Qur'an (Trans. **Ali AY**). Ware, UK: Wordsworth Editions; 2000.

71. **Aljazoli A.** Islam Position on Disability. Morocco: ISESCO; 2004.

72. **Ibrahim I, Ismail MF.** Muslims with disabilities: psychosocial reforms from an Islamic perspective. Journal of Disability & Religion 2018;**22**(1):1–4.

73. **Samadi SA.** Comparative policy brief: status of intellectual disabilities in the Islamic Republic of Iran. Journal of Policy and Practice in Intellectual Disabilities 2008;**5**(2):129–32.

74. **Handoyo RT.** A Multimethod Exploration of Stigma Towards people with Intellectual Disability in Indonesia. Doctoral dissertation, University College London; 2019. Available from: https://discovery.ucl.ac.uk/id/eprint/10086659/

75. **Masood AF, Turner LA, Baxter A.** Causal attributions and parental attitudes toward children with disabilities in the United States and Pakistan. Exceptional Children 2007;**73**(4):475–87.

76. **Rohwerder B.** Disability Stigma in Developing Countries. K4D Helpdesk Report. Brighton: Institute of Development Studies; 2018.

77. **Krahn GL.** WHO World Report on Disability: a review. Disability and Health Journal 2011;**4**(3):141–2.

78. **Disability Rights Commission.** Equal Treatment: Closing the Gap-Interim Report of a Formal Investigation into Health Inequalities. London: Disability Rights Commission; 2006.

79. **Michael J, Richardson A.** Healthcare for all: the independent inquiry into access to healthcare for people with learning disabilities. Tizard Learning Disability Review 2008;**13**(4):28–34.

80. **Hasnain R, Shaikh LC, Shanawani H.** Disability and the Muslim Perspective: An Introduction for Rehabilitation and Health Care Providers. Buffalo, NY: Center for International Rehabilitation Research Information and Exchange; 2018.

81. **Wahyuningsih S.** Inclusive education for persons with disabilities: the Islamic perspective. QIJIS (Qudus International Journal of Islamic Studies) 2016;**4**(1):1–8.

82. **Gaad E.** Inclusive Education in the Middle East. London: Routledge; 2010.

83. **Hart W.** The Art of Living: Vipassana Meditation as Taught by SN Goenka. Onalaska, WA: Pariyatti; 2011.

84. **Ambedkar B.** The Buddha and His Dhamma. Reprinted and donated by the Corporate Body of the Buddha Educational Foundation. Taipei, Taiwan: Buddha Educational Foundation; 1997.

85. **Sri Dhammananda K.** What Buddhists Believe. Taipei, Taiwan: Buddha Educational Foundation; 1993.

86. **Miles M.** Buddhism and responses to disability, mental disorders and deafness in Asia: a bibliography of historical and modern texts with introduction and partial annotation, and some echoes in western countries. 2013. Available from: http://cirrie.buffalo.edu/bibliography/buddhism/index.php

87. **Fischer N.** What Is Zen Buddhism and how do you practice it? Lions Roar; 2022 Available from: https://www.lionsroar.com/what-is-zen-buddhism-and-how-do-you-practice-it/

88. **Miles M.** Disability on a different model: glimpses of an Asian heritage. Disability & Society 2000;**15**(4):603–18.

89. **Miles M.** Disability in South Asia—millennium to millennium. Journal of Religion, Disability & Health 2002;**6**(2-3):109–15.

90. **Bejoian LM.** Nondualistic paradigms in disability studies & Buddhism: creating bridges for theoretical practice. Disability Studies Quarterly 2006;**26**(3).

91. **Harischandra D, Harischandra T.** Psychiatric Aspects of Jātaka Stories: A Modern Analysis of the Ancient Stories of the Buddha's Past Lives, 2nd edition. Colombo: Vijitha Yapa Publications; 2015.

92. **Browne C, Brown G, Smith IC.** Adapting dialectical behaviour therapy in forensic learning disability services: a grounded theory informed study of 'what works'. Journal of Applied Research in Intellectual Disabilities 2019;**32**(4):792–805.

93. **Taylor JL, Lindsay WR, Willner P.** CBT for people with intellectual disabilities: emerging evidence, cognitive ability and IQ effects. Behavioural and Cognitive Psychotherapy 2008;**36**(6):723–33.

94. **Visuddhācāra B.** Curbing Anger Spreading Love. Sri Lanka: BPS; 2007.

95. **Kuruppuarachchi KA, Rajakaruna RR.** Psychiatry in Sri Lanka. Psychiatric Bulletin 1999;**23**(11):686–88.

96. **Avasthi A, Kate N, Grover S.** Indianization of psychiatry utilizing Indian mental concepts. Indian Journal of Psychiatry 2013;**55**(Suppl 2):S136.

97. **Kang C.** Hinduism and mental health: engaging British Hindus. Mental Health, Religion & Culture 2010;**13**(6):587–93.

98. **Wilson A.** Barriers and enablers provided by Hindu beliefs and practices for people with disabilities in India. Christian Journal for Global Health 2019;**6**(2):12–25.

99. **Bhaumik S, Gumber R, Gangavati S, Gangadharan SK.** Intellectual disabilities across cultures. In: **Bhugra D, Bhui K**, editors. Textbook of Cultural Psychiatry, 2nd edition. Cambridge: Cambridge University Press; 2018: 493–502.

100. **Gabel S.** South Asian Indian cultural orientations toward mental retardation. Mental Retardation 2004;**42**(1):12–25.

101. **Sheridan JC.** Attitudes Towards Intellectual Disabilities Across Cultures. Doctoral thesis, University College London; 2007. Available from: https://discovery.ucl.ac.uk/id/eprint/1445086/

102. **Miles M.** Disability in an Eastern religious context: historical perspectives. Disability & Society 1995;**10**(1):49–70.

103. **Narayan J.** Commentary: persons with disabilities in India: a special educator's personal perspective. Disability Studies Quarterly 2004;**24**(2).

104. **Kenyon M.** Attitudes Towards People with Learning Disabilities Within the UK South Asian Hindu Community. Doctoral Thesis, University College London; 2008. Available from: https://discovery.ucl.ac.uk/id/eprint/1445086/1/U592399.pdf

105. **McKenzie K, Milton M, Smith G, Ouellette-Kuntz H.** Systematic review of the prevalence and incidence of intellectual disabilities: current trends and issues. Current Developmental Disorders Reports 2016;**3**(2):104–15.

106. **Maulik PK, Mascarenhas MN, Mathers CD, Dua T, Saxena S.** Prevalence of intellectual disability: a meta-analysis of population-based studies. Research in Developmental Disabilities 2011;**32**(2):419–36.

107. **Siperstein GN.** Multinational Study of Attitudes Towards Individuals with Intellectual Disabilities: General Findings and Calls to Action. Washington, DC: Special Olympics; 2003.

108. **Bardon JN, Siperstein GN, Parker RC, Corbin S.** Attitudes of the Public in South Africa Toward People with Intellectual Disabilities. Washington, DC: Special Olympics; 2006.

109. **Nyangweso M.** Disability in Africa: a cultural/religious perspective. In: **Falola T, Hamel N,** editors. Disability in Africa: Inclusion, Care, and the Ethics of Humanity (Rochester Studies in African History and the Diaspora). Martlesham, UK: Boydell & Brewer; 2021: 115–36.

110. **Kromberg J, Zwane E, Manga P, Venter A, Rosen E, Christianson A.** Intellectual disability in the context of a South African population. Journal of Policy and Practice in Intellectual Disabilities 2008;**5**(2):89–95.

111. **Mulatu MS.** Perceptions of mental and physical illnesses in north-western Ethiopia: causes, treatments, and attitudes. Journal of Health Psychology 1999;**4**(4):531–49.

112. **Hartley SO, Ojwang P, Baguwemu A, Ddamulira M, Chavuta A.** How do carers of disabled children cope? The Ugandan perspective. Child: Care, Health and Development 2005;**31**(2):167–80.

113. **Mung'omba J.** Comparative policy brief: status of intellectual disabilities in the Republic of Zambia. Journal of Policy and Practice in Intellectual Disabilities 2008;**5**(2):142–44.

114. **Adegbindin O.** Disability and human diversity: a reinterpretation of Ẹni-òòṣà philosophy in Yorùbá belief. Yoruba Studies Review 2018;**3**(1):1–30.

115. **Torre M.** Santería: The Beliefs and Rituals of a Growing Religion in America. Grand Rapids, MI: WB Eerdmans; 2004.

116. **Stainton T.** Reason and value: the thought of Plato and Aristotle and the construction of intellectual disability. Mental Retardation 2001;**39**(6):452–60.

117. **Munyi CW.** Past and present perceptions towards disability: a historical perspective. Disability Studies Quarterly 2012;**32**(2).

118. **Mckenzie JA, McConkey R, Adnams C.** Intellectual disability in Africa: implications for research and service development. Disability and Rehabilitation 2013;**35**(20):1750–5.

119. **Eiesland NL.** The Disabled God: Toward a Liberatory Theology of Disability. Nashville, TN: Abingdon Press; 1994.

120. **Mugeere AB, Omona J, State AE, Shakespeare T.** 'Oh God! Why did you let me have this disability?': religion, spirituality and disability in three African countries. Journal of Disability & Religion 2020;**24**(1):64–81.

121. **Opoku MP, Gyamfi N, Badu E, Kwadwo W.** 'They think we are all beggars': the resilience of a person with disability in Ghana. Journal of Exceptional People 2017;**2**(11):7–18.

122. **Gara NM.** Effects of caring on mothers of intellectually disabled children in Alice, Eastern Cape, South Africa. Doctoral dissertation, University of Cape Town.

123. Shodipo RO. Culture, African Traditional Religion, and Disability: Implications for Pastoral Care Ministry in Nigeria. Disability and Disciplines: International Conference on Educational, Cultural, and Disability Studies, 3–4 July. Centre for Culture and Disability Studies, Liverpool Hope University, Liverpool, UK; 2019.

124. **Gaventa B.** Lessons in community building from including the 'other': caring for one an-other. Journal of Religion, Disability & Health 2012;**16**(3):231–47.

125. **Griffin MM, Kane LW, Taylor C, Francis SH, Hodapp RM.** Characteristics of inclusive faith communities: a preliminary survey of inclusive practices in the United States. Journal of Applied Research in Intellectual Disabilities 2012;**25**(4):383–91.

126. **Emerson E, Hatton C.** Deinstitutionalization in the UK and Ireland: outcomes for service users. Journal of Intellectual and Developmental Disability 1996;**21**(1):17–37.

127. **Department of Health.** Valuing People: A New Strategy for Learning Disability for the 21st Century A White Paper. London: Department of Health; 2001.

128. **Cummins RA, Lau AL.** Community integration or community exposure? A review and discussion in relation to people with an intellectual disability. Journal of Applied Research in Intellectual Disabilities 2003;**16**(2):145–57.

129. **Swinton J.** From inclusion to belonging: a practical theology of community, disability and humanness. Journal of Religion, Disability & Health 2012;**16**(2):172–90.

Chapter 14

People with intellectual disability in the criminal justice system

Ayomipo J. Amiola, Harm Boer,
Chikkanna Manju, Sowmya Srikumar, and
Regi T. Alexander

Introduction

Intellectual disability (ID) is defined as significant impairment of intellectual functioning and adaptive behaviour originating before the age of 18 years (1). Little is known about the needs and prevalence of people with ID in the criminal justice system (CJS) internationally, although there have been several studies attempting to estimate the number of people with ID in prisons.

Cultural attitudes to crime

Culture broadly defined is a common heritage or set of beliefs, norms, and values (2). Tylor (3), who established the theoretical principles of Victorian anthropology, defined culture as 'that complex whole which includes knowledge, beliefs, acts, morals, laws, customs and any other capabilities and habits acquired by man as a member of society'. Crime as defined by social anthropologists are usually those acts that are universally disapproved of by the members of the society in which they are committed; crime therefore is generally defined, understood, and sanctioned in relation to the sociocultural dynamics within societies. The intersection between culture and crime is often complex; in some cases, acts that may be defined as criminal on one hand may also be linked to specific cultural beliefs on the other, which can lead to complexities in the clear articulation of such acts as crimes (4).

Following Europe's colonization of Africa and international migration, contemporary societies are culturally diverse and the attitudes to crime in most communities are also diverse. In many communities, the CJS is modelled after

Western concepts, values, systems, and structures. Nevertheless, research has established the prevalence and functionality of traditional structures such as family courts, royal courts, and other forms of culturally sensitive, community-based crime prevention practices in checking crime in the African continent (5,6). In the UK, the Muslim Arbitration Tribunal, an Alternate Dispute Resolution organization dealing with Sharia law, is recognized under the Arbitration Act (1996).

Cultural attitudes to criminal activity by the mentally disordered

Attitudes towards mental illness vary among individuals, families, ethnicities, cultures, and countries. Cultural and religious teachings often influence beliefs about the origins and nature of mental illness, and shape attitudes towards the mentally ill. In India, for example, culturally, disabilities may be explained as karmic phenomena—someone is disabled because of the bad deeds they did in their previous life. Hence disability is viewed negatively and people with ID go through various forms of abuse (7). In many parts of Africa, mental disorder is a taboo subject that attracts stigma and arouses suspicion, fear, and avoidance (8,9).

Stigma associated with mental illness and negative attitudes towards the mentally ill are a global reality (10–12); in Europe, as late as the twentieth century, the association between low intelligence and crime remained and influenced public thought, models of care, medical education, and public policy. Nee and Watt's research (13) on the public perceptions of crime risk in the mentally ill suggest that perceptions of an individual's propensity to commit crime continue to be somewhat negatively affected by that individual's history of mental illness. With no real evidence base for a link between mental illness and criminal behaviour, this could be described as a stereotypical, discriminatory response.

Intellectual disability and crime

Historically, ID has been described as associated with crime and offending behaviour, a finding reported in studies from different parts of the world, until very recently. Using the Swedish administrative birth cohort sample, Hodgins (14) concluded that men with ID were three times more likely to offend than those without ID. Likewise, Nixon et al. (15) in Australia suggested that people with ID were twice as likely to be charged with a criminal offence with them being 15 times more likely than those without ID to be charged with a sexual offence and three times more likely to be charged with a violent offence. Subsequent studies have suggested that conclusions of this nature could be explained by methodological limitations (16). The suggestion now is that the relationship between intelligence and crime is curvilinear. There is an inverse relationship between rates of criminal activity and the intelligence quotient (IQ), but this disappears when the IQ level is below 70. Thus, while those near the border-lines of normal intellectual functioning seem more likely to be implicated in criminal activity, this finding does not necessarily extend to those with an ID whose IQ levels may be below 70. Indeed, most people with ID are law abiding (17–20). Nevertheless, for the minority of them who encounter the CJS, there are unique challenges, difficulties, vulnerabilities, and needs which often go un-recognized at various levels of the CJS (21–25).

Prevalence

People with ID are over-represented at different stages of the CJS such as police stations and prisons in the UK and internationally (24,26–30). Many studies have reported prevalences of ID in forensic settings; however, due to incon-sistent use of terminology and research methods or flawed research designs, the rates vary widely (31). The highest was in an Israeli study where the prevalence rate of ID in a prison was 69.9% (32) and the lowest was among remand pris-oners in South London, UK, where none of the men had an IQ in the ID range, although the mean Verbal IQ, mean Full Scale IQ, mean reading age, and mean numeracy age were all significantly lower in the index group than in the control group (33).

In English police stations, the prevalence of ID has been reported to be be-tween 6.7% and 8.6% (34,35). Scott et al. (36) found a prevalence of 1% when screening 9000 police records in Northern Ireland. In a sample drawn from accused persons aged over 18 years appearing before four Magistrates Courts in an Australian city, Vanny et al. (37) found that the proportion of participants with an IQ score of less than 70 and significant deficits in adaptive behaviour was more than three times and four times the rate in the general population, respectively.

Chaplin et al. (38) estimated the prevalence of ID in prisoners to be 11% of remand and 5–7% of sentenced prisoners. Hellenbach et al. (39) reported that people with borderline ID (IQ 70–85) constitute between 25% and 30% of in-mates, while another 10% of inmates have mild ID (IQ 50–69). Fazel et al. (40), in looking at ten prison surveys across four countries involving almost 12,000 inmates, suggested that typically 0.5% and 1.5% of prisoners were diagnosed with ID (range 0–2.8% across studies). Søndenaa et al. (41) suggested that up to 10% of sentenced prisoners in Norway had ID. In Australia, it is estimated 9–10% of prisoners about to be released experience ID (42). This high prevalence compares to 1–3% of people in the general population with ID (43,44).

Chester et al. (45) found the prevalence of ID to be 16.5% among 401 long-stay patients in high secure settings and a representative sample of those in medium secure settings in England; and a prevalence rate of 9.2% was found in a large forensic programme of a tertiary psychiatric hospital in Toronto, Ontario, Canada (46).

In non-Western countries, Ghubash and El- Rufaie (47) in the United Arab Emirates found that 4 out of 142 prisoners had an ID in 1999. There are relatively few psychiatrists in many African countries including Nigeria (48); however, Agbahowe et al. (49) in 1998 reported one person with probable mild mental retardation among a sample of 100 prisoners in a medium security prison in Nigeria. While the prevalence of ID in forensic settings in Egypt is not known, El-Khanka is a large forensic psychiatry hospital on the outskirts of Cairo (in the desert) with imposing walls and gates, including armed guards with a specific ward for people with learning disability (50). In India, prevalence rates of the intellectually disabled in the CJS is difficult to obtain as these convictions are made under several other acts such as the Juvenile justice Act (Care and Protection of Children) Act, 2015, the Protection of Children from sexual Offences (POCS0), 2012 and the Mental Health Care Act, 2017 (51–53); hence there are no clear estimates of the number of convicted intellectually disabled people.

Identification of people with intellectual disability in prisons or in police custody

Evidence suggests that in general the types of offences committed by people with ID are comparable to those of other offenders (54). Offenders with ID are like the general offender population especially in their psychological characteristics, social adversities, and other risk factors for offending. Nevertheless, those with ID are likely to experience greater difficulty when they encounter the CJS. Cognitive impairments make them more vulnerable to criminogenic environments (55), they have a lesser ability to conceal their actions, and are more likely to be caught and arrested for their crimes when they do occur (56). Being interviewed can be an extremely frightening and overwhelming experience for people with ID, hence they may be particularly prone in certain circumstances to provide information which is unreliable, misleading, or self-incriminating (57). Increased suggestibility, confabulation, acquiescence, and compliance also increase the vulnerability to making false confessions (59–61).

During court sessions, communication impairments make it difficult for defendants with ID to understand what is being said in court or to make themselves understood and hence effective participation in court proceedings is difficult (62). In prison, communication difficulties can also limit access to services, support, and therapeutic approaches, thus they are likely to experience greater difficulty in coping (63). Individuals with ID are also more vulnerable to bullying, financial, physical, and sexual abuse, and are at greater risk of attempted suicide (21,40).

Due to these vulnerabilities all people who encounter the CJS should be assessed for the presence of ID. The dividing line between 'challenging behaviour' and 'offending behaviour' is often blurred (64). Eliciting intention to commit crime (*mens rea*) is important in legally determining the difference between challenging behaviour and criminal behaviour and when ascertaining legal responsibility (20). Even for experienced professionals working with people with ID, it is not always easy to recognize those with ID, particularly in a setting away from home, such as prison or a police station (21). Identifying ID in the CJS is complicated by the wide range of diagnostic and classification criteria used, as well as the variety of assessment tools utilized by clinicians and researchers (18).

In India, there are many recommendations in the Juvenile Justice Act for care, psychological evaluation, and treatment of all offenders. This will help to identify those with mental illness, borderline intelligence levels, personality disorders, or other mental health conditions, thus ensuring their care and treatment. However, this ideal contrasts very sharply with the current conditions in Indian remand homes with inadequate and unqualified staff.

Making a diagnosis of ID involves formal assessments of intelligence and adaptive functioning including taking a developmental history to establish onset before the age of 18 years. This involves qualified personnel, can be time intensive, and often is not done in the early stages of contact with the CJS; referrals for full-scale diagnostic assessment generally only occur when intellectual difficulties are suspected, leading to an underestimation of the prevalence of ID in these settings (65,66). Therefore, the use of reliable screening tools that suggest the possibility of ID and help professionals decide about the need for more formal diagnostic assessments is encouraged (67).

Screening questions have some utility, but even when used, it is suggested that some people with ID are not being identified (68). Screening questions such as whether the person had 'reading problems or learning difficulties' or 'had been to special school' (33) may unwittingly sample many people with borderline ID. Also, like formal, psychometric, and IQ tests, they are largely irrelevant in many developing countries and more seriously may prove to be culturally biased against minority groups (69).

The Hayes Ability Screening Index (HASI) was developed by Susan Hayes (70) as a screening tool; it is a brief instrument that can be administered and scored by any trained staff in 10–15 minutes. It consists of three short tests measuring spelling, visuospatial, and visuo-constructional abilities including collecting background information about learning difficulties that are already known. The HASI has been shown to be a valid, user-friendly, and time-saving instrument for screening ID in the Australian CJS and among offender and non-offender samples in Norway, and it was found to be a suitable, time-efficient, and resource-conscious way to detect ID in persons with a substance problem among a Dutch speaking sample (66,71–73). However, in an adolescent offender sample in the UK the HASI was reported as not having adequate specificity to be helpful in identifying possible ID (74).

The 'Learning Disability Screening Questionnaire' was originally developed to screen people for ID when they were referred to community learning disability teams (75); it is brief, requires no special equipment, can be used by prison staff with minimal training, needs no formal psychology qualification (76), and has been validated in three forensic settings: a community ID forensic service, a forensic in-patient secure unit, and a prison—although using a relatively small sample of just 94 individuals (77). Though it has been considered the best available validated screening tool suitable for use by prison staff (78), since it is a screening tool, it is limited in rating ID (21).

More recently, the Glasgow Level of Ability and Development Scale (GLADS) (79) has been shown to be able to categorize ID accurately and to have good psychometric properties. It is quick to administer and popular with professionals. The GLADS may therefore be particularly useful in lower- and middle-income countries where specialist services are not available (21).

Boer et al. (21) suggested some simple (untested) screening questions such as:

1. Does the interviewer think the person has ID?
2. Does the person, the family, or carers think he or she has ID?
3. Does the person have any problems in reading, writing, or filling in forms?
4. Has he or she been to special school or special educational support in mainstream school, or has he or she had to drop out of mainstream school?
5. Is there any history of ID or of contact with ID services (community services, hospital)?
6. Is the person capable of living independently? Does the person need support from family or carers to support him- or herself?
7. Is the person able to travel independently?
8. (If applicable) Is the person able to use technology such as mobile phones, the Internet, television, radio, and so on?

Associated conditions

Mental disorders are common in people with ID. People with ID can experience the full range of mental disorders that occur in the general population and some mental disorders that are infrequent in the general population (79). About a third of people with ID have a mental health comorbidity (80). In hospital settings, rates of major mental illness may be as high as 50% (81). This is in addition to other comorbid neurodevelopmental conditions (such as autism spectrum disorders and attention deficit hyperactivity disorder), personality disorders, substance misuse, and physical conditions such as epilepsy, visual impairments, hearing impairments, gastro-oesophageal reflux disorder, dysphagia, constipation, diabetes, thyroid dysfunction, osteoporosis, contractures, mobility and balance impairments, injuries, eczema, xerosis, obesity, heart failure, and possibly asthma (79,82–85).

Whereas among mainstream prisoners a systematic review reported a prevalence of 3.7% and 11.4% for psychotic illness and major depression, respectively (86), for prisoners with ID, the estimated lifetime and current prevalence of co-occurring mental disorders was 52.5% and 37.2%, respectively (16). For individuals treated within or referred to forensic (i.e. secure) hospital services for those with ID, similarly high figures are reported. Comorbid personality disorder may be present in up to 50%, up to a third have an autism spectrum disorder, the prevalence of comorbid major mental illness and substance misuse/dependence is similar at about 30–50%, and about a fifth have epilepsy (87,88).

Thus, the presentation of ID is even more complex than that of patients without ID with significant multimorbidity of major mental illness, neurodevelopmental conditions, personality disorders, substance misuse, and physical health conditions. Often these conditions are unrecognized because the symptoms are attributed to ID (diagnostic overshadowing). Contact with the CJS may be due to a new presentation of one of these conditions, and professionals dealing with offenders should consider this (21).

Pathways of care

Offenders with ID, like the general population, have a right to be held accountable for intentional actions, to have fair boundaries set, and to have the full range of sentencing options available to them (21), and a balance should be struck between diverting people with ID and significant mental health problems from the CJS and those factors favouring prosecution and safeguarding the public (89). 'Appropriate Diversion' was described by Lord Bradley as 'a process whereby people are assessed and their needs identified as early as possible in the offender pathway (including prevention and early intervention), thus informing subsequent decisions about where an individual is best placed to receive treatment, taking into account public safety, safety of the individual and punishment of an offence' (90).

In the UK, the journey of an offender with ID (unlike that of non-disabled offenders) can often be complex, but there are various opportunities for support and diversion into more suitable and appropriate systems of care. In Australia, there also exist a variety of court and other diversion and transitional schemes, albeit their long-term success in keeping people with cognitive disorders already arrested by police out of ongoing CJS enmeshment and reoffending appears to be limited (91). In Ireland, mental health assessment is provided by the prison primary care staff with some input from forensic psychiatrists but screening for ID is lacking (92).

In Norwegian criminal law, criminal responsibility is determined by the defendant's mental health status at the time of the crime and causal or correlational relationship between the mental condition and the crime is not required. Persons above the age of 15 years who commit crimes and are found to have moderate ID (with an intellectual functioning level corresponding to an IQ of <55) are absolved from criminal responsibility and punishment while offenders with an IQ higher than 55 are viewed as criminally responsible and are thus given a regular sentence, to be served either in prison or in society (e.g. community service). In cases of very serious and life-threatening offences or where the risk of reoffending is high, rather than being fully acquitted, offenders with an IQ less than 55 can be sentenced to so-called mandatory care where the person is under the responsibility of the specialist health services (93).

In many former colonies of the British empire like Nigeria and India, the judicial system has a lot of similarities with the British system; the doctrine of *mens rea* presupposes that for an act (*actus reus*) to be criminal, there needs to be a criminal intent motivating it. In India, the Rights of People with Disabilities Act, 2016, has rights-based perspective advocating for rights, privileges of the disabled, and prevention of discrimination (94). This piece of legislation allows for the assessment of severity of disability (95,96) which is used during the conviction and trial. In Nigeria, the 1999 Constitution contains an extensive list of human rights, including due process rights, which should be accorded to every citizen of Nigeria regardless of their mental capabilities. Although there is no specific legislation to ensure that people with intellectual disability who commit crimes are redirected from the CJS and referred to mental healthcare, anecdotal evidence suggests that most are resolved through community based, culturally informed alternative dispute resolution structures.

Within the UK, the Bradley report (90) recommends early identification of people with ID when they encounter the CJS, clear referral protocols, appropriate training for those working within the CJS, and appropriate community-based treatment and care packages for those at risk. Those who have screened positive using a screening questionnaire should be referred to mental healthcare staff, with expertise in assessment and treatment of ID. Where there are comorbid mental disorders or needs, referral to a psychiatric team able to deal with people with ID is warranted. In cases where there is doubt that the person has ID, a referral to a psychologist for formal psychological testing may be necessary; thus, it is important that the professional working with offenders with developmental disorders has a good relationship with local health and social services providing for those with ID (7).

Conclusion

In conclusion, people with ID should have rights which are comparable to the general population. In view of their vulnerability and limited understanding, they may have difficulty in exercising their rights within CJSs, and they may consequently need extra support at all levels of the CJS. Screening for ID should be adopted by police stations, courts, and prisons, such that people with ID can be recognized early and where possible diverted from custody. Governmental departments, agencies, and organizations working with offenders with ID need to work together to create local pathways of care. Community and inpatient services should be available such that they can be managed safely in the least restrictive setting.

References

1. **American Association on Intellectual and Developmental Disabilities**. Intellectual Disability. Definition, Classification, and System of Supports. The 11th Edition of the ASIDD Definition Manual. Washington, DC: American Association on Intellectual and Developmental Disabilities; 2010.
2. **US Department of Health and Human Services**. Mental Health: A Report of the Surgeon General. Rockville, MD: US Department of Health and Human Services; 1999.
3. **Tylor EB.** Primitive Culture. London: John Murray; 1871.
4. **Petrus T.** Cultural beliefs, witchcraft and crimes in South Africa. In: **Sadique K, Stanislas P**, editors. Religion, Faith and Crime. London: Palgrave Macmillan; 2016: 137–66.
5. **Ojebode A, Ojebuyi BR, Onyechi NJ, Oladapo O, Oyedele OJ, Fadipe IA.** Explaining the Effectiveness of Community-Based Crime Prevention Practices in Ibadan, Nigeria. Enugu, Nigeria: Institute of Development Studies; 2016.
6. **Tade O, Olaitan F.** Traditional structures of crime control in Lagos, Nigeria. African Security Review 2015;**24**(2):138–52.
7. **Chaturvedi S.** Culture and disability. Indian Anthropologist 2019;**49**(1):67–82.

8. **Gureje OY, Lasebikan VO, Ephraim-Oluwanuga O, Olley BO, Kola L.** Community study of knowledge of and attitude to mental illness in Nigeria. British Journal of Psychiatry 2005;**186**(5):436–41.

9. **Adewuya AO, Makanjuola RO.** Social distance towards people with mental illness in southwestern Nigeria. Australian & New Zealand Journal of Psychiatry 2008;**42**(5):389–95.

10. **Jorm AF, Korten AE, Jacomb PA, Christensen H, Henderson S.** Attitudes towards people with a mental disorder: a survey of the Australian public and health professionals. Australian & New Zealand Journal of Psychiatry 1999;**33**(1):77–83.

11. **Furnham A, Wong L.** A cross-cultural comparison of British and Chinese beliefs about the causes, behaviour manifestations and treatment of schizophrenia. Psychiatry Research 2007;**151**(1–2):123–38.

12. **Ng CH.** The stigma of mental illness in Asian cultures. Australian & New Zealand Journal of Psychiatry 1997;**31**(3):382–90.

13. **Nee C, Witt C.** Public perceptions of risk in criminality: the effects of mental illness and social disadvantage. Psychiatry Research 2013;**209**(3):675–83.

14. **Hodgins S.** Mental disorder, intellectual deficiency, and crime: evidence from a birth cohort. Archives of General Psychiatry 1992;**49**(6):476–83.

15. **Nixon M, Thomas SD, Daffern M, Ogloff JR.** Estimating the risk of crime and victimisation in people with intellectual disability: a data-linkage study. Social Psychiatry and Psychiatric Epidemiology 2017;**52**(5):617–26.

16. **Taylor JL, Lindsay WR, Devapriam J.** Offending behaviours in people with intellectual disabilities. In: **Baumik S, Alexander R,** editors. Oxford Textbook of Psychiatry of Intellectual Disability. Oxford: Oxford University Press; 2020: 169–70.

17. **Holland T, Clare IC, Mukhopadhyay T.** Prevalence of criminal offending by men and women with intellectual disability and the characteristics of offenders: implications for research and service development. Journal of Intellectual Disability Research 2002;**46**(Suppl 1):6–20.

18. **Jones J.** Persons with intellectual disabilities in the criminal justice system: review of issues. International Journal of Offender Therapy and Comparative Criminology 2007;**51**(6):723–33.

19. **Fazel S, Xenitidis K, Powell J.** The prevalence of intellectual disabilities among 12000 prisoners—a systematic review. International Journal of Law and Psychiatry 2008;**31**(4):369–73.

20. **Chester V.** People with intellectual and developmental disorders in the United Kingdom criminal justice system. East Asian Archives of Psychiatry 2018;**28**(4):150–8.

21. **Boer H, Alexander R, Devapriam J, Torales J, Ng R, Castaldelli-Maia J,** et al. Prisoner mental health care for people with intellectual disability. International Journal of Culture and Mental Health 2016;**9**(4):442–6.

22. **Taylor JL, McKinnon I, Thorpe I, Gillmer BT.** The impact of transforming care on the care and safety of patients with intellectual disabilities and forensic needs. BJPsych Bulletin 2017;**41**(4):205–8.

23. **Brolan CE, Ware RS, Gomez MT, Lennox NG.** The right to health of Australians with intellectual disability. Australian Journal of Human Rights 2011;**17**(2):1–32.

24. **Shepherd SM, Ogloff JR, Shea D, Pfeifer JE, Paradies Y.** Aboriginal prisoners and cognitive impairment: the impact of dual disadvantage on Social and Emotional Wellbeing. Journal of Intellectual Disability Research 2017;**61**(4):385–97.

25. **Maxwell Y, Day A, Casey S.** Understanding the needs of vulnerable prisoners: the role of social and emotional wellbeing. International Journal of Prisoner Health 2013;**9**(2):57–67.

26. **Silva D, Gough K, Weeks H.** Screening for learning disabilities in the criminal justice system: a review of existing measures for use within liaison and diversion services. Journal of Intellectual Disabilities and Offending Behaviour 2015;**6**(1):33–43.

27. **Cockram J.** Justice or differential treatment? Sentencing of offenders with an intellectual disability. Journal of Intellectual and Developmental Disability 2005;**30**(1):3–13.

28. **Hayes S.** Suicide and Offenders with Intellectual Disability—What Do We Know? Disability and the Criminal Justice System: Achievements and Challenges. Conference presented by the Australian Community Support Organisation, Department of Justice Victoria and Office of the Public Advocate.

29. **Hayes S, Shackell P, Mottram P, Lancaster R.** The prevalence of intellectual disability in a major UK prison. British Journal of Learning Disabilities 2007;**35**(3):162–7.

30. **Talbot J.** No One Knows. London: Prison Reform Trust; 2008.

31. **McBrien J.** The intellectually disabled offender: methodological problems in identification. Journal of Applied Research in Intellectual Disabilities 2003;**16**(2):95–105.

32. **Einat T, Einat A.** Learning disabilities and delinquency: a study of Israeli prison inmates. International Journal of Offender Therapy and Comparative Criminology 2008;**52**(4):416–34.

33. **Murphy GH, Harnett H, Holland AJ.** A survey of intellectual disabilities amongst men on remand in prison. Mental Handicap Research 1995;**8**(2):81–98.

34. **Young S, Goodwin EJ, Sedgwick O, Gudjonsson GH.** The effectiveness of police custody assessments in identifying suspects with intellectual disabilities and attention deficit hyperactivity disorder. BMC Medicine 2013;**11**:248.

35. **Gudjonsson GH, Clare IC, Rutter S, Pearse J.** Persons at Risk During Interviews in Police Custody: The Identification of Vulnerabilities. London: HM Stationery Office; 1992.

36. **Scott D, McGilloway SI, Donnelly M.** The mental health needs of people with a learning disability detained in police custody. Medicine, Science and the Law 2006;**46**(2):111–14.

37. **Vanny KA, Levy MH, Greenberg DM, Hayes SC.** Mental illness and intellectual disability in magistrates courts in New South Wales, Australia. Journal of Intellectual Disability Research 2009;**53**(3):289–97.

38. **Chaplin E, McCarthy J, Underwood L, Forrester A, Hayward H, Sabet J,** et al. Characteristics of prisoners with intellectual disabilities. Journal of Intellectual Disability Research 2017;**61**(12):1185–95.

39. **Hellenbach M, Karatzias T, Brown M.** Intellectual disabilities among prisoners: prevalence and mental and physical health comorbidities. Journal of Applied Research in Intellectual Disabilities 2017;**30**(2):230–41.

40. **Fazel S, Xenitidis K, Powell J.** The prevalence of intellectual disabilities among 12 000 prisoners—a systematic review. International Journal of Law and Psychiatry 2008;**31**(4):369–73.

41. **Søndenaa E, Palmstierna T, Iversen VC.** A stepwise approach to identify intellectual disabilities in the criminal justice system. European Journal of Psychology Applied to Legal Contex 2010;**2**(2):183–98.

42. **Dias S, Ware RS, Kinner SA, Lennox NG.** Co-occurring mental disorder and intellectual disability in a large sample of Australian prisoners. Australian & New Zealand Journal of Psychiatry 2013;**47**(10):938–44.

43. **Harris JC.** Intellectual Disability: Understanding its Development, Causes, Classification, Evaluation, and Treatment. Oxford: Oxford University Press; 2006.

44. **Maulik PK, Mascarenhas MN, Mathers CD, Dua T, Saxena S.** Prevalence of intellectual disability: a meta-analysis of population-based studies. Research in Developmental Disabilities 2011;**32**(2):419–36.

45. **Chester V, Völlm B, Tromans S, Kapugama C, Alexander RT.** Long-stay patients with and without intellectual disability in forensic psychiatric settings: comparison of characteristics and needs. BJPsych Open 2018;**4**(4):226–34.

46. **Ray I, Simpson AI, Jones RM, Shatokhina K, Thakur A, Mulsant BH.** Clinical, demographic, and criminal behavior characteristics of patients with intellectual disabilities in a Canadian forensic program. Frontiers in Psychiatry 2019;**10**:760.

47. **Ghubash R, El-Rufaie O.** Psychiatric morbidity among sentenced male prisoners in Dubai: transcultural perspectives. Journal of Forensic Psychiatry 1997;**8**(2):440–6.

48. **Ogunlesi AO, Ogunwale A, De Wet P, Roos L, Kaliski S.** Forensic psychiatry in Africa: prospects and challenges: guest editorial. African Journal of Psychiatry 2012;**15**(1):3.

49. **Agbahowe SA, Ohaeri JU, Ogunlesi AO, Osahon R.** Prevalence of psychiatric morbidity among convicted inmates in a Nigerian prison community. East African Medical Journal 1998;**75**(1):19–26.

50. **Boer H, O'Brien G.** Offenders with learning disability in Egypt. Learning Disability Psychiatry 2010; **12**(2):8–9.

51. **Gazette of India.** The juvenile justice (care and protection of children) Act, 2015. Available from https://cara.nic.in/PDF/JJ%20act%202015.pdf (accessed 7 July 2023).

52. **Ministry of Law and Justice.** The Protection of Children from Sexual Offences Act, 2012. 2012. Available from: https://wcd.nic.in/sites/default/files/POCSO%20 Act%2C%202012.pdf

53. **The Gazette of India.** Mental Healthcare Act 2017. Available from https://web.archive.org/web/20191012072136/http://www.prsindia.org/uploads/media/Mental%20Health/Mental%20Healthcare%20Act,%202017.pdf (accessed 7 July 2023).

54. **Murphy G, Mason J.** Forensic and offending behaviours. In: **Tsakanikos E, McCarthy J,** editors. Handbook of Psychopathology in Intellectual Disability. New York: Springer; 2014: 281–303.

55. **Salekin KL, Olley JG, Hedge KA.** Offenders with intellectual disability: characteristics, prevalence, and issues in forensic assessment. Journal of Mental Health Research in Intellectual Disabilities 2010;**3**(2):97–116.

56. **Alexander RT, Chester V, Green FN, Gunaratna I, Hoare S.** Arson or fire setting in offenders with intellectual disability: clinical characteristics, forensic histories,

and treatment outcomes. Journal of Intellectual and Developmental Disability 2015;**40**(2):189–97.

57. **Home Office.** Police and Criminal Evidence Act. London: Home Office; 1985.

58. **Gudjonsson GH.** The relationship of intelligence and memory to interrogative suggestibility: the importance of range effects. British Journal of Clinical Psychology 1988;**27**(2):185–7.

59. **Clare IC, Gudjonsson GH.** The vulnerability of suspects with intellectual disabilities during police interviews: a review and experimental study of decision-making. Mental Handicap Research 1995;**8**(2):110–28.

60. **Gudjonsson GH, Clare IC.** The relationship between confabulation and intellectual ability, memory, interrogative suggestibility and acquiescence. Personality and Individual Differences 1995;**19**(3):333–8.

61. **Finlay WM, Lyons E.** Acquiescence in interviews with people who have mental retardation. Mental Retardation 2002;**40**(1):14–29.

62. **Talbot J.** No one knows: offenders with learning disabilities and learning difficulties. International Journal of Prisoner Health 2009;**5**(3):141–52.

63. **Talbot J.** Prisoners' voices: experiences of the criminal justice system by prisoners with learning disabilities. Tizard Learning Disability Review 2010;**15**(3):33–41.

64. **Douds F, Bantwal A.** The 'forensicisation' of challenging behaviour: the perils of people with learning disabilities and severe challenging behaviours being viewed as 'forensic' patients. Journal of Learning Disabilities and Offending Behaviour 2011;**2**(3):110–13.

65. **Hayes S.** Missing out: offenders with learning disabilities and the criminal justice system. British Journal of Learning Disabilities 2007;**35**(3):146–53.

66. **Herrington V, Hunter G, Harvey S.** Meeting the healthcare needs of offenders with learning disabilities. Learning Disability Practice 2005;**8**(4):28–32.

67. **To WT, Vanheule S, Vanderplasschen W, Audenaert K, Vandevelde S.** Screening for intellectual disability in persons with a substance abuse problem: exploring the validity of the Hayes Ability Screening Index in a Dutch-speaking sample. Research in Developmental Disabilities 2015;**36**:498–504.

68. **McKinnon IG, Grubin D.** Health screening of people in police custody—evaluation of current police screening procedures in London, UK. European Journal of Public Health 2013;**23**(3):399–405.

69. **Roy M, Balaratnasingam S.** Intellectual disability and indigenous Australians: an overview. Asia-Pacific Psychiatry 2014;**6**(4):363–72.

70. **Hayes SC.** Hayes Ability Screening Index: HASI: Manual. Sydney: University of Sydney; 2000.

71. **Hayes SC.** Early intervention or early incarceration? Using a screening test for intellectual disability in the criminal justice system. Journal of Applied Research in Intellectual Disabilities 2002;**15**(2):120–8.

72. **Søndenaa E, Bjørgen TG, Nøttestad JA.** Validation of the Norwegian version of Hayes ability screening index for mental retardation. Psychological Reports 2007;**101**(3 Suppl):1023–30.

73. **Søndenaa E, Rasmussen K, Palmstierna T, Nøttestad J.** The prevalence and nature of intellectual disability in Norwegian prisons. Journal of Intellectual Disability Research 2008;**52**(12):1129–37.

74. **Ford G, Andrews R, Booth A, Dibdin J, Hardingham S, Kelly TP.** Screening for learning disability in an adolescent forensic population. Journal of Forensic Psychiatry & Psychology 2008;**19**(3):371–81.

75. **McKenzie K, Paxton D.** Learning disability screening questionnaire. Edinburgh: GCM Records; 2005.

76. **Murphy GH, Gardner J, Freeman MJ.** Screening prisoners for intellectual disabilities in three English prisons. Journal of Applied Research in Intellectual Disabilities 2017;**30**(1):198–204.

77. **McKenzie K, Michie A, Murray A, Hales C.** Screening for offenders with an intellectual disability: the validity of the Learning Disability Screening Questionnaire. Research in Developmental Disabilities 2012;**33**(3):791–5.

78. **Cooray S, Cooper SA, Weber G, Bhaumik S, Roy A, Gangadharan S,** et al. The clinical utility of the Glasgow Level of Ability and Development Scale in screening for disorders of intellectual development: a multicentre international study. Journal of Intellectual Disability Research 2016;**60**(7–8):775.

79. **Cooper SA.** Types of mental disorders in people with intellectual disability In: **Baumik S, Alexander R,** editors. Oxford Textbook of Psychiatry of Intellectual Disability. Oxford: Oxford University Press; 2020: 169–70.

80. **Cooper SA, Smiley E, Morrison J, Williamson A, Allan L.** Mental ill-health in adults with intellectual disabilities: prevalence and associated factors. British Journal of Psychiatry 2007;**190**(1):27–35.

81. **Alexander RT, Piachaud J, Singh I.** Two districts, two models: in-patient care in the psychiatry of learning disability. British Journal of Development Disabilities 2001;**47**(93):105–10.

82. **Bowley C, Kerr M.** Epilepsy and intellectual disability. Journal of Intellectual Disability Research 2000;**44**(5):529–43.

83. **McCarron M, Swinburne J, Burke E, McGlinchey E, Carroll R, McCallion P.** Patterns of multimorbidity in an older population of persons with an intellectual disability: results from the intellectual disability supplement to the Irish longitudinal study on aging (IDS-TILDA). Research in Developmental Disabilities 2013;**34**(1):521–7.

84. **Böhmer CJ, Niezen-de Boer MC, Klinkenberg-Knol EC, Devillé WL, Nadorp JH, Meuwissen SG.** The prevalence of gastroesophageal reflux disease in institutionalized intellectually disabled individuals. American Journal of Gastroenterology 1999;**94**(3):804–10.

85. **Robertson J, Chadwick D, Baines S, Emerson E, Hatton C.** Prevalence of dysphagia in people with intellectual disability: a systematic review. Intellectual and Developmental Disabilities 2017;**55**(6):377–91.

86. **Fazel S, Seewald K.** Severe mental illness in 33 588 prisoners worldwide: systematic review and meta-regression analysis. British Journal of Psychiatry 2012;**200**(5):364–73.

87. **Alexander RT, Crouch K, Halstead S, Piachaud J.** Long-term outcome from a medium secure service for people with intellectual disability. Journal of Intellectual Disability Research 2006;**50**(4):305–15.

88. **Plant A, Mcdermott E, Chester V, Alexander RT.** Substance misuse among offenders in a forensic intellectual disability service. Journal of Learning Disabilities and Offending Behaviour 2011;**2**(3):127–35.

89. **Royal College of Psychiatrists**. Forensic care pathways in people with learning disabilities. 2014. Available from: https://www.rcpsych.ac.uk/docs/default-source/members/faculties/intellectual-disability/id-fr-id-04.pdf?sfvrsn=ba5ce38a_4

90. **Department of Health**. The Bradley Report: Lord Bradley's Review of People with Mental Health Problems or Learning Disabilities in the Criminal Justice System. London: Department of Health; 2009.

91. **Baldry E, Dowse L, Clarence M.** People with mental and cognitive disabilities: pathways into prison. In: Background Paper for Outlaws to Inclusion Conference UNSW, Sydney, February 2012.

92. **Gulati G, Quigley S, Murphy VE, Yacoub E, Bogue J, Kearns A,** et al. A novel care pathway for prisoners with intellectual disability designed through a Delphi process. International Journal of Prisoner Health 2018;**14**(4):276–86.

93. **Søndenaa E, Friestad C, Storvik B, Johnsen B.** Criminal responsibility and challenges in the criminal justice system for people with intellectual disability in Norway. Bergen Journal of Criminal Law & Criminal Justice 2019;**7**(1):97–109.

94. **Sundaray NK.** Annual Report. National Trust for People with Autism, Cerebral Palsy, Intellectual disabilities and Multiple disabilities. Department of Empowerment for People with Disabilities. Delhi: Ministry of Justice and Social Welfare; 2021.

95. **Kishore MT, Udipi GA, Seshadri SP.** Clinical practice guidelines for assessment and management of intellectual disability. Indian Journal of Psychiatry 2019;**61**(Suppl 2):194.

96. **Chavan BS, Rozatkar AR.** Intellectual disability in India: charity to right based. Indian Journal of Psychiatry 2014;**56**(2):113–16.

Part 4

Service models in different parts of the world

Chapter 15

Intellectual disability services in North America

Anupam Thakur, Ruth Chau,
Muhammad Irfan Jiwa, Prabhleen Jaggi, and
Yona Lunsky

Introduction

North America includes the countries of Canada, the US, and Mexico. Most of the authors who contributed to this chapter are from Canada and so naturally the chapter has more details and emphasis on services in Canada but relevant information from the US and Mexico is included in separate sections.

Mental health care of adults with intellectual and developmental disabilities in Canada
Introduction

> Michael is a 36-year-old male diagnosed with intellectual disability (ID), moderate in severity, living with his elderly parents in suburban Toronto. He has limited vocabulary and communicates in small sentences. He has an underlying genetic syndrome and several physical health conditions including epilepsy, diabetes mellitus, and hypertension. Michael has long-standing difficulties related to aggression and self-injurious behaviours, which have resulted in numerous emergency room visits and several hospitalizations lasting days to weeks. He has taken multiple antipsychotic medications over the years and, lately, has developed dyskinetic movements around his lips and hands. He receives support from a community agency and is on the waitlist for a specialized residential setting.

Nearly one in every 100 adults in Ontario, Canada, have an intellectual or developmental disability (IDD) (1). Similar to Michael, many people with IDD have a chronic and complex clinical presentation, which has been associated with poorer health outcomes. In a cross-sectoral linked data study in Ontario, Canada, Lin et al. (2019) found that adults with IDD were twice as likely to have repeat emergency room visits, more likely to be re-hospitalized within a month of discharge, and 17.5 times more likely to be living in a long-term care facility at a young age (2). People with IDD have higher rates of mental health issues (1), with one population-based study reporting that 44% of adults with IDD had a diagnosis of mental illness (3). Lunsky et al. (2018) reported the high use of psychotropic drugs in this population (4). Lin and colleagues (2016) reported a greater incidence of chronic physical health conditions, such as diabetes, hypertension, and chronic obstructive pulmonary disease, in the IDD population compared to those without IDD (5). In addition, people with IDD are four times more likely to die before the age of 75 as compared to those who do not have IDD (2). These numbers suggest that people with IDD have high mental health comorbidity, are high users of healthcare resources, and are at a higher risk of dying prematurely (6). The COVID-19 pandemic has further exposed the vulnerabilities of this population with studies from around the world suggesting a greater likelihood of COVID hospitalizations and death in those with IDD relative to other adults (7–10). It can be a challenge to bridge this wide gap in healthcare of people with IDD. This section describes the mental healthcare of Canadian adults with IDD from a health system perspective.

A macro–meso–micro-level perspective

This section reviews the mental healthcare of adults with IDD at the level of healthcare policy (macro), healthcare organizations (meso), and patient care (micro) (11). Canada is a federation of ten provinces and three territories, with a population of 38.3 million (12). At a *macro level*, health and social care are a responsibility of the provinces and territories. The Canada Health Act (R.S.C 1985) (13) lays down the framework for insurance-based healthcare services provided by the individual provinces and territories of Canada.

Federal disability legislation includes the Accessibility Canada Act of 2019, which lays down the provisions to support equality for people with disability, including IDD (14). The Act recognizes the Canadian Charter of Rights and Freedoms, the Canadian Human Rights Act, and Canada's commitment to the United Nations Convention on the Rights of Persons with Disabilities. The priority areas covered in the Act include employment, built environments such as buildings and public spaces, and transportation for supporting people with disability. However, federal legislation does not dictate how healthcare services are provided, which means there is extensive variability across the country. Most provinces and territories have health ministries responsible for healthcare delivery and a separate ministry responsible for social services. This can lead to a siloing of services for people with IDD. In the province of Ontario, the Developmental Disabilities Act, 2008, lays down the foundation for supporting people with IDD in adulthood (15). The law includes supports for person-directed planning and direct funding support to help people with developmental disabilities have more choice and flexibility in alignment with their needs. The Community Living Authority Act, 2004 in British Columbia governs how services are provided to people with IDD in British Columbia (16). Similar legislation in other provinces, such as the Persons with Developmental Disabilities Services Act in Alberta, ensures the provision of programmes, resources, and services for people with IDD (17). The eligibility for such services varies by province, and the age groups targeted can also vary. These three provinces have additional legislation which focuses on accessibility across disabilities, which should help with access to services, including healthcare.

In Canada, programmes have been developed to help coordinate interprofessional health services for adults with IDD. In some cases, clinical health services can be provided as part of the social services offered to this population. In others, these services are strictly the responsibility of healthcare providers. At a *meso level*, Developmental Services Ontario is the point of access for services for adults with IDD (18). As part of its role, it carries out eligibility assessments and acts as a gateway to government-funded services, including specialist and clinical services, respite services, and housing support. Similar programmes also exist for care coordination in other provincial jurisdictions, such as Community Living British Columbia (19) and the Persons with Developmental Disabilities programme in Alberta (20). Mental health services for people with IDD in British Columbia, 12 years and older, are directed through Developmental Disabilities Mental Health Services (21) which are delivered through one of several regional specialized mental health teams. The services include behavioural, psychological, psychiatric assessment and treatment, and counselling. Inpatient care for adults with IDD is mostly provided in general psychiatry units although some hospitals have tertiary-level specialist inpatient units for adults with IDD, such as Ontario Shores (Whitby, Canada) (22). Adults with IDD and forensic issues are supported within the general forensic services, and are grossly over-represented in these settings (23–25). There are other legislations at a provincial level that lay down provisions for quality clinical care. The Public Hospitals Act (26), Excellent Care for All Act (27), and Mental Health Act (28) in Ontario are some examples of legislation that support best governance practice of hospital-based mental healthcare.

Primary care practitioners are at the core of the circle of care for people with IDD at a *micro level*. Family physicians and nurse practitioners are often the most consistent care provider for screening, identification, and management of mental health needs. These needs are further compounded by factors related to the social determinants of health, such as housing, relationships, poverty, and culture. Grier and colleagues (2018) describe a 'generalist expert' approach in addressing complexities related to mental health and physical health in this population, including needs related to communication and care coordination

(29). In Ontario, there are a select number of specialized interdisciplinary teams that may include a behaviour therapist, an occupational therapist, a social worker, a nurse, a clinical psychologist, and a psychiatrist. The teams work collaboratively to provide person-centred care, either through a hospital or a community social services agency. There are not enough of these specialized teams to meet the needs of the entire population, however, and huge service gaps remain (2). Along with the care provided by the health sector, service providers from the social services sector form the backbone of support for mental health issues in adults with IDD. The frontline staff who tend to provide most of the care receive 1–2 years of community college training with some introductory education about mental health and IDD.

Understanding mental health needs at a systems level

The Canadian Survey on Disability (30), a national cross-sectional survey in Canada, illuminates the needs of the IDD population. The survey is administered annually for people 15 years and older who have functional limitations due to a health-related problem or condition. While not specific to people with IDD, the results of the survey have provided important systems-level information about health and social care needs of those with disabilities. The findings from the 2017 survey were not surprising, showing that people with disabilities are less likely to finish high-school or post-secondary education, participate in the labour force or be employed, and earn on average less per year in total income. Over the years, cross-sectoral collaborations such as the Health Care Access Research and Developmental Disabilities (H-CARDD) programme have led to a better understanding of the care needs of the IDD population. H-CARDD was launched to bring scientists, clinicians, patients, and families together to understand and respond to the most pressing healthcare needs experienced by the IDD population (31). The goal of this programme is to monitor and improve the health of people with IDD in Ontario, Canada. The programme weaves through the macro, meso, and micro levels by actively engaging researchers, policymakers, healthcare planners, clinicians, adults with IDD, and caregivers.

In its first phase (2010–2013), the programme focused on assessing the quality of primary care for people with IDD through the creation of a linked data set across Ontario's social services and health sectors (1). The initiative found that within a cohort of over 66,000 adults with developmental disabilities, those with IDD had higher rates of morbidity, were more likely to be diagnosed with chronic diseases, had higher rates of preventable hospitalization, received less preventative screening, and were prescribed higher rates of antipsychotics, compared to adults without disabilities (32–34).

In the second phase (2013–2016), the programme identified four areas of care for people with IDD that needed attention: those with mental health needs, care for women with IDD, transitional youth, and ageing adults (31). Regarding mental health, H-CARDD found that adults with IDD who had a mental illness or addiction had the highest rates of physician, hospital, or emergency room care compared to adults with only IDD or those without IDD. They also had higher repeat service use, including 30-day readmissions and 30-day repeat emergency room visits (3). Healthcare utilization data generated in this programme provide helpful system-level information for policymakers and programme planners as they determine programme development.

Barriers in intellectual and developmental disabilities mental healthcare

Siloed systems

H-CARDD and other initiatives have assisted in the recognition of key issues in the care of people with IDD, including a need to strengthen primary care, improve coordinated interprofessional care in the community, and develop a more patient- and family-centred approach. While the prevalence of need has been better understood, there remains a dearth of effective mental healthcare and supports for individuals with IDD. One of the barriers to IDD care in Canada include the siloed nature of the government systems responsible for IDD supports and services. For people with IDD, particularly those with a dual diagnosis and complex care needs, there is significant overlap in health, mental health, and social care needs. In Ontario there are two separate ministries primarily involved in IDD care: the Ministry of Health and Long-Term Care, which oversees health services delivery (35), and the Ministry of Children, Community and Social Services (MCCSS), which oversees developmental services (36). Funding support streams are separated, with the Ministry of Health and Long-Term Care providing funding for healthcare, and the MCCSS providing funding for the Ontario Disability Support Program and funding for community participation (called the Passport Program) through Developmental Services Ontario (18). Similar siloing has also been identified in other parts of the country (37). Collaborative efforts across ministries can help with integration of clinical and psychosocial care needs.

Canada can seek solutions to this issue by looking to other jurisdictions which have successfully integrated services across sectors. This leads to better coordination of services based on needs of the patient, and a simpler experience navigating the system from the patient's perspective. For example, the Health and Care Bill in the UK promotes greater integration between health and social care services and covers all of England as part of an integrated care system (38).

Lack of IDD-specific training among healthcare providers

Another issue is the lack of exposure and training surrounding IDD in health education curricula. Despite the significant prevalence of IDD, the core curricula of health professionals' education do not sufficiently expose students to the needs that come with IDD care and how these needs should be addressed. Studies have shown that many healthcare providers, at various levels of training, feel inadequately prepared to care for people with IDD (39,40). There is also evidence that healthcare providers may have negative attitudes and perceptions towards people with IDD (41–43), which impacts the quality of care this population receives.

To address this need for exposure and training, McMaster University (Hamilton, Ontario) integrated IDD competencies into its medical school curricula through the Curriculum of Caring programme (44). This programme involves direct interaction and clinical skills development through working with the IDD population. Similarly, enhanced learning opportunities in the medical school curriculum at the University of Toronto have been introduced in various stages. The genetics week (year 1), advanced communications in clinical skills week (year 1), and complexities week (year 2) are a few examples. Seminars for medical students transitioning to residency programmes and elective interprofessional workshops for nurses and medical students are additional examples of educational innovations. In addition, the Centre for Addiction and Mental Health and the University of Toronto developed Extension for Community Healthcare Outcomes (ECHO) Ontario Mental Health, which is a virtual education and capacity building model for continuing professional education (45). ECHO uses video conferencing to link expert interdisciplinary teams with frontline care providers to share best practices and discuss recommendations for complex cases. ECHO also hosts training session specifically related to adult IDD for mental health, primary care, and developmental service providers (46).

Managing transitions in care

Yet another crucial issue facing the care of people with IDD are transitions in care. These include the transition from paediatric to adult care, the transition from adult to older adult care, and from the community to hospital and back (47). Transitions are a challenging period for any individual, with a need to adapt to changing expectations and social roles. Focusing on the transition from paediatric to adult care, it can be difficult for people with IDD and their families given that people with IDD may not be developmentally ready to fulfil the roles and responsibilities of a neurotypical adult (48,49). In Ontario, many youths with IDD remain in the publicly funded school education system until the age of 21, but they must transfer from child to adult health services after their 18th birthday (49). They also become eligible for additional community supports through Developmental Services Ontario at that age (50). There is often a gap when the individual is without services, between the time children's services end and when families find suitable community programmes, as they must also contend with long waitlists. There is also the added challenge of navigating eligibility criteria for adult developmental programmes. Unfortunately, this gap in services during the transitional period can negatively impact the progress that the individual with IDD has been making towards independence (51). These changes can be a stressful life change for people with IDD and can have impacts on their mental well-being.

To address this need for a more seamless transition, in 2013 the Ontario MCCSS and Ministry of Education collaborated to promote integrated transition planning, requiring each region in the province to be responsible for developing transition planning protocols for people with IDD (52). Specific to mental health, there are also the Transitional-Age Youth programmes in many centres across Ontario which address the mental health needs of individuals aged 16–24 (53). These programmes, while not specific to people with IDD, do work to ensure successful transition to adult care and assist with linkage to community services.

Systems-level enablers of mental healthcare

Primary care guidelines

Some capacity-building efforts have led to improvements in care. In 2005, the first set of national guidelines on primary care for adults with IDD were published (49). About one-third of the guidelines focused on mental health, recognizing that primary care providers are the first people to deal with mental health in this population. These guidelines were updated in 2011 (49) and again in 2018 (51), and as part of the programme, a series of clinical tools were developed to assist healthcare providers in guideline implementation.

The guidelines are supported by several tools that focus on different aspects of healthcare (such as healthcare communication and planning, decision-making, approaches to common health issues in IDD, and symptom monitoring) and are targeted to people with IDD, their family and caregivers, as well as healthcare providers (54). Additional tools have also been developed during the COVID-19 pandemic to address accommodations for administering vaccines, putting together an advance care plan, and preparing for hospital admissions (17). In addition to guideline and clinical tool development, the Developmental Disabilities Primary Care Program (DDPCP) has also been involved with providing primary care training and the establishment of clinical support networks with continuing medical education opportunities (55). Continuing education in this regard leads to greater changes than the provision of guidelines and resources alone.

Several teams across Ontario and in other jurisdictions have taken the initiative to implement these guidelines and embed the clinical tools into team structures and processes (56,57). A recent example comes from two Ontario family health teams, who implemented a Health Check protocol for patients with IDD in their practice (58,59). The annual health check is recommended by the guidelines to improve preventative care in this population (60). Staff rated higher comfort and skill with the IDD population following the implementation of guidelines and tools in practice (58). While there were positive results, the study also identified staff's need for more support, and have recommended using an electronic medical record-based process to alert staff before health checks so that accommodations can be arranged (61). The study also suggested that incentive payments may be needed to increase uptake, to account for the extra time required to conduct health checks in this population. Efforts have been made to integrate guideline recommendations into a family medicine residency curriculum (62,63). A teaching programme was developed at Queen's University (Kingston, Ontario) which involves mentored clinical encounters with adults with IDD involving a Health Check (62). The programme also provided access to various IDD learning resources, including tools developed by the DDPCP, and involved a reflective exercise. Experiential training was shown to lead to a greater increase in reported comfort and skill than didactic training alone (63).

Going forward, it would be important to continue identifying successful implementation strategies for the guidelines. Furthermore, while the guidelines recognize that the optimal standards of care involve a broad range of interprofessional services, some clinical settings may not have these resources readily available. Physicians and healthcare professionals can play a role in advocating for more interprofessional primary care services. More research would also be needed to determine the best way to implement interprofessional health teams and would require investigating the scope of interprofessional primary care services required by this population (64).

Interprofessional care in the community

Another Ontario-based programme is the Community Networks of Specialized Care (CNSC), which was developed specifically to assist adults with IDD who require high support and have complex care needs (65). Such complexities in care often involve mental health issues and behavioural crises situations.

CNSC links specialized services and professionals to collaborate and develop complex support plans, as well as acting as a resource for service agencies and Developmental Services Ontario. The programme also facilitates cross-sectoral collaboration between developmental services, health, research, education, and justice to improve navigation, access, and quality of services. Similarly, the Complex Needs Initiative in Alberta is a partnership between Alberta Health Services and Disability Services to help people with IDD and a mental illness receive coordinated and integrated care (66). This programme utilizes Community Support Teams, which consist of an interprofessional group of service providers. Another such example is Developmental Disabilities Mental Health Services in British Columbia, which provides interprofessional support for IDD mental health needs (21). Other provinces have similar programmes. The age cut-off can range from as early as 12 years to 19 years.

Virtual mental healthcare

The delivery of mental health services in Canada, given its vast geography and shortage of specialists in remote regions, has invested in various models of telemedicine or virtual care. The Mashkikiiwininiwag Mazinaatesijigan Wichiiwewin (MMW) is an example of a programme that offers interprofessional care services through videoconferencing to adults with IDD in Northwestern Ontario (67). Virtual healthcare services using video-conferencing technology started in 2004–2005 in the MMW programme, a long time before the potential of virtual mental health was leveraged during the COVID-19 pandemic. This programme collaborates with community partners, including the Sioux Lookout First Nation Health Authority and Community Living Dryden Sioux Lookout. The MMW team is primarily based in Toronto and provides services for people with IDD in Northwestern Ontario, including fly-in services to communities such as Weagamow and Sandy Lake. For context, Toronto is situated more than 800 miles away from Weagamow. This liaison model was critical in terms of building trusted relationships between service users, local staff, and remote providers, and to help clinicians with understanding cultural realities in these communities. Together, the multidisciplinary team offers psychiatric and psychological assessment and consultation, behaviour therapy and consultation, individual counselling, service coordination/case management, therapeutic groups, and educational activities (e.g. workshops and courses for staff, families, and other professionals).

Fig. 15.1 gives an overview of the programme and its services.

The COVID-19 pandemic saw virtual care as an important tool to support mental health of adults with IDD remotely. Selick et al.'s (2021) scoping review

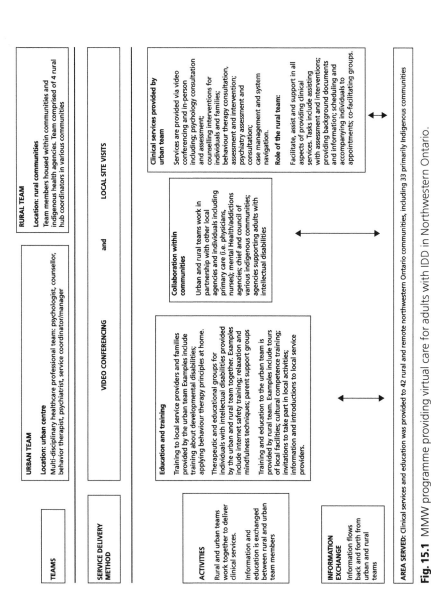

Fig. 15.1 MMW programme providing virtual care for adults with IDD in Northwestern Ontario.

found that most studies reported positive feedback from patients and caregivers regarding virtual care (68). The benefits included saving time and reducing challenges for patients who could not tolerate waiting in the waiting room, as well as the possibility of improved quality of care by allowing providers insight into the patient's home environment. Both the MMW programme and early reports from the COVID-19 virtual care experience suggest virtual mental healthcare is a promising avenue for delivering accessible, high-quality care to people with IDD even within the post-pandemic landscape.

Caregiver involvement

A person-centred approach is paramount in the care of individuals with IDD, and often involves engaging family members or caregivers who know the patient well. The caregiver plays a crucial role in helping to support the individual, coordinate care, and monitor needs (60,69). Caregivers are essential when it comes to understanding and supporting behaviours that challenge. They can play a role in delivering positive behaviour supports, as well as monitoring and evaluating the efficacy of medications (70), and the delivery of psychological interventions (71). Additionally, caregivers have an important role to play as educators. For example, the aforementioned ECHO Ontario Mental Health programme involves family advisors in its curriculum development and delivery (72). Furthermore, caregivers have a role in advocacy, with the MCCSS engaging family members of people with IDD in working groups as relevant stakeholders in policymaking decisions (73).

ECHO-AIDD: a national initiative during the COVID-19 pandemic

ECHO is a community-based virtual capacity-building model that has been used worldwide in over 23 countries to share best clinical practices and create communities of practice (74). This is a 'hub-and-spoke' model that connects content experts (hub) with geographically spread out participants and has four guiding principles: (i) use of technology to leverage scarce resources, (ii) share best practices, (iii) case-based learning, and (iv) monitoring outcomes to increase impact (75).

During COVID-19, the ECHO framework was used to engage with people with IDD, family caregivers, and service providers to address their needs and mental health concerns (ECHO Ontario Adult Intellectual and Developmental Disabilities: ECHO-AIDD). ECHO-informed 6-week virtual courses were developed and implemented in Ontario and later scaled up to be delivered across Canada for each of the groups (46). Notably, adults with IDD, family caregivers, and healthcare professionals co-produced and taught the curriculum. Participants in all the three groups reported some improvements in knowledge and self-efficacy, maintained at 8-week follow-up (72,76). Families also reported significant improvement in their well-being, maintained at follow-up (72). The model, which follows the 'all teach, all learn' philosophy, has great potential for building resource capacity and reducing gaps in skill base to support the mental health of people with IDD.

A bright future ahead

> Through a central programme that coordinates interprofessional services for adults with IDD, Michael is connected to a speech language pathologist to help improve his expressive language skills. He is also connected to behavioural services who assist with developing a behaviour support plan to manage his aggression and self-injurious behaviours, as well as a psychiatrist to reassess his antipsychotic medication prescriptions. Michael's elderly parents are provided with respite care while he is on the waitlist for a specialized residential setting. His primary care physician follows up with Michael yearly for health checks, and assists with the management of his epilepsy, diabetes mellitus, and hypertension. With these supports in place, Michael is able to avoid recurrent emergency room visits and hospitalizations and continues to live a full life in the community.

As illustrated with Michael, optimizing care for people with IDD will need strengthening of primary care as well as improvement of out-of-hospital services. Health and social services within the community need to be integrated to better support the needs of people with dual diagnoses and complex needs. By breaking down the walls of bureaucratic and organizational silos, there will be room for collaborative care that is patient and family centred. Other important considerations for IDD care include the need for more seamless transitions in care, adequate training of health professionals to care for this population, and the potential use of new methods of care delivery such as virtual care. Furthermore, in the diverse multicultural landscape of Canada, it is also important that mental healthcare is delivered with a culturally competent framework (77). A commitment to diversity and equity will involve increased access and availability of culturally appropriate services, including for Indigenous, Black, and other racialized minorities. Work in Canada has already begun about understanding the needs of adults with IDD from Indigenous communities through the MWW programme. Goyal et al. (2018) found that Indigenous individuals with IDD had stronger visual–spatial abilities compared to verbal, and thus may benefit from a more visual, hands-on approach (78). The Adaptive Behaviour Scale for Northern Communities (ABS-NC) is an example of a tool that has been adapted to create more culturally and geographically relevant questions for the assessment of adaptive daily living skills in Indigenous people (79).

While there appears to be positive changes in policy and best practices, the real change is still required to be implemented at the organizational and personal levels. Often change plans are unsuccessful because they fail to consider the motivations and behaviours of individuals and long-term sustainability. Therefore, it is important that change efforts be backed by the principles of change management. Kotter has provided a model for organizational change, which includes eight steps: convey urgency; gather a steering committee with core stakeholders; develop a roadmap for the change initiative; communicate upcoming changes; make change steps easy and clear; create short-term wins; build on quick wins and learn from challenges; and ensure that change is supported long-term (80). The buy-in of staff is also crucial, and thus it is important to consider how individuals psychologically react to change. Chip and Dan Heath have created a framework that considers the human factors of implementing change, which includes motivating, directing, and shaping (81: p 8). 'Motivating' appeals to people's emotions by turning negative feelings towards change, such as pessimism and anxiety, into positive feelings of excitement and hope. 'Directing' involves the creation of a vision that appeals to people's logic, and 'shaping' involves a consideration of external reinforcements such as creating prompts or adjusting the environment. Being able to understand and apply change management principles will help create tangible and lasting improvements in IDD service delivery.

While there is still much left to do to improve IDD care, the Canadian examples illustrate successful models that can inspire work in other jurisdictions, as well as provide learning points around existing gaps. The global community can work together to continue learning from each other and share new insights.

The United States

The US, a federal republic, shares borders with Canada to the north and Mexico to the south.

Prevalence of intellectual disability in the US

Despite varying methodologies, operational definitions, and differing demographics, the prevalence of intellectual disability (ID) in the US is similar to the rest of the world. The estimates of prevalence of ID in adults in the US vary from 0.7% (82) to 1.2% (83) whereas in children, the prevalence is higher at 1.36% (84). The most common causes of ID have been identified as birth defects and genetic conditions such as Down syndrome, fetal alcohol syndrome, and fragile X syndrome. Certain demographic characteristics such as older maternal age and low socioeconomic status, appear to be associated with ID, more so with mild ID (85).

Brief history of intellectual disability in the US

The American evolution of nomenclature and nosology of ID has mirrored the prevailing attitudes and understanding of the American scientific community and the general public. In 1904, Martin W. Barr, the chief physician at the Pennsylvania Training School for the Feeble-Minded, noted how the use of the terms 'idiot' and 'imbecile' for centuries had resulted in oppression and exclusion (86).

In the history of ID in the US, the changes have not only been in the name—the American Psychiatric Association's *Diagnostic and Statistical Manual of Mental Disorders* (DSM) which first called the condition 'mental deficiency' in its first iteration in 1952, 'mental retardation' in the DSM-II in 1968 (which was used until the DSM IV-TR in 2000), and finally as 'intellectual disability' in the DSM-5 in 2013, but also in the methods used in the treatment and care for people with ID (87–89).

Evolution of services

The institutional model period

The American institutional model was a self-sufficient agrarian model in which residents would work the fields growing sustenance to support other residents and themselves. The idea was to remove people with ID from the 'stresses and tribulations of urban life' (86). One of the first such institutions was the Massachusetts School for Idiot and Feeble-Minded Youth, started in 1848 by Samuel Gridley Howe and the renowned advocate for the mentally ill, Dorothea Dix (90). Although designed as a protective and humane model, with its success, it inadvertently convinced its reviewers that people with ID should permanently live there despite Howe's calls for their reintegration into society, and for their rights to participate in the community (86). Public attitudes towards people with ID became more unfavourable with the eugenics movement in the early twentieth century—Henry Goddard's 1912 review of the Kallikak family erroneously linked mental defects and criminality (91). Physicians encouraged families to institutionalize children with mental defects as, according to them, there would be no benefit for the child to live with their family and could rather endanger the family unit. This eventually led to overcrowding of institutions and worsening of their conditions. Lack of funding due to the Great Depression and the two World Wars only exacerbated the problems (86).

Community-based care

In the 1960s, President Kennedy created the President's Commission on Mental Retardation (92). The commission's panel of clinical experts and advocates, after reviewing existing evidence from US and from Scandinavian countries that did not rely on the institutional model, concluded that institutions must be closed, and community-based support must be developed to enable integration of people with ID into the society. Funding for these measures was obtained from the federal and state Medicaid programmes. This led to the start of the Intermediate Care Facilities/Mental Retardation programme under which states received funding in return for meeting some basic quality standards (93). However, the improved quality of care had the opposite effect—slowing the deinstitutionalization process. Still, community supports became available and the community mental health centre model made mental health services affordable (94). Litigations against the gross mistreatment of residents at institutions such as New York's Willowbrook State Center and Pennsylvania's Pennhurst State School and Hospital, further ushered the end of the institutional era (95).

Community services model and civil rights for the disabled

In Pennsylvania, when the closure of Pennhurst, a state institution for people with ID was ordered, the federal government used this opportunity to study the effect of closure of such institutions. In his government-commissioned research, Dr Jim Conroy found an increase in skills regarding domestic activities, overall happiness, and satisfaction of both the people with ID and their families, and opportunities to exercise choice, along with decrease in costs, while no significant effect on mortality (96).

The Independent Living Movement in the 1970s advocated for a community model rather than a medical model espousing the idea that if an individual needs support in the community, then these supports should be provided (97). The first such centre arising from this movement, the Berkeley Centre for Independent Living, was founded by Ed Roberts in 1978 (98). Today, community-based homes are funded under Medicaid waiver plans and are the dominant form of residential support for people with ID. They have been found to promote growth, integration, and consumer satisfaction (99). Other alternatives being examined are adult foster care or 'life sharing' and increased funding for family members to take care of their family (100). This has led to a change in focus to a 'strength-based approach': accommodation, to help them achieve their personally selected goal, rather than change to the life of a typical person, is the aim of the interventions (101). However, problems such as high cost, and long waitlists still exist (102). The future might see technology-supported homes that rely less on staff to cut costs (103) and more financial support from alternative funding streams to pay families to take care of their family members (104).

Psychiatric training

The Accreditation Council for Graduate Medical Education, the body responsible for accrediting all graduate medical programmes in the US, requires training in developmental disabilities, especially to help trainees recognize the role of community placements and prolongation of lifespan; however, the council does not stipulate a minimum duration of such training. Therefore, there exists a great variation in the amount of training provided in general psychiatry and child and adolescent psychiatry programmes in the US, ranging from limited exposure to autism spectrum disorder and ID patients across all settings, to more intensive placements along with extensive didactics (105). These more rigorous programmes that prioritize ID, however, are a minority. There is a recognition of this patient group thus being underserved, as well as the benefits of more psychiatry training in IDD such as multidisciplinary teamwork, increased skills with diagnostic complexity, treatment, and rehabilitation, and non-cognitive aspects of psychotherapy. Some of the strategies being implemented to fulfil the unmet needs of people with ID and their families are evaluating the fund of knowledge regarding ID of psychiatric trainees to inform curricula, examining trainees' attitudes towards ID and autism spectrum disorder, investigation of barriers between primary and secondary care, and increased advocacy from psychiatrists, training institutions, and the public (106).

Mexico

Mexico is the southern portion of North America and is bordered at its north by the US.

It is estimated that the prevalence of IDD in Mexico is about 3% (107), though attempts to quantify them have proven to be difficult as most psychiatric hospitals for adults do not refer to ID as a primary diagnosis and instruments that have been used for psychiatric surveys in Mexico such as the Composite International Diagnostic Interview, do not have a validated questionnaire for ID (108). This problem of estimation of prevalence is further complicated by social exclusion and deprivation, and lack of empowerment of people with ID (109). Mexico is one of the 96 countries that have ratified the United Nations Convention on the Rights of Persons with Disabilities in 2006. However, several barriers exist for people living with disabilities due to a lack of effective implementation of specialized mental health programmes, resulting in challenges in establishing primary care centres for mental health, inadequate training of health workers, and a lack of facilities for patient rehabilitation and reinsertion (110). Moreover, institutionalization of people with ID has led to considerable human rights violations according to a report by Disability Rights

International. This discrimination also appears to extend to the criminal justice system as challenges also exist in access to treatment or diversion (111).

Of late, the government has prioritized mental health with the Specific Action Program for Mental Health 2013–2018 which aims at increasing quality of care and reducing costs, apart from strengthening pathways to early diagnosis and early prevention through a community-based network (110). This mental health programme which also mentions ID gives emphasis to staff training for promoting the human rights and fundamental freedoms of people with mental disabilities and preventing cruel and inhuman treatment (112). Recent literature has identified the need for change in public policy in providing holistic care for people with ID, specifically towards personal skills development, providing more opportunities for vocational training and jobs, community inclusion, and empowerment through economic autonomy (113).

References

1. **Lunsky Y, Klein-Geltink JE, Yates EA.** Atlas on the Primary Care of Adults with Developmental Disabilities in Ontario. Toronto: Institute for Clinical Evaluative Sciences and Centre for Addiction and Mental Health; 2013.

2. **Lin E, Balogh RS, Durbin A, Holder L, Gupta N, Tiziana V,** et al. Addressing Gaps in the Health Care Services Used by Adults with Developmental Disabilities in Ontario. Toronto: Institute for Clinical Evaluative Sciences; 2019.

3. **Lin E, Balogh R, Selick A, Dobranowski K, Wilton AS, Lunsky Y.** Adults with Developmental Disabilities Plus a Mental Illness or Addiction (DD-Plus). Toronto: Health Care Access Research and Developmental Disabilities Program; 2016. Available from: https://www.porticonetwork.ca/documents/38160/99698/DD+Plus_fi nal+report+%28August+17+2016%29.pdf/c70a84ae-ea20-42c7-abfb-c2091e8cc5c8

4. **Lunsky Y, Khuu W, Tadrous M, Vigod S, Cobigo V, Gomes T.** Antipsychotic use with and without comorbid psychiatric diagnosis among adults with intellectual and developmental disabilities. Canadian Journal of Psychiatry/Revue Canadienne de Psychiatrie 2018;**63**(6):361–9.

5. **Lin E, Balogh R, McGarry C, Selick A, Dobranowski K, Wilton AS,** et al. Substance-related and addictive disorders among adults with intellectual and developmental disabilities (IDD): an Ontario population cohort study. BMJ Open 2016;**6**(9):e011638.

6. **Ouellette-Kuntz H, Shooshtari S, Balogh R, Martens P.** Understanding information about mortality among people with intellectual and developmental disabilities in Canada. Journal of Applied Research in Intellectual Disabilities 2015;**28**(5):423–35.

7. **Landes SD, Turk MA, Formica MK, McDonald KE, Stevens JD.** COVID-19 outcomes among people with intellectual and developmental disability living in residential group homes in New York State. Disability and Health Journal 2020;**13**(4):100969.

8. **Public Health England.** Deaths of people identified as having learning disabilities with COVID-19 in England in the spring of 2020. 2020. Available from: https://assets.publish ing.service.gov.uk/government/uploads/system/uploads/attachment_data/file/933612/ COVID-19__learning_disabilities_mortality_report.pdf

9. Lunsky Y, Lai MC, Balogh R, Chung H, Durbin A, Jachyra P, et al. Premature mortality in a population-based cohort of autistic adults in Canada. Autism Research 2022;**15**(8):1550–9.

10. Landes SD, Turk MA, Bisesti E. Uncertainty and the reporting of intellectual disability on death certificates: a cross-sectional study of US mortality data from 2005 to 2017. BMJ Open 2021;**11**(1):e045360.

11. Sawatzky R, Kwon JY, Barclay R, Chauhan C, Frank L, van den Hout WB, et al. Implications of response shift for micro-, meso-, and macro-level healthcare decision-making using results of patient-reported outcome measures. Quality of Life Research 2021;**30**(12):3343–57.

12. Government of Canada. Canada's population clock (real-time model). Statistics Canada; 2018. Available from: https://www150.statcan.gc.ca/n1/pub/71-607-x/71-607-x2018005-eng.htm

13. Government of Canada. Canada Health Act. 1985. Available from: https://laws-lois.justice.gc.ca/eng/acts/c-6/page-1.html

14. Government of Canada. Accessible Canada Act. 2019. Available from: https://laws-lois.justice.gc.ca/eng/acts/A-0.6/

15. Ontario Government. Services and Supports to Promote the Social Inclusion of Persons with Developmental Disabilities Act, 2008. Queen's Printer for Ontario; 2008. Available from: https://www.ontario.ca/laws/statute/08s14

16. Government of British Columbia. Community Living Authority Act. Queen's Printer; 2004. Available from: https://www.bclaws.gov.bc.ca/civix/document/id/complete/statreg/04060_01

17. Government of Alberta. Persons with Developmental Disabilities Services Act. Queen's Printer; 2000. Available from: https://open.alberta.ca/publications/p09p5

18. Developmental Services Ontario. Funded services. 2022. Available from: https://www.dsontario.ca/funded-services

19. Community Living British Columbia. Homepage. 2018. Available from: https://www.communitylivingbc.ca/

20. Government of Alberta. Persons with developmental disabilities (PDD). 2022. Available from: https://www.alberta.ca/persons-with-developmental-disabilities-pdd.aspx

21. Fraser Health. Developmental disabilities mental health services. Fraser Health Authority; 2021. Available from: https://www.fraserhealth.ca/health-topics-a-to-z/developmental-disabilities-mental-health-services#.YkC38ufMLIU

22. Ontario Shores. Dual Diagnosis Service. Ontario Shores Centre for Mental Health Sciences; 2021. Available from: https://www.ontarioshores.ca/services/dual-diagnosis-service

23. Lin E, Whittingham L, Busch L, Calzavara A, Kouyoumdjian F, Durbin A, et al. Intensive use of forensic inpatient services by people with intellectual and developmental disabilities in Ontario, Canada: prevalence and associated characteristics. International Journal of Forensic Mental Health 2022. Published online: 20 Jan.

24. Woodbury-Smith M, Furimsky I, Chaimowitz GA. Point prevalence of adults with intellectual developmental disorder in forensic psychiatric inpatient services in Ontario, Canada. International Journal of Risk and Recovery 2018;**1**(1):4–11.

25. **Ray I, Simpson AIF, Jones RM, Shatokhina K, Thakur A, Mulsant BH.** Clinical, demographic, and criminal behavior characteristics of patients with intellectual disabilities in a Canadian forensic program. Frontiers in Psychiatry 2019;**10**:760.

26. **Ontario Government.** Public Hospitals Act. Queen's Printer for Ontario; 1990. Available from: https://www.ontario.ca/laws/statute/90p40

27. **Ontario Government.** Excellent Care for All Act. Queen's Printer for Ontario; 2010. Available from: https://www.ontario.ca/laws/statute/10e14

28. **Ontario Government.** Mental Health Act. Queen's Printer for Ontario; 1990. Available from: https://www.ontario.ca/laws/statute/90m07

29. **Grier E, Abells D, Casson I, Gemmill M, Ladouceur J, Lepp A,** et al. Managing complexity in care of patients with intellectual and developmental disabilities: natural fit for the family physician as an expert generalist. Canadian Family Physician/Medecin de Famille Canadien 2018;**64**(Suppl 2):S15–22.

30. **Cloutier E, Chantal G, Levesque A.** Canadian Survey on Disability, 2017: concepts and methods guide. 2018. Available from: https://www150.statcan.gc.ca/n1/pub/89-654-x/89-654-x2018001-eng.htm

31. **Health Care Access Research and Developmental Disabilities.** What is H-CARDD? Centre for Addiction and Mental Health; n.d. Available from: https://www.porticonetwork.ca/web/hcardd/about/mission

32. **Australian Institute of Health and Welfare.** Disability Services national minimum data set 2010–11. 2011. Available from: https://meteor.aihw.gov.au/content/index.phtml/iteMid/428708

33. **Hourigan S, Fanagan S, Kelly C.** Annual report of the National Intellectual Disability Database Committee 2017 main findings. Health Research Board; 2017. Available from: https://www.hrb.ie/fileadmin/2._Plugin_related_files/Publications/2018_pubs/Disability/NIDD/NIDD_Annual_Report_2017.pdf

34. **Public Health England.** Improving Health and Lives Learning Disabilities Observatory. n.d. Available from: https://improvinghealthandlives.org.uk/

35. **Ontario Government.** Ministry of Health. Queen's Printer for Ontario; 2021. Available from: https://www.ontario.ca/page/ministry-health

36. **Ministry of Children, Community and Social Services.** Adults with developmental disabilities in Ontario. Queen's Printer for Ontario; 2022. Available from: https://www.ontario.ca/page/adults-developmental-disabilities-ontario

37. **Gough H, Morris S.** Dual diagnosis public policy in a federal system: the Canadian experience: dual diagnosis public policy. Journal of Policy and Practice in Intellectual Disabilities 2012;**9**(3):166–74.

38. **Puntis J.** Health and Care Bill: the government does not want to limit privatisation or integrate services. BMJ 2021;**374**:n2139.

39. **Wilkinson J, Dreyfus D, Cerreto M, Bokhour B.** 'Sometimes I feel overwhelmed': educational needs of family physicians caring for people with intellectual disability. Intellectual and Developmental Disabilities 2012;**50**(3):243–50.

40. **Boreman CD, Thomasgard MC, Fernandez SA, Coury DL.** Resident training in developmental/behavioral pediatrics: where do we stand? Clinical Pediatrics 2007;**46**(2):135–45.

41. **Lewis S, Stenfert-Kroese B.** An investigation of nursing staff attitudes and emotional reactions towards patients with intellectual disability in a general hospital setting. Journal of Applied Research in Intellectual Disabilities 2010;**23**(4):355–65.

42. **Lunsky Y, Gracey C, Gelfand S.** Emergency psychiatric services for individuals with intellectual disabilities: perspectives of hospital staff. Intellectual and Developmental Disabilities 2008;**46**(6):446–55.

43. **Iezzoni LI, Rao SR, Ressalam J, Bolcic-Jankovic D, Agaronnik ND, Donelan K,** et al. Physicians' perceptions of people with disability and their health care: study reports the results of a survey of physicians' perceptions of people with disability. Health Affairs (Millwood) 2021;**40**(2):297–306.

44. **Boyd K.** The curriculum of caring: fostering compassionate, person-centered health care. AMA Journal of Ethics 2016;**18**(4):384–92.

45. **The Centre for Addiction and Mental Health**. Project ECHO Ontario Mental Health at CAMH & The University of Toronto. Available from: https://camh.echoontario.ca/

46. **The Centre for Addiction and Mental Health**. ECHO Ontario Adult Intellectual & Developmental Disabilities (AIDD). Available from: https://camh.echoontario.ca/programs-aidd/

47. **Health Care Access Research and Developmental Disabilities (H-CARDD)**. Summary of Proceedings: 'Making the Invisible Visible' H-CARDD Provincial Meeting, February 23, 2016, Toronto, Canada. 2016. Available from: https://www.porticonetwork.ca/documents/38160/99698/Provincial+Meeting+Report/5b4d97ed-301d-447c-a58f-8121e4ff36d0

48. **Tencza M, Forsythe L.** Transition-of-care planning: preparing for the future care of the individual with intellectual and developmental disabilities. Journal of Intellectual Disabilities 2021;**25**(2):277–89.

49. **Ally S, Boyd K, Abells D, Amaria K, Hamdani Y, Loh A,** et al. Improving transition to adulthood for adolescents with intellectual and developmental disabilities: proactive developmental and systems perspective. Canadian Family Physician/Medecin de Famille Canadien 2018;**64**(Suppl 2):S37–43.

50. **Developmental Services Ontario**. How to access services. 2022. Available from: https://www.dsontario.ca/how-to-access-services

51. **Ministry of Children, Community and Social Services**. Report on consultations regarding the transformation of developmental services: issues and recommendations. 2006. Available from: https://www.mcss.gov.on.ca/en/mcss/publications/developmentalServices/reportOnConsultation/issues.aspx

52. **McKay K.** A new approach to transition planning for transitional aged youth with intellectual and developmental disabilities. Journal on Developmental Disabilities 2019;**24**(1):27–42.

53. **Canadian Mental Health Association Ontario**. Transitioning from Youth to Adult Mental Health Services. n.d. Available from: https://ontario.cmha.ca/documents/transitioning-from-youth-to-adult-mental-health-services/

54. **Surrey Place**. Tools for the primary care of adults with intellectual and developmental disabilities. n.d. Available from: https://ddprimarycare.surreyplace.ca/tools-2/

55. **Balogh R, Wood J, Lunsky Y, Isaacs B, Ouellette-Kuntz H, Sullivan W.** Care of adults with developmental disabilities: effects of a continuing education course for

primary care providers. Canadian Family Physician/Medecin de Famille Canadien 2015;**61**(7):e316–23.

56. **Lepp A, Casson I, Griffiths J.** Program description: implementing the Canadian Consensus Guidelines for the Primary Care of Adults with Developmental Disabilities: clinical and educational enhancements in an academic family medicine practice. Clinical Bulletin of the Developmental Disabilities Division 2012;**23**(4). Available from: https://www.schulich.uwo.ca/ddp/about_us/2012_Winter.pdf

57. **Vanderebilt Kennedy Center.** Primary care for adults with IDD addressed with Health Care E-Toolkit. n.d. Available from: https://iddtoolkit.vkcsites.org/

58. **Durbin J, Selick A, Casson I, Green L, Perry A, Chacra MA,** et al. Improving the quality of primary care for adults with intellectual and developmental disabilities: value of the periodic health examination. Canadian Family Physician/Medecin de Famille Canadien 2019;**65**(Suppl 1):S66–72.

59. **Durbin J, Selick A, Casson I, Green L, Spassiani N, Perry A,** et al. Evaluating the implementation of health checks for adults with intellectual and developmental disabilities in primary care: the importance of organizational context. Intellectual and Developmental Disabilities 2016;**54**(2):136–50.

60. **Sullivan WF, Diepstra H, Heng J, Ally S, Bradley E, Casson I,** et al. Primary care of adults with intellectual and developmental disabilities: 2018 Canadian consensus guidelines. Canadian Family Physician/Medecin de Famille Canadien 2018;**64**(4):254–79.

61. **Selick A, Durbin J, Casson I, Lee J, Lunsky Y.** Barriers and facilitators to improving health care for adults with intellectual and developmental disabilities: what do staff tell us? Health Promotion and Chronic Disease Prevention in Canada: Research, Policy and Practice 2018;**38**(10):349–57.

62. **Casson I, Abells D, Boyd K, Bradley E, Gemmill M, Grier E,** et al. Teaching family medicine residents about care of adults with intellectual and developmental disabilities. Canadian Family Physician/Medecin de Famille Canadien 2019;**65**(Suppl 1):S35–40.

63. **Selick A, Durbin J, Casson I, Green L, Abells D, Bruni A,** et al. Improving capacity to care for patients with intellectual and developmental disabilities: the value of an experiential learning model for family medicine residents. Disability and Health Journal 2022;**15**(3):101282.

64. **Bobbette N, Lysaght R, Ouellette-Kuntz H, Tranmer J, Donnelly C.** Organizational attributes of interprofessional primary care for adults with intellectual and developmental disabilities in Ontario, Canada: a multiple case study. BMC Family Practice 2021;**22**(1):157.

65. **Community Networks of Specialized Care.** About us. n.d. Available from: https://www.community-networks.ca/about-us-2/

66. **Alberta Health Services.** Intellectual/developmental disability (IDD) & mental health supports - complex needs initiative. 2022. Available from: https://www.albertahealths ervices.ca/info/page9213.aspx

67. **Surrey Place.** MMW clinical videoconferencing program. 2022. Available from: https://www.surreyplace.ca/services/mmw-clinical-videoconferencing-program/

68. **Selick A, Bobbette N, Lunsky Y, Hamdani Y, Rayner J, Durbin J.** Virtual health care for adult patients with intellectual and developmental disabilities: a scoping review. Disability and Health Journal 2021;**14**(4):101132.

69. Selick A, Durbin J, Salonia C, Volpe T, Orr E, Hermans H, et al. The nuts and bolts of health care: evaluating an initiative to build direct support professional capacity to support the health care of individuals with intellectual disabilities. Journal of Applied Research in Intellectual Disabilities 2022;**35**(2):623–32.

70. Deb SS, Limbu B, Unwin G, Woodcock L, Cooper V, Fullerton M. Short-Term Psycho-Education for Caregivers to Reduce Overmedication of People with Intellectual Disabilities (SPECTROM): development and field testing. International Journal of Environmental Research and Public Health 2021;**18**(24):13161.

71. Jahoda A, Hastings R, Hatton C, Cooper SA, Dagnan D, Zhang R, et al. Comparison of behavioural activation with guided self-help for treatment of depression in adults with intellectual disabilities: a randomised controlled trial. Lancet Psychiatry 2017;**4**(12):909–19.

72. Thakur A, Pereira C, Hardy J, Bobbette N, Sockalingam S, Lunsky Y. Virtual education program to support providers caring for people with intellectual and developmental disabilities during the COVID-19 pandemic: rapid development and evaluation study. JMIR Mental Health 2021;**8**(10):e28933.

73. Ministry of Children, Community and Social Services. Journey to belonging: choice and inclusion. Queen's Printer for Ontario; 2022. Available from: https://www.ontario.ca/page/journey-belonging-choice-and-inclusion

74. Struminger B, Arora S, Zalud-Cerrato S, Lowrance D, Ellerbrock T. Building virtual communities of practice for health. Lancet 2017;**390**(10095):632–4.

75. Project ECHO. About the ECHO model. The University of New Mexico. Available from: https://hsc.unm.edu/echo/what-we-do/about-the-echo-model.html

76. St. John L, Volpe T, Jiwa MI, Durbin A, Safar Y, Formuli F, et al. 'More together than apart': the evaluation of a virtual course to improve mental health and well-being of adults with intellectual disabilities during the COVID-19 pandemic. Journal of Applied Research in Intellectual Disabilities 2022;**35**(6):1360–9.

77. Fung K, Lo HTT, Srivastava R, Andermann L. Organizational cultural competence consultation to a mental health institution. Transcultural Psychiatry 2012;**49**(2):165–84.

78. Goyal S, Temple V, Sawanas C, Brown D. Cognitive profile of adults with intellectual disabilities from indigenous communities in Ontario, Canada. Journal of Intellectual and Developmental Disabilities 2020;**45**(1):59–65.

79. Temple V, Sawanas C, Brown D. Measuring daily living skills in First Nations communities: development and validation of the Adaptive Behaviour Scale for Northern Communities (ABS-NC). Journal on Developmental Disabilities 2014;**20**(3):4–18.

80. Kotter J. The 8-Step Process for Leading Change. 2013. Available from: https://www.kotterinc.com/8-step-process-for-leading-change/

81. Heath C, Heath D. Switch: How to Change Things When Change is Hard. Toronto: Random House Canada; 2010.

82. United States Department of Health and Human Services, Centers for Disease Control and Prevention, National Center for Health Statistics. National Health Interview Survey on Disability, 1995: phase II, child followback. ICPSR Data Holdings; 1999. Available from: https://www.icpsr.umich.edu/web/NACDA/studies/2577

83. Fujiura GT. Continuum of intellectual disability: demographic evidence for the 'forgotten generation'. Mental Retardation 2003;**41**(6):420–9.

84. Van Naarden Braun K, Christensen D, Doernberg N, Schieve L, Rice C, Wiggins L, et al. Trends in the prevalence of autism spectrum disorder, cerebral palsy, hearing loss, intellectual disability, and vision impairment, Metropolitan Atlanta, 1991–2010. PLoS One 2015;**10**(4):e0124120.

85. Karam SM, Riegel M, Segal SL, Félix TM, Barros AJ, Santos IS, et al. Genetic causes of intellectual disability in a birth cohort: a population-based study. American Journal of Medical Genetics Part A 2015;**167**(6):1204–14.

86. Spreat S. Brief history and future of intellectual disability services in America. Social Innovations Journal 2017;**32**. Available from: https://socialinnovationsjournal.org/74-what-works-what-doesn-t/2325-brief-history-and-future-of-intellectual-disability-services-in-america

87. American Psychiatric Association. Diagnostic and Statistical Manual of Mental Disorders. Washington, DC: American Psychiatric Association; 1952.

88. American Psychiatric Association. Diagnostic and Statistical Manual of Mental Disorders, 4th edition, text revision. Washington, DC: American Psychiatric Association; 2000.

89. American Psychiatric Association. Diagnostic and Statistical Manual of Mental Disorders, 5th edition. Arlington, VA: American Psychiatric Association; 2013.

90. Chamberlain CD. Challenging custodialism: families and eugenic institutionalization at the Pennsylvania Training School for Feeble-Minded Children at Elwyn. Journal of Social History 2021;**55**(2):484–509.

91. Liscum M, Garcia ML. You can't keep a bad idea down: dark history, death, and potential rebirth of eugenics. Anatomical Record 2021;**305**(4):902–37.

92. Harris JC. Intellectual Disability: Understanding its Development, Causes, Classification, Evaluation, and Treatment. Oxford: Oxford University Press; 2006.

93. Rochefort DA. Origins of the 'third psychiatric revolution': the Community Mental Health Centers Act of 1963. Journal of Health Politics, Policy and Law 1984;**9**(1):1–30.

94. Drake RE, Latimer E. Lessons learned in developing community mental health care in North America. World Psychiatry 2012;**11**(1):47–51.

95. Rothman DJ, Rothman SM. The Willowbrook Wars: Bringing the Mentally Disabled into the Community. New Brunswick, NJ: Aldine Transaction; 2009.

96. Conroy JW. The Pennhurst Longitudinal Study and public policy: how we learned that people were better off. In: Downey DB, Conroy JW, editors. Pennhurst and the Struggle for Disability Rights. University Park, PA: Penn State University Press; 2020:150–76.

97. Deegan PE. The Independent Living Movement and people with psychiatric disabilities: taking back control over our own lives. Psychosocial Rehabilitation Journal 1992;**15**(3):3–19.

98. White GW, Lloyd Simpson J, Gonda C, Ravesloot C, Coble Z. Moving from independence to interdependence: a conceptual model for better understanding community participation of Centers for Independent Living Consumers. Journal of Disability Policy Studies 2010;**20**(4):233–40.

99. McLean KJ, Hoekstra AM, Bishop L. United States Medicaid Home and community-based services for people with intellectual and developmental disabilities: a scoping review. Journal of Applied Research in Intellectual Disabilities 2020;**34**(3):684–94.

100. **Munly K, Roberto KA, Allen KR.** Understanding resilience of adult foster care providers. In: **Resnick B, Gwyther L, Roberto K,** editors. Resilience in Aging: Concepts, Research, and Outcomes. Cham: Springer; 2018: 367–83.

101. **Garwood JD, Ampuja AA.** Inclusion of students with learning, emotional, and behavioral disabilities through strength-based approaches. Intervention in School and Clinic 2018;**55**(1):46–51.

102. **Mollica RL, Check M, Farnharm J, Reinhard S, Simms-Kastelein K, Baldwin C,** et al. Building Adult Foster Care: What States Can Do. Washington, DC: AARP; 2009: 25–9.

103. **Wehmeyer ML, Tassé MJ, Davies DK, Stock S.** Support needs of adults with intellectual disability across domains: the role of technology. Journal of Special Education Technology 2012;**27**(2):11–21.

104. **Williamson HJ, Perkins EA, Acosta A, Fitzgerald M, Agrawal J, Massey OT.** Family caregivers of individuals with intellectual and developmental disabilities: experiences with Medicaid managed care long-term services and supports in the United States. Journal of Policy and Practice in Intellectual Disabilities 2016;**13**(4):287–96.

105. **Marrus N, Veenstra-VanderWeele J, Hellings JA, Stigler KA, Szymanski L, King BH,** et al. Training of child and adolescent psychiatry fellows in autism and intellectual disability. Autism 2013;**18**(4):471–5.

106. **Werner S, Stawski M.** Mental health: knowledge, attitudes and training of professionals on dual diagnosis of intellectual disability and psychiatric disorder. Journal of Intellectual Disability Research 2011;**56**(3):291–304.

107. **Katz G, Márquez-Caraveo ME, Lazcano-Ponce E.** Perspectives of intellectual disability in Mexico: epidemiology, policy, and services for children and adults. Current Opinion in Psychiatry 2010;**23**(5):432–35.

108. **Harley DA.** People with disabilities and mental health disorders in Mexico: rights and practices. In: **Harley D, Ysasi N, Bishop M, Fleming A,** editors. Disability and Vocational Rehabilitation in Rural Settings. Cham: Springer; 2017: 367–81.

109. **Emerson E.** Poverty and people with intellectual disabilities. Mental Retardation and Developmental Disabilities Research Reviews 2007;**13**(2):107–13.

110 **Gonzalez D, Alvarez M.** Depression in Mexico: stigma and its policy implications. Yale Global Health Review 2016;**4**(1):13–16.

111. **Rodriguez P, Rosenthal E, Guerrero H, Abott M, Boychuk C, Ahern L,** et al. No Justice: Torture, Trafficking and Segregation in Mexico. Washington, DC: Disability Rights International; 2015: 7–18.

112. **Comisión Coordinadora de Institutos Nacionales de Salud y Hospitales de Alta Especialidad.** Programa de Acción Específico Atención Psiquiátrica: Programa Sectorial de Salud 2013–2018. Mexico City: Gobierno de Mexico; 2014: 45–52.

113. **Miguel-Esponda G, Bohm-Levine N, Rodríguez-Cuevas FG, Cohen A, Kakuma R.** Implementation process and outcomes of a mental health programme integrated in primary care clinics in rural Mexico: a mixed-methods study. International Journal of Mental Health Systems 2020;**14**:21.

Chapter 16

Intellectual disabilities across cultures: The case of South America

Julio Torales, Marcelo O'Higgins, and João Mauricio Castaldelli-Maia

Introduction

Intellectual disability (ID) is characterized by significant limitations that affect intellectual functioning, adaptive behaviour, and practical skills, which directly interfere with interpersonal relationships and the environment (1). ID is one of the disabilities with the greatest variation in terms and definitions. The World Health Organization (WHO) uses the term 'intellectual disability', and defines it as follows: a disorder defined by the presence of incomplete or arrested mental development, which may occur with or without any other physical or mental disorder, and it is characterized by the impairment of skills and intelligence in areas such as cognitive, language, and social and motor skills. The WHO reports that the aetiology of ID is unknown in 60% of cases. In cases where it can be determined, it can be grouped into four categories, namely genetic disorders, chromosomal disorders, biological and organic causes, and environmental causes (2).

This condition is particularly difficult to assess and address in developing countries due to its stigma and the scarcity of appropriate resources to offer to these patients by public and private entities. With regard to South America, this is accentuated by the particularities of each country and the amount of funding that can be assigned to the management of programmes related to this subject and to support access to the services that the legislation grants to people with disability. According to the WHO, 10% of the population of South America has some type of disability (3).

Information is scarce about the stigma towards people with ID. Few studies have been done, and most were qualitative with small samples. It appears that stigma is common in South America, but there is no information about the influence of sociodemographic variables such as age and educational level (4).

General situation and administrative institutions related to people with intellectual disability in South America

South America consists of 12 countries (Argentina, Bolivia, Brazil, Chile, Colombia, Ecuador, Guyana, Paraguay, Peru, Suriname, Uruguay, and Venezuela) with different backgrounds and levels of development. There is a variety of cultural groups in each country and different ways of engaging the difficulties that come with ID. There is a lack of uniformity in access to medical, mental, and rehabilitation centres, and they have particular features in each of these countries (5).

In general, there is a lack of studies related to ID, and most of the data come from the national census and specific governmental studies in this regard (6).

Argentina

In Argentina, around 13% of the population had some kind of disability at the time of the last census. This represents 5,114,190 individuals. In a more recent survey in 2018, the results have shown that 10% of the population aged 6 years and older has some type of disability, reaching 25.3% of households (7). Regarding the most frequent disability, it was reported that motor impairment represented the main presentation, followed by visual impairment, hearing impairment, and mental cognitive impairment. The age distribution indicates that 72% of people with disabilities are 65 years of age or older (8).

In recent years, there have been efforts to give individuals with disabilities more accessibility to the different programmes recognized by the law. This was translated in the use of the Single Disability Certificate (Certificado Único de Discapacidad). However, only 33% of the total disabled population has acquired this document, even with an extensive media campaign by the government (9).

In Argentina, the agency overseeing compliance with state plans related to people with disabilities is the National Disability Agency (Agencia Nacional de Discapacidad) (10). Argentina is among the countries that have ratified the United Nations Convention on the Rights of Persons with Disabilities the fastest and has sought to have an interinstitutional collaboration between the different agencies of the Argentinean state in order to have better policies in terms of rights and guarantees for people with disabilities (11).

In Argentina, since the 1960s, there has been an increase in the participation of civil society in the quest to obtain rights for people with disabilities. Changes have been considered in the legal and administrative provisions regarding the institutionalization of this type of person (12). It is well known that in recent years, both from the academic and family sectors and people with disabilities themselves, greater participation in decision-making about the health of people with ID has been requested. These sectors speak of the fact that the state, particularly the Argentine state, has had a policy of infantilization of minority sectors until very recently, among them especially the group of people with disabilities. They say that before autonomy, there is a heteronomy promoted by the state sectors and that the direct participation of people with disabilities in the design, implementation, and control of policies related to their group should be favoured (13). However, the public policies regarding this have been limited, isolated, and although significant resources have been invested in areas of health and rehabilitation services, there has been a lack of policies aimed to reduce the stigma and approach the social demands of this population (14).

With regard to some specific disorders, some studies have been performed to measure the burden of these conditions in the country and the people who live with them. In the case of Down syndrome, the birth prevalence in Argentina, from a study in 2019, is about 17.26 per 10,000 births. This study also showed that the prevalence was higher in private sector hospitals, which the researchers interpreted as being influenced by differences in the structure of maternal age and a greater proportion of prenatal diagnosis (15).

From a legal aspect, the National University of La Plata designed a project to identify and support systems for decision-making based on the daily experience of people with ID (16). This and other projects (17) have been undertaken in order to give people living with ID more possibilities in decision-making and a more autonomous range of activities in their day-to-day routines.

From this context, movements of people with disabilities emerged that sought to obtain guarantees of their rights. An example of this is the 'Movimiento de Vida Independiente' (MVI; 'Independent Living Movement'), that arose in the US in the 1970s. In Argentina, the experience of MVI forms the basis of the project 'Independent Living for People with Intellectual Disabilities' carried out by various foundations and non-governmental organizations. This project began to be developed in 2007, making it possible for several people with ID to live together independently (18).

Bolivia

In a study in 2011, the prevalence rate of ID in the Plurinational State of Bolivia was 0.22 people per 100 inhabitants. The most prevalent type of ID was found to be moderate ID in 41.82%, followed by severe ID in 21.02%, while 20.12% of the people were classified as having a mild degree of ID. In 34.39% of the cases, a prenatal aetiology was found, followed by a perinatal cause in 30.69%, and 18.92% of cases were classified as having a postnatal aetiology (19).

In Bolivia, the entity in charge of promoting the defence of the rights of people with disabilities is the National Committee for Persons with Disabilities (Comité Nacional de Personas con Discapacidad (CONALPEDIS)). This body was created to comply with the General Law for Persons with Disabilities (20).

Brazil

In Brazil, the agency in charge of assisting people with disabilities is the National Secretariat for the Rights of People with Disabilities (Secretaria Nacional dos Direitos da Pessoa com Deficiência (SNDPD)), which in turn reports to the Ministry of Women, Family and Human Rights (Ministério da Mulher, da Família e dos Direitos Humanos) (21).

The supply of mental health professionals in Brazil has great variation in access by geographic region. For example, the number of psychiatrists is roughly 5 per 100,000 inhabitants in the Southeast region, and the Northeast region has less than one psychiatrist per 100,000 inhabitants. There is a lack of psychiatric nurses in all geographical areas. By 2006, there were 848 Community Psychosocial Centers (CAPS) registered in Brazil, a ratio of 0.9 CAPS per 200,000 inhabitants, with the Northeast and the North regions having lower figures than the South and Southeast regions (22).

A study in Brazil on the diagnostic status among individuals with moderate and severe ID in special schools showed that clear aetiological explanations were limited (24%); most diagnoses indicated only the type and the degree of impairment, and for the majority (61.4%) the cause was unknown. About half were sporadic cases within their families. For 44.2%, there was another ID case in the extended family, and 34.5% presented potential familial cases (1). In another study carried out in the south of Brazil, where the genetic causes that could be related to the presence of ID were studied, a prevalence of intellectual genetic disability of 0.82% was found, including Cornelia de Lange, Noonan, Williams, Moebius, fragile X, and Down syndromes, tuberous sclerosis, autosomal dominant microcephaly (proband, mother, and two siblings), abnormal microarrays, and multifactorial disorders such as schizencephaly, porencephalic cyst, and myelomeningocele (23). With regard to Down syndrome, it is estimated to have a prevalence of 14 per 10,000 live births. A study following births between 2012 and 2018 showed an incidence of 4 in 10,000 live births. That study stated a significant association ($p < 0.05$) with maternal age of 35 years or older, paternal age of 30 years or older, the performance of six or more prenatal consultations, prematurity, and low birth weight (24).

With regard to the participation of people with ID in different activities, there are many reasons that motivate a person to take part in different groups or activities. For example, in a study in which included more than 200 athletes from Special Olympics Brazil, the most frequent answers were in part mainly to get ribbons and medals, to play with other people from the team, to go to new and different places, and to feel like an important person (25).

Chile

In Chile, the institution in charge of promoting equal opportunities for people with disabilities, seeking their social inclusion, and eliminating any form of discrimination based on disability is the National Disability Service (Servicio Nacional de la Discapacidad (SENADIS)). Its functions include coordinating the actions of the state in the implementation of policies, programmes, and strategies for inclusive local development. It was created through Law No. 20.422, which establishes rules on Equal Opportunities and Social Inclusion of Persons with Disabilities, published in the Official Gazette on 10 February 2010 (26).

Unemployment among people with disabilities in Chile stands at 70.8%. It has been pointed out that the training centres for people with disabilities have tried to increase employment insertion but that many training centres have not yet systematically put into practice insertion systems that would allow a higher level of employment for those people with disabilities who can or wish to enter the labour market (27).

Regarding the educational integration of people with disabilities in Chile, a 2005 investigation shows that one in eight people has some type of disability, 9.8% do not have access to education, and one in two people with disabilities has not completed basic education (3). In Chile, laws have been approved on the integration of students with special educational needs, ensuring compliance with the principle of equal opportunities, particularly for those children with learning difficulties. Enrolment in the school integration service has increased by 616% due to the school integration policy implemented in 1997, increasing the coverage of students who receive specific school support. Despite these advances, various challenges remain that hinder the educational processes of these people, among which are a lack of reliable statistics by state or private institutions, continuity of studies for these students is not ensured, regular education teachers have no guidelines, and that there are no clear promotion criteria (6).

In a study on caregivers of children with disabilities in Curiacó, the prevalence of intense levels of overload was 48.1%, with caregivers of children with multiple disabilities having a greater burden (p = 0.015) (28).

In a study about the impact of the COVID-19 pandemic on this population, comparing groups in the US and Chile, there was an increase in mental health problems, with about 50% of the Chilean individuals indicating that they experienced an increase of mental health resources demand during this period (29).

Colombia

In Colombia, Law 1145 of 2007 created the National Disability System (Sistema Nacional de Discapacidad), which is a set of programmes and institutions related to the task of promoting the formulation and implementation of public policy on disability in a coordinated manner. It consists of a series of levels, starting with the Ministry of Social Protection as the lead agency at the first level, followed by the National Council on Disability (Consejo Nacional de Discapacidad, CND) as a consulting and advisory body. Then comes the third level with Departmental and District Disability Committees and a fourth level integrated by the Municipal and Local Disability Committees. The latter function as spaces for the consolidation and follow-up of public policies (30).

A 2005 study found that 2.6 million people had some type of disability, which equates to 6.4% of the Colombian population: 9.1% of people with disabilities had motor disabilities, 14% sensory disabilities, 34.8% cognitive disabilities, and 19.8% mental disabilities. From these results, it was also determined that 22.5% of people with disabilities were illiterate, which contrasts with 8.7% of illiteracy among people without disabilities (31).

Ecuador

In Ecuador, the National Council for the Equality of Disabilities (Consejo Nacional para la Igualdad de Discapacidades (CONADIS)) is the entity in charge of formulating, monitoring, and evaluating public policies on disability issues. Its scope of action covers both the public and private levels (32).

Regarding the population with disabilities, a 2004 study found that 12.14% of the population had disabilities. The same study indicated that, at that time, there was no record of information on people with disabilities living in institutions between psychiatric hospitals, asylums, and orphanages. It was found that 40% of people with disabilities do not attend an educational centre and that 93.4% of people with disabilities live with their families (33).

Guyana

In Guyana, the National Commission on Disability (NCD) is an executive branch agency. It officially began operating on 10 December 1997. In 2010, the Guyana Act No. 11 of 2010 Persons with Disability Act 2010 was enacted. While progress has been made, there is still a need for additional efforts related to the education of individuals with disabilities in Guyana before their full potential is realized (34).

Paraguay

Paraguay has a national entity in charge of taking care of different kinds of disabilities called the National Secretary for the Human Rights of Persons with Disabilities (Secretaria Nacional por los Derechos Humanos de las Personas con Discapacidad (SENADIS)). It was created in 1979 and, since its origin, aims to provide assistance and rehabilitation services to this population (35).

In Paraguay, it is estimated that approximately 15% of the population has some type of disability. However, there is an official undercount since less than 1% of them appear in the National Population and Housing Census 2002 (55,000 individuals), thus preventing visibility to the state. Paraguay has a national accessibility law that seeks universal accessibility criteria for public and private spaces and a labour inclusion law that establishes benefits for companies that seek to incorporate people with disabilities (36).

Peru

Peru has a body in charge of developing strategies to care for people with disabilities called the National Council for the Integration of Persons with Disabilities (Consejo Nacional de Integración de la persona con Discapacidad (CONADIS)) (37).

A national evaluation called the National Specialized Survey on Disability (ENEDIS) in 2012 showed that 5.2% of the Peruvian population had a disability. Peru also has a National Registry of Persons with Disabilities (RNPCD), which as of March 2022, only included 21% of these people (38).

A study aiming to profile patients with congenital hypothyroidism resulted in the majority of patients showing a borderline intellectual quotient (38.5%), the most frequent social category was educable (88.7%), and most of the patients presented delay in developing speech (88.5%). In addition, the neuropsychological developmental delay was more frequent in patients with congenital hypothyroidism diagnosed and treated after 21 days of age (39).

Of the population registered in these registries, 65.3% had communication limitations, 76.2% had self-care limitations, 53.2% had behavioural limitations, and 79.5% had dexterity limitations. The most prevalent type of disability corresponded to 'generalized, sensory and other' disability, which was found in 39.6%, followed by ID in 33.9% and musculoskeletal disability in 28.5% of people (37).

Uruguay

In Uruguay, the National Honorary Commission on Disability (Comisión Nacional Honoraria de la Discapacidad (CNHD)) was created by Article 10 of Law No. 16.095 on 26 October 1989, and ratified by Article 13 of Law No. 18,651 of February 2010, operating under the jurisdiction of the Ministry of Social Development (MIDES). Currently, MIDES has a National Secretary of Care and Disability who is the entity in charge of the National Registry of Persons with Disabilities (40).

In the National Census of 2011 carried out by the National Institute of Statistics Uruguay, it was observed that 15.9% of the population had at least some type of disability. Of these, in the range of 0–14 years of age, there were 36,730 people with disabilities, of whom approximately 50% had some permanent difficulty in understanding and/or learning (41).

Venezuela

In Venezuela, the National Council for Persons with Disabilities (Consejo Nacional para las Personas con Discapacidad, Conapdis) is an entity attached to the Ministry of People's Power of the office of the Presidency and Monitoring of Government Management. Its purpose is to promote comprehensive care for people with disabilities and seek cultural changes in relation to disability within the territory of the Bolivarian Republic of Venezuela. From a study carried out in 2001, it was found that the prevalence of ID corresponded to 9.3% (42). The small number of publications in this regard in the country is striking.

Efforts and experiences related to the well-being of people with intellectual disability

In recent years there has been a substantial increase in efforts to integrate people with ID into different social environments, whether educational, work, sports, and so on. In this sense, multiple efforts have been made by public and private entities and they have had different levels of response.

Programmes to provide preventive healthcare for people with ID have received increased attention, associated with the now accepted definition of health as a state of complete well-being in a biopsychosocial paradigm. The WHO suggested in multiple reports that special attention is required to meet the needs of those ageing with ID, particularly in developing countries. It was concluded that there is a significant need for national health and social policies that provide inclusive lifespan services and supports to people with ID in healthcare, housing, employment, and education (43).

Family involvement is a critical component of health promotion programmes in South America. It is well established that family is a central component of Latin American culture, and many people with ID are cared for by family members throughout their lives (44).

There are more than 200,000 Special Olympics athletes in Latin America. There are different sports categories, including football, alpine and cross-country skiing, team handball, tennis, and bocce, in which these athletes take part. There is an increase in this participation and in almost all countries of South America, there is an increasing amount of interest in these activities. This growth may be indicative of the increased awareness of the benefits of physical activity for people with ID (45).

Conclusion

Although ID represents a major challenge for people living with this condition, with adequate support in a favourable context, many of the associated difficulties can be overcome. Unfortunately, in South America, there is still a long way to go in terms of developing adequate support networks and ensuring access to rights for people with ID. In addition, although there are a series of strategies put into practice by the governments of each country, there is still a lack of unified policies in each country that could develop public and private resources that could allow better development of the capacities of these people.

References

1. **Oliveira LF, Chaves TF, Baretto N, de Luca GR, Barbato IT, Barbato Filho JH,** et al. Etiology of intellectual disability in individuals from special education schools in the south of Brazil. BMC Pediatrics 2020;**20**(1):506.
2. **Suárez-Escudero JC.** Discapacidad y neurociencias: la magnitud del déficit neurológico y neuro psiquiátrico. Acta Neurológica Colombiana 2014;**30**(4):290–9.
3. **Romero R, Lauretti P.** Integración educativa de las personas con discapacidad en Latinoamérica. Educere 2006;**10**(33):347–56.
4. **Tenorio M, Donoso J, Ali A, Hassiotis A.** Stigma toward persons with intellectual disability in South America: a narrative review. Journal of Policy and Practice in Intellectual Disabilities 2020;**17**(4):346–63.
5. **Torales JC, Castaldelli-Maia JM, O'Higgins MG, Florio L, Almirón Santacruz J, Barrios JI,** et al. Índice de vulnerabilidad CAPE: Compasión, Acción Asertiva, Pragmatismo y Evidencia—Versión para América Latina y el Caribe (CAPE VI—LAC)

'Globalización, conflicto, cambio climático, desastres naturales: poner la salud mental en la política exterior'. Anales de la Facultad de Ciencias Médicas (Asunción) 2021;**54**(1):21–50.

6. **Mercadante MT, Evans-Lacko S, Paula CS.** Perspectives of intellectual disability in Latin American countries: epidemiology, policy, and services for children and adults. Current Opinion in Psychiatry 2009;**22**(5):469–74.

7. **Meijide SS.** Infancia, discapacidad y pobreza en contexto de pandemia. Ciudadanías. Revista De Políticas Sociales Urbanas 2021;**9**. Available from: http://revistas.untref.edu. ar/index.php/ciudadanias/article/view/1290

8. **Mareño Sempertegui M.** Transformaciones normativas recientes en el derecho a la seguridad social de las personas con discapacidad en Argentina. Legal transformations in Social Security entitlements for people with disabilities in Argentina. 9 Nov 2020. Riberdis. Available from: http://riberdis.cedid.es/handle/11181/6161

9. **Puga C, Pagotto V, Giunta D, Vicens J, Leist M, Vaucheret Paz E**, et al. Prevalencia e incidencia de discapacidad a partir del Certificado Único de Discapacidad en un hospital universitario del Área Metropolitana de Buenos Aires. Archivos Argentinos de Pediatría 2019;**117**(3):183–7.

10. **Roma MC, Gastaldo Z.** Los derechos de las Personas con Discapacidad durante la Pandemia en Argentina. Revista Científica Arbitrada de la Fundación MenteClara 2021;**6**. Available from: https://fundacionmenteclara.org.ar/revista/index.php/RCA/arti cle/view/244

11. **Venturiello MP, Palermo MC, Tiseyra MV.** La discapacidad bajo sospecha: políticas públicas en discapacidad en la Argentina durante el período 2016–2019. Revista Argentina de Sociología 2020;**16**(27):28–34. from: https://ri.conicet.gov.ar/handle/ 11336/151367

12. **Lentini E.** La institucionalización de la discapacidad intelectual en perspectiva histórica. En Facultad de Psicología, Universidad de Buenos Aires; 2013. Available from: https://www.aacademica.org/000-054/577

13. **Contino AM, Micheletti A.** Niñez eterna. La infantilización en la discapacidad intelectual. F@ro: revista teórica del Departamento de Ciencias de la Comunicación 2019;**1**(29):5.

14. **Venturiello MP.** Políticas sociales en discapacidad: una aproximación desde las acciones del Estado en Argentina. Revista Española de Discapacidad 2017;**5**(2):149–69. Available from: https://ri.conicet.gov.ar/handle/11336/73154

15. **Martini J, Bidondo MP, Duarte S, Liascovich R, Barbero P, Groisman B.** [Birth prevalence of Down syndrome in Argentina]. Salud Colectiva 2019;**15**:e1863.

16. **Vásquez Encalada A, Bialik K, Stober K.** Supported decision making in South America: analysis of three countries' experiences. Int J Environ Res Public Health 2021;**18**(10):5204.

17. **Barani M, Kopitowski K, Carrara C, Yanzi MVR.** Shared decision making in Argentina in 2017. Z Evid Fortbild Qual Gesundhwes 2017;**123–124**:12–16.

18. **Rucci AC.** El surgimiento del Movimiento de Vida Independiente (MVI) en América Latina y su repercusión en la legislación de los países del Mercado Común del Sur (MERCOSUR). Informe Integrar 2015;**92**:2–16. Available from: http://sedici.unlp.edu. ar/handle/10915/72409

19. Lugo NT, Téllez OB, Rodríguez MAL, Camacho OA, Estévez OP, Serraniega RD, et al. Discapacidad intelectual. Aproximación a las principales causas en el Estado Plurinacional de Bolivia. Revista Cubana de Genética Comunitaria 2011;**5**(2):50–6.

20. Díaz-Aristizabal U, Sanz-Victoria S, Sahonero-Daza M, Ledesma-Ocampo S, Cachimuel-Vinueza M, Torrico M. Reflexiones sobre la estrategia de rehabilitación basada en la comunidad (RBC): la experiencia de un programa de RBC en Bolivia. Ciência & Saúde Coletiva 2012;**17**(1):167–77.

21. da Fonseca IF, De Souza Dias F. A convenção da Organização dos Estados Americanos para as pessoas com deficiência e as políticas federais brasileiras: Indicadores de monitoramento e ações do governo federal. Texto para Discussão No. 2602. Instituto de Pesquisa Econômica Aplicada (IPEA), Brasília; 2020. Available from: https://www.econstor.eu/handle/10419/240796

22. Mateus MD, Mari JJ, Delgado PG, Almeida-Filho N, Barrett T, Gerolin J, et al. The mental health system in Brazil: policies and future challenges. International Journal of Mental Health Systems 2008;**2**(1):12.

23. Karam SM, Riegel M, Segal SL, Félix TM, Barros AJD, Santos IS, et al. Genetic causes of intellectual disability in a birth cohort: a population-based study. American Journal of Medical Genetics Part A 2015;**167**(6):1204–14.

24. Laignier MR, Lopes-Júnior LC, Santana RE, Leite FMC, Brancato CL. Down Syndrome in Brazil: occurrence and associated factors. International Journal of Environmental Research and Public Health 2021;**18**(22):11954.

25. Pedrinelli VJ, Brandão MRF, Shapiro D, Fugita M, Gomes SS. Motives for sport participation of athletes with intellectual disability at the Special Olympics Brazil Program. Motricidade 2012;**8**(Supppl. 2):1005–12.

26. Tenorio M, Aparicio A, Arango PS, Fernández AK, Fergusson A, Turull J, et al. PaísDI: feasibility and effectiveness of an advocacy program for adults with intellectual disability and their stakeholders' groups in Chile. Journal of Applied Research in Intellectual Disabilities 2022;**35**(2):633–8.

27. Vidal RE, Cornejo CV, Arroyo LH. La inserción laboral de personas con discapacidad intelectual en Chile. Convergencia Educativa 2013;(2):93–102.

28. Arias Reyes C, Muñoz-Quezada MT. Calidad de vida y sobrecarga en cuidadores de escolares con discapacidad intelectual. Interdisciplinaria 2019;**36**(1):257–72.

29. Rosencrans M, Arango P, Sabat C, Buck A, Brown C, Tenorio M, et al. The impact of the COVID-19 pandemic on the health, wellbeing, and access to services of people with intellectual and developmental disabilities. Research in Developmental Disabilities 2021;**114**:103985.

30. Gómez-Aristizábal LY, Avella-Tolosa A, Morales LA. Observatorio de Discapacidad de Colombia. Revista Facultad Nacional de Salud Pública 2015;**33**(2):277–85.

31. Hurtado LT. Inclusión educativa de las personas con discapacidad en Colombia. CES Movimiento y Salud 2014;**2**(1):45–55. Available from: http://riberdis.cedid.es/handle/11181/4889

32. Salinas-Escobar J, Panamá-Mazhenda K, Robles-Bykbaev Y, Robles-Bykbaev V, Tenorio-Carpio H. ITaCaS: a serious game and an expert system to support the teaching of sexual-health and hygiene for youth with intellectual disability. 2020 6th International Conference on Science in Information Technology (ICSITech), Palu, Indonesia. 2020: 80–5.

33. **Galarza HM.** Discapacidad intelectual: demanda por un análisis cultural y social crítico en Ecuador. Intersticios Revista sociológica de pensamiento crítico 2008;2(2). Available from: https://intersticios.es/article/view/2711

34. **Cheong KA, Kellems RO, Andersen MM, Steed K.** The education of individuals with disabilities in Guyana: an overview. Intervention in School and Clinic 2019;**54**(4):246–50.

35. **Giménez AR.** Empleabilidad de personas con discapacidad desde el marco rector de SENADIS, Paraguay. Revista Internacional de Investigación en Ciencias Sociales 2015;**11**(2):209–22.

36. **Pérez Bejarano NM, Alarcón Gónzalez VS, Ferreira Gaona MI, Díaz Reissner CV, Duré P, Andriotti N,** et al. Estado de Salud Oral en Discapacitados Residentes en la Fundación Pequeño Cottolengo Don Orione, Paraguay. International Journal of Odontostomatology 2016;**10**(1):69–74.

37. **Panclas GM, Meléndez ML.** ¿Qué factores favorecen el conocimiento sobre los derechos de las personas con discapacidad? CASUS: Revista de Investigación y Casos en Salud 2017;**2**(3):147–55.

38. Ruralidad y uso de servicios informales de salud en personas con discapacidad de Perú: Análisis de una encuesta nacional. Universidad Peruana de Ciencias Aplicadas (UPC), Lima, Peru; 2018. Available from: https://repositorioacademico.upc.edu.pe/handle/10757/624896

39. **Herrera-Chinchay L, Silva-Ocas I, Castro-Silva N, Del Águila Villar C.** Social, cognitive and psychomotor development in Peruvian children with congenital hypothyroidism. Andes Pediatrica 2021;**92**(2):235–40.

40. **Mancebo Castro M.** el accionar colectivo en torno a la discapacidad en Uruguay. Revista Uruguaya de Ciencia Política 2016;**25**(SPE):79–98.

41. **Obando D, Elaine M.** Aprendizaje cooperativo para la inclusión educativa de niños/as con discapacidad intelectual en una escuela común uruguaya. Final degree project. University of the Republic (Uruguay). Faculty of Psychology; 2016. Available from: https://www.colibri.udelar.edu.uy/jspui/handle/20.500.12008/8471

42. **Ministerio de Educación Superior, Pestana Correia L.** Integración de personas con discapacidad en educación superior en Venezuela. Caracas: UNESCO; 2005.

43. **Frey GC, Temple VA.** Health promotion for Latin Americans with intellectual disabilities. Salud Publica de Mexico. 2008;**50**(S2):167–77.

44. **Blacher J, Baker BL.** Positive impact of intellectual disability on families. American Journal on Mental Retardation 2007;**112**(5):330–48.

45. **Temple VA, Stanish HI.** Physical activity and persons with intellectual disability: some considerations for Latin America. Salud Publica de Mexico 2008;**50**(S2):185–93.

Chapter 17

Intellectual Disability Services in the United Kingdom and Ireland

Samuel J. Tromans, Verity Chester, Avinash Hiremath, and Rohit Gumber

Epidemiology

A 2015 report by Public Health England (1) estimated that around 1,087,100 people with intellectual disability (ID) were living in England, of whom 930,400 were adults. When also considering Wales, Scotland, and Northern Ireland, there are an estimated 1.4 million people with ID in the entirety of the UK, of whom approximately 1.1 million are adults (2). In terms of the prevalence of mental illness among adults with ID, a population-based study by Cooper et al. (3), involving 1023 Scotland-based adults, reported a point prevalence of 40.9% for mental illness,[1] based on clinical diagnosis, representing a high rate relative to their non-ID peers. Furthermore, mental illness was significantly associated with female sex, increased severity of ID, receiving paid carer support, increased number of life events in the past year, increased number of general practitioner appointments in the past year, urinary incontinence, and being a smoker. This increased prevalence of mental illness in adults with ID is likely attributable to a myriad of biopsychosocial factors, including genetic syndromes causal of ID, and health inequality.

Emerson (2012) (4) conducted a cross-sectional survey to investigate ID in different ethnic groups, based on the educational records of children aged 7–15 years (n = 5.18 million). He reported a general trend of lower rates of identified people with ID among minority ethnic groups. However, exceptions to this trend were higher rates of less severe ID among Gypsy/Romany and Irish Traveller groups, and higher rates of more severe ID among Pakistani and Bangladeshi groups. As the author pointed out, however, it is unclear whether these differences correspond to genuine differences in true prevalence, or are instead reflective of other issues, such as inequities in access to diagnostic assessment (5).

A literature review on autism identification across ethnic groups similarly reported that identification appears to be generally lower in minority ethnic groups relative to the majority population, and that individuals presenting with autism from minority groups appear to have more severe forms of the condition (6). Possible explanations for inter-ethnicity differences in autism identification included reduced access to or quality of healthcare services, fear or being stigmatized leading to reduced help-seeking, or higher rates of parental consanguinity in certain cultural groups (6).

History

The UK and Ireland represent the only countries in the world where the psychiatry of ID is treated as a distinct psychiatric subspecialty, with an associated training pathway (7) and linked services. This is in contrast to other countries, where training may take the form of a specific time-limited placement or simply lecture-based teaching only (8), and where in practice people with ID are treated by general psychiatrists and other medical professionals as necessary. Nevertheless, it is essential for all doctors in patient-facing roles to receive both under- and postgraduate training in the psychiatry of ID, as all will be working with patients with these conditions (7).

Intrinsically linked to the UK and Ireland model of treating ID as a psychiatric speciality are debates related to 'mainstreaming' versus 'specialization', both of which are viewed to have benefits and drawbacks for the ID population. Mainstream services meet aims related to normalization and inclusion, while specialization is conversely viewed as excluding. Conversely, while the equity of access that mainstreaming brings is commendable, it is meaningless if not accompanied by equity of outcome, which can be variable depending on the ID experience and expertise of the treating generic professionals.

The origins of having psychiatric specialists in ID in the UK is rooted in the 1913 Mental Deficiency Act (9), where 'mental deficiency colonies', analogous to mental asylums, were set up for people with ID (10). This act was linked with the eugenics movement, alongside broadly negative attitudes to those with ID and/or mental health problems. Reports of all types of abuse were widespread in relation to such institutions. Publication of the Better Services for the Mentally Handicapped government white paper in 1971 (11) outlined the vision to move away from caring for people with 'mental handicap' in institutional settings and to increase the provision of local and community care, while noting the shortage of appropriate residential accommodation, of social workers, and of training centres, which were more pronounced in certain parts of the country, causing pressure to admit more patients to overcrowded and unsuitable facilities. The 1980s saw the deinstitutionalization programme, defined as the process that led to widespread closure of long-stay hospitals, with people with ID moving back into the community (12). This movement was given impetus by increasing public and political pressure to reject 'institutionalization' and the negative consequences of institutional life for patients, such as passivity, loss of autonomy, and stigma. Congruently, the findings of an Irish study suggested that government funding should aim to promote individualized supports by redistributing funds from traditional, congregated service delivery to individualized models (13). Psychiatric care of this group then shifted to community clinics and general hospitals on an as-required basis (14).

The second phase of the strategy was intended to be a much more complex process than simply closing institutions, but to substantially improve care quality in community settings, providing comprehensive support to patients and their families, fuelled by ideals such as normalization and participation. The government set out its proposals for improving the lives of people with ID and their families and carers in its 2001 report, entitled *Valuing People: A New Strategy for Learning Disability for the 21st Century* (15), emphasizing the rights of those with ID as citizens, social inclusion in local communities, choice in their daily lives, and real opportunities to be independent. The strategy highlighted the importance of personalization and person-centred approaches.

Different forms of community living models were set up to improve the lives of people with ID. Supported independent houses and transitional residential homes with three to ten residents were the main two models (16). In some places, supported-living houses and small residential homes were clustered in a locality. Positive effects of deinstitutionalization include improved quality of life and improvement in skills. While the move of deinstitutionalization was largely positive for people with mild or moderate ID, people with more severe ID and/or behaviours that challenge still resided in specialist hospitals or large residential facilities, leading to a difference in outcome between the groups.

Prior to deinstitutionalization, colonies had a 'visiting medical officer', usually a general practitioner, and were originally operated by local authorities. The expectation that medical officers had specialist expertise in ID, as well as the National Health Service (NHS) eventually taking over such institutions and the 1959 Mental Health Act (17), led to the then-called psychiatrists of mental handicap becoming the central medical figure for this patient group (10). Their role was quite broad at this time, involving management of both the physical and mental health of people with ID. The deinstitutionalization movement led to the role of psychiatrists of mental handicap evolving into its modern-day equivalent, the psychiatrist of ID, with a corresponding narrowing of professional focus to management of mental health problems and challenging behaviour (12). Recruitment of psychiatrists into psychiatry of ID has been low in recent years (18); however, most trainees working within the speciality feel satisfied and well supported with respect to their training (19). A 2011 faculty report by the Royal College of Psychiatrists described the future role of psychiatrists of ID (20), in the form of a tiered care model, summarized in Fig. 17.1. This tiered approach provides clarity concerning the roles of professionals residing on the respective tiers, as well as supporting efficient commissioning of specialist services.

Psychiatrists in ID are principally employed by either community or inpatient teams, or a hybrid arrangement. Their role includes the treatment of mental illnesses in people with ID, as well as support with neurodevelopmental conditions, such as ID and autism, and liaising with other professionals with a view to advocating for their health and social care needs, as well as the needs of the carers who support them (21).

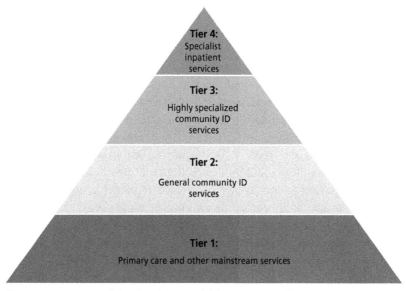

Fig. 17.1 A summary of the tiered care model for psychiatry of ID. Please note that tier 1 involves limited direct contact with psychiatrists of ID (20).
Royal College of Psychiatrists. Future role of psychiatrists working with people with learning disability: Royal College of Psychiatrists Faculty Report FR/LD/1. 2011; Available from: https://www.rcpsych.ac.uk/docs/default-source/members/faculties/intellectual-disability/id-futureroleofpsychiatristsinld-services.pdf?sfvrsn=33500689_4

A small number of UK- and Ireland-based psychiatrists are also involved in academia or are in clinical academic roles, managing a caseload and conducting research. Research recommendations for adults with ID have been identified by the National Institute of Health and Care Excellence and pertain to mental illness as well as challenging behaviour. These are summarized in Table 17.1.

However, while important research involving people with ID is being conducted in the UK, they are often excluded from clinical research. Spaul and colleagues (25) conducted a review of 26,293 England-based studies. They reported that 60.3% ($n = 15,853$) of sampled studies excluded ID groups, and that only 1.4% ($n = 368$) of studies were specifically related to people with ID. Such exclusion of people with ID from clinical research carries a significant opportunity cost, as it impedes development of valuable new clinical evidence for this patient group that could be used to improve their care and quality of life.

Table 17.1 Current research priorities for mental disorder and/or behaviours the challenge in people with intellectual disability

Category	Subcategory	Research priorities
Prevention		• Preventing behaviours that challenge from developing in children aged under 5 years with ID (23)
Diagnosis		• Development of case identification tools for common mental health problems (24)
Interventions	General	• Interventions to reduce the frequency and extent of moderate to severe behaviours that challenge within community settings (23)
	Psychological	• Children and young people with internalizing disorders (24) • Depression and anxiety in adults with mild to moderate ID (24)
	Pharmacological	• Anxiety disorders in people with ID and autism (24)
	Other	• Psychosocial interventions for people with more severe ID (24)
Care provision		• Understanding the experiences of people with ID and mental disorders within services (24) • Locally accessible care (23) • Factors associated with sustained, high quality residential care (24)

Reproduced with permission from Thurston R, Tromans S, Chester V, Cooper SA, Strydom A, Bhaumik S, et al. Current and Future Research Priorities in the Psychiatry of Intellectual Disability. In: Bhaumik S, Alexander R, editors. Oxford Textbook of the Psychiatry of Intellectual Disability, Oxford: Oxford University Press; 2020. p. 275–288.

Community care model

The deinstitutionalization movement has relocated the care of the many specialized healthcare needs of the ID population in the UK to the community (26). Community learning disability (ID) teams were created to provide a diverse range of clinical services to meet the comprehensive mental and some physical health needs of people with ID. Such teams are made up of psychiatrists, clinical psychologists, community ID nurses, speech and language therapists, occupational therapists, behaviour therapists, physiotherapists, and may include social workers. They provide an diverse range of direct clinical services to a very heterogeneous population (from people with mild ID to individuals with profound and multiple disabilities), including specialist mental health services, forensic services, challenging behaviour services, health advocacy and education, communication and social skills training, and rehabilitative programmes (27,28).

This model of care has been criticized for frequently bypassing mainstream primary care services and resulting in those with ID being excluded from local mental health strategies (27). It is a statutory requirement under the Equality Act 2010 (29) and the Health and Social Care Act 2008 (30) that public sector agencies make reasonable adjustments to their practice that will make them as accessible and effective for people with autism, ID, mental health issues, or a combination of these. However, there remains a need for improved staff training in the assessment of those with a dual diagnosis of ID and mental illness within mainstream mental health services and also improved expertise within forensic community teams for the care of offenders with ID (28). The 'Reasonably Adjusted? Mental Health Services and Support for People with Autism and People with Learning Disabilities' report in 2012 (31) highlighted shortcomings and recommendations for mental health services to take specific action in relation to this requirement. Government and charitable organizations continue to drive this agenda through campaigns, such as the Royal Mencap Society's 'Treat Me Well' campaign (32).

The lives of people with intellectual disability

The community care model was intended to drastically improve the lives of those with ID in the UK and Ireland, in terms of every aspect of life, including residence, employment, and social contact. In terms of the residences of people with ID today, 78% of adults in England who receive long-term support for ID live in their own home or with family, with some living in residential care facilities, primarily supported living settings (33). Over time, this proportion has increased, driven by the development of supported living services that aim to enhance social inclusion, networks, and belonging, alongside enhancing well-being and mental health.

The principles of supported living are that people with ID own or rent their home and have control over the support they get, who they live with (if anyone), and how they live their lives. Supported living assumes that all people with ID, regardless of the level or type of disability, can make choices about how to live their lives even if the person does not make choices in conventional ways (34). For most people with ID, support is intrinsically linked with people being able to live successfully in their own homes. This support may vary from a low level to help manage a tenancy and aspects of daily life, to an intensive package of support to help manage all areas of life (34). Even in those with severe ID, positive effects of the move to supported living have been reported including improvement in mood and a decrease in their challenging behaviours.

Education and employment

Research indicates that the perceived benefits of work for people with ID are similar to those of the non-disabled population; namely, the sense of feeling productive and staying busy, having relationships with co-workers, feeling important, increased income, and having opportunities for continued growth and advancement (35). At the time of publication of *Valuing People* (15), less than 10% of those with ID nationally were in work, with most people heavily dependent on social security benefits.

Sheltered employment was the preferred model for those with ID until relatively recently. Such provisions offered opportunities for increasing the number of workers with disabilities who otherwise could not enter mainstream employment (35). However, themes of normalization have affected this provision too, with the trend toward moving people into mainstream employment. In the UK, the largest such provider was Remploy, which at its height in the late 1980s, employed more than 10,000 people at 94 non-profit factory sites, the last of which closed in 2013 (36). Despite the goal of mainstreaming, the Adult Social Care Outcomes Framework for 2017/2018 (37) reported that 6% of adults with ID in England were in paid employment. In Scotland, the proportion in employment was lower, with just 4.2% in employment as of 2018 (38). Of this group, 42.9% were reported to be in open employment,[2] 31.0% in non-open employment,[3] 0.6% were self-employed, and for 25.5% the precise nature of their employment arrangements were not known. The NHS Long Term Plan (39) notes that employment rates for those with ID have remained low for many years and proposed several measures to rectify this situation, such as increasing the uptake of supported internship programmes, a 1-year study programme which takes place in the workplace. It remains to be seen whether advancements in employment will be made for this population in the coming years.

Leisure, social contact, and relationships

For decades, services for people with ID were heavily reliant on large, often institutional, day centres (15), which provided a range of social and occupational activities, primarily for those with disabilities. Policy in the UK for adults with ID no longer supports such day care services, which were criticized for failing to promote social inclusion, independence, or opportunities to develop individual interests or the skills and experience they need in order to move into employment (15). Personalized care and support under individuals' control with choice of community-based opportunities is now promoted (40).

Despite governmental commitments and strategies, evidence as to whether social inclusion and participation have increased is unclear, possibly related to the quality of community placements (16). Numerous studies have suggested that people with ID have few friends (41). Social networks of those with ID have been described as limited, mainly composed of other disability service users, staff, and family members (42). Subsequently, it has been reported that loneliness is a common experience in ID (42). Access to activities can depend on the quality of provision (43). Developments have been seen in certain areas through the provision of initiatives such as 'Gig Buddies' which was established to help people with ID overcome some of the barriers they face to going out in the evening, such as not having anyone to go out with, limited access to support workers, limited access to transport, and concerns about safety issues (44).

Current service provision

Following the deinstitutionalization movement, long-stay beds reduced from approximately 64,000 in 1970, to around 3954 as of 2012–2013, representing a 93.8% reduction (12). As such, the majority of the ID population were residing in community facilities, with some availability of specialist mental health inpatient beds for those who required them, funded via taxation, and principally provided by the NHS (7).

This was the care model status quo until a 2011 undercover investigation for the British Broadcasting Corporation's *Panorama* documentary series found a litany of appalling abuses of people with ID and autism within Winterbourne View, a private hospital based in Gloucestershire, England (45). These abuses, including physical assault (slapping, and misuse of physical restraint), as well as verbal threats and humiliation, led to the imprisonment of multiple staff members and closure of the hospital (45). In the wake of the events at Winterbourne

View, the UK government published *'Transforming care: a national response to Winterbourne View hospital'* (46), alongside a corresponding programme of action (47). One of the conclusions of these reports was that people with ID were spending too long in these hospitals (12), effectively providing the outdated institutional care of the past (48). Thus, in the subsequent years there has been a move to further reduce inpatient beds for patients with ID, a trend that is set to continue, as outlined in the NHS Long Term Plan (39), which has ambitions for a further 50% reduction in inpatient bed provision by 2023/2024, relative to 2015. However, there is a need to ensure the necessary infrastructure is in place to support people with ID and complex needs in the community in order to safely achieve this ambition (48).

Historically, patients with ID and/or autism could be detained in hospital under the 1983 Mental Health Act (49) by virtue of these conditions. However, this legislation has been scrutinized in recent years (50), and the 2021 UK government report entitled *Reforming the Mental Health Act* (51) has proposed that patients with ID and/or autism will no longer be able to detained under Section 3 of the act (detention for treatment) on the basis of these conditions, though they could still be detained in the presence of co-occurring mental illness. With respect to Section 2 (detention for assessment), the report proposes that patients with ID and/or autism could be detained when 'their behaviour is so distressed that there is a substantial risk of significant harm to self or others and a probably mental health cause to that behaviour that warrants assessment in hospital' (51). Concerns have been raised about the unintended consequences of such legislative change (52), pointing to the case of New Zealand, where equivalent changes led to a limited options for people with ID and offending behaviours, who risked ending up in prison or community placements that were inappropriate for their needs, leading to further legislative changes to address this issue (53).

Another concern raised in the inquiry into Winterbourne View was that of over-prescription of psychotropic medications (46,54). A multi-site UK-based cohort study by Sheehan et al. (55) supported this view, reporting that antipsychotic drug prescribing for people with ID was 'disproportionate to the level of recorded severe mental illness', and was associated with 'challenging behaviour, older age, and diagnoses of autism and dementia'. A similar trend was reported in a Public Health England study of primary care databases (56).

In response to this, in 2015 the NHS England-led stopping overmedication of people with a learning disability, autism, or both (STOMP) initiative was born, with a view to reducing the prescribing of psychotropic medication (57). A previous 'Call to Action' with respect to antipsychotic prescribing in people with dementia had led to a reported 51.8% reduction in inappropriate prescribing

(54,58), and it was hoped that STOMP would yield a similar response (54). Indeed, a subsequent report by Public Health England (59,60) suggests that patterns in psychotropic prescribing are moving in the right direction, though it is unclear whether this is a direct consequence of the STOMP initiative.

People with ID die prematurely relatively to their non-ID peers, frequently of preventable causes (61). The *'Treat Me Right!'* Report (62), published by the charity Mencap, outlined the poorer health of people with ID, including a summary of recommendations on what needs to be done. This was followed by the *'Death by Indifference'* report (63), describing six case reports of people with ID whereby neglect and substandard care led to their premature deaths.

The 'Death by Indifference' report resulted in an independent inquiry (64), of which the recommendations led to the 'Confidential Inquiry into the deaths of people with learning disabilities' (CIPOLD) (65). This population-based study reviewed the deaths of 247 people with ID who had died between June 2010 and May 2012. The median age of death within the study population was just 64 years, with 22% ($n = 54$) being below 50 years of age. CIPOLD found that 37% of the deaths were considered avoidable through good-quality healthcare, compared to just 13% in the general population of England and Wales. Factors significantly associated with premature death included problems with advanced care planning, adherence to the Mental Capacity Act (66), inappropriate accommodation, adjustment of care in response to changing needs, and carers feeling that they were not being listened to. These findings clearly demonstrated that issues pertaining to care service provision were contributing to the premature deaths of patients with ID. The authors set out a series of recommendations intended to address this situation (65).

The findings of CIPOLD resulted in the development of the Learning from Life and Death Reviews (LeDeR) programme (67). This is a standardized review process for deaths of all people with ID and/or autism aged 4 years and above, whereby episodes of previous receipt of health and social care are considered (67,68). This done to identify areas of both good practice and where improvements are required, with a view to both improving the care and preventing the premature deaths of people with ID and/or autism.

Future plans

The NHS Long Term Plan (39), published in 2019, sets out plans to improve the health and lives of people with ID and autism over the coming years. These include addressing morbidity and preventable deaths, improving understanding of the needs of this group, reducing waiting list times for specialist services, further reducing inpatient care provision (with a corresponding increased

Table 17.2 A summary of the targets for improving the lives of persons with intellectual disability and autism, as described in the NHS Long Term Plan

Goal[a]	Example of related strategy
'Action will be taken to tackle the causes of morbidity and preventable deaths in people with a learning disability and for autistic people'	Ensuring ≥75% of people with ID of >14 years of age receive an annual health check within primary care services
'The whole NHS will improve its understanding of the needs of people with learning disabilities and autism, and work together to improve their health and well-being'	By 2023/2024, patients with ID and/or autism will have a 'digital flag' in their electronic healthcare records
'Autism diagnosis will be included alongside work with children and young people's mental health services to test and implement the most effective ways to reduce waiting times for specialist services'	By 2023/2024, children and young people with ID and/or autism with complex needs will have their own keyworker
'Children, young people, and adults with a learning disability, autism or both, with the most complex needs, have the same rights to live fulfilling lives'	By 2023/2024 inpatient care provision will have reduced to 50% of that of 2015
'Increased investment in intensive, crisis and forensic community support'	Local healthcare providers will be required to have utilized this investment to provide a 7-day service that provides specialist multidisciplinary care support
'We will focus on improving the quality of inpatient care across the NHS and independent sector'	By 2023/2024, all care provided or commissioned by the NHS will have to satisfy the Learning Disability Improvement Standards (69).

[a] Transcribed verbatim from the NHS Long Term Plan document (39).

Data from National Health Service. The NHS Long Term Plan. 2019. Available at: https://www.longtermp lan.nhs.uk/wp-content/uploads/2019/08/nhs-long-term-plan-version-1.2.pdf

investment in community support), and improving the quality of remaining inpatient care services. Further detail pertaining to these goals are provided in Table 17.2.

Summary

This chapter has summarized the historical and present care of those with ID in the UK and Ireland. Like other countries, this began with an institutional approach to care, with those with ID segregated in asylums, leading unfulfilling lives, and often suffering various forms of abuse. This was followed by the deinstitutionalization movement, prioritizing community care based on ideologies of personalization, mainstreaming, and inclusion. Some inpatient services did remain, for the assessment and treatment of mental illness when it did occur. However, these services were subject to similar criticism as institutional care, and these bed numbers are again under scrutiny and review, with changes in legislation to further support reduced inpatient provision. Deinstitutionalization has seen an increased presence of those with ID in community-based residences, but whether it has fully achieved its aims of full inclusion in society is unclear, with low numbers of those with ID reporting satisfaction with their social lives, and life opportunities. The role of the psychiatrist in care for this population remains prominent in the UK and Ireland, with ongoing involvement in both community and inpatient service provision, as well as practice-based and academic projects aiming to improve various health and lifestyle outcomes.

Notes

1. The authors included the following conditions within this prevalence estimate: psychotic disorders, affective disorders, anxiety disorders (excluding specific phobias), obsessive–compulsive disorders, organic disorders, alcohol/substance abuse disorders, pica, sleep disorders, attention deficit hyperactivity disorder, autistic spectrum disorders, problem behaviour, personality disorder, and 'other mental health'.

2. Defined by the authors as 'Employment in a workplace that is not specifically set up for people with learning disabilities. People with learning disabilities are paid the going rate for the job.'

3. Defined by the authors as 'the workplace is specifically set up for people with learning disabilities. Non-open posts are not usually advertised.'

References

1. **Public Health England**. Learning Disabilities Observatory: people with learning disabilities in England 2015: main report. 2016. Available from: https://assets.publishing.service.gov.uk/government/uploads/system/uploads/attachment_data/file/613182/PWLDIE_2015_main_report_NB090517.pdf

2. **Mencap**. How common is learning disability? n.d. Available from: https://www.mencap.org.uk/learning-disability-explained/research-and-statistics/how-common-learning-disability

3. **Cooper SA, Smiley E, Morrison J, Williamson A, Allan L.** Mental ill-health in adults with intellectual disabilities: prevalence and associated factors. British Journal of Psychiatry 2007;**190**:27–35.

4. **Emerson E.** Deprivation, ethnicity and the prevalence of intellectual and developmental disabilities. Journal of Epidemiology and Community Health 2012;**66**(3):218–24.

5. **Tromans S, Brugha T.** Autism epidemiology: distinguishing between identification and prevalence. Progress in Neurology and Psychiatry 2022;**26**(1):4–6.

6. **Tromans S, Chester V, Gemegah E, Roberts K, Morgan Z, Yao GL, et al.** Autism identification across ethnic groups: a narrative review. Advances in Autism 2020;**7**(3):241–55.

7. **Perera B, Courtenay K.** Mental health services for people with intellectual disability in the United Kingdom. Advances in Mental Health and Intellectual Disabilities 2018;**12**(3):91–8.

8. **Dias MC, Perera B, Riese F, De Picker L, da Costa MP, Petricean A, et al.** Are we training psychiatrists to develop skills in intellectual disability psychiatry? Current European context and future directions. European Psychiatry 2020;**63**(1):e99.

9. **Leach R.** The Mental Deficiency Act, 1913. London: The Local Government Press Company; 1914. Available from: https://wellcomecollection.org/works/h7ykpfbw/items?canvas=5

10. **Carpenter P.** Should there be a faculty of learning disability psychiatry? Psychiatric Bulletin 2002;**26**(3):83–4.

11. **Department of Health and Social Security.** Better Services for the Mentally Handicapped. London: Department of Health and Social Security; 1971.

12. **Devapriam J, Rosenbach A, Alexander R.** In-patient services for people with intellectual disability and mental health or behavioural difficulties. BJPsych Advances 2015;**21**(2):116–23.

13. **Fleming P, McGilloway S, Barry S.** Day service provision for people with intellectual disabilities: a case study mapping 15-year trends in Ireland. Journal of Applied Research in Intellectual Disabilities 2017;**30**(2):383–94.

14. **Kritsotaki D, Long V, Smith M.** Introduction: deinstitutionalisation and the pathways of post-war psychiatry in the western world. In: **Kritsotaki D, Long V, Smith M,** editors. Deinstitutionalisation and After: Post-War Psychiatry in the Western World. London: Palgrave Macmillan Ltd; 2016: 1–36.

15. **Department of Health.** Valuing People: A New Strategy for Learning Disability for the 21st Century. London: UK Department of Health; 2001.

16. **Bredewold F, Hermus M, Trappenburg M.** 'Living in the community' the pros and cons: a systematic literature review of the impact of deinstitutionalisation on people with intellectual and psychiatric disabilities. Journal of Social Work 2020;**20**(1):83–116.

17. **Gov.UK.** Mental Health Act, 1959. 1959. Available from: https://www.legislation.gov.uk/ukpga/1959/72/pdfs/ukpga_19590072_en.pdf

18. **Health Education England.** ST4 psychiatry guidance documents. 2022. Available from: https://www.nwpgmd.nhs.uk/st4_psy_train_guidance_docs

19. **Walton C, Williams F, Bonell S, Barrett M.** The current state of training in psychiatry of intellectual disability: perspectives of trainees and trainers. BJPsych Bulletin 2021;**45**(1):59–65.

20. **Royal College of Psychiatrists.** Future role of psychiatrists working with people with learning disability: Royal College of Psychiatrists Faculty Report FR/LD/1. 2011. Available from: https://www.rcpsych.ac.uk/docs/default-source/members/faculties/intellectual-disability/id-futureroleofpsychiatristsinld-services.pdf?sfvrsn=33500689_4

21. **Royal College of Psychiatrists.** Intellectual disability psychiatrist. n.d. Available from: https://www.rcpsych.ac.uk/become-a-psychiatrist/choose-psychiatry/what-is-psychiatry/types-of-psychiatrist/intellectual-disability

22. **Thurston R, Tromans S, Chester V, Cooper SA, Strydom A, Bhaumik. S.**, et al. Current and future research priorities in the psychiatry of intellectual disability. In: **Bhaumik S, Alexander R**, editors. Oxford Textbook of the Psychiatry of Intellectual Disability. Oxford: Oxford University Press; 2020: 275–88.

23. **National Institute for Health and Care Excellence**. Challenging behaviour and learning disabilities: prevention and interventions for people with learning disabilities whose behaviour challenges (NG11). 2015. Available from: https://www.nice.org.uk/guidance/ng11

24. **National Institute for Health and Care Excellence**. Mental health problems in people with learning disabilities: prevention, assessment and management (NG 54). 2016. Available from: https://www.nice.org.uk/guidance/ng54

25. **Spaul SW, Hudson R, Harvey C, Macdonald H, Perez J.** Exclusion criterion: learning disability. Lancet 2020; **395**(10223):e29.

26. **Balogh R, McMorris CA, Lunsky Y, Ouellette-Kuntz H, Bourne L, Colantonio A**, et al. Organising healthcare services for persons with an intellectual disability. Cochrane Database of Systematic Reviews 2016;4:CD007492.

27. **O'Hara J.** Learning disabilities services: primary care or mental health trust? Psychiatric Bulletin 2000;**24**(10):368–9.

28. **Royal College of Psychiatrists.** Community-based services for people with intellectual disability and mental health problems. 2015. Available from: https://www.rcpsych.ac.uk/docs/default-source/members/faculties/intellectual-disability/id-fr-id-06.pdf?sfvrsn=5a230b9c_2

29. **HM Government**. Equality Act 2010. 2010. Available from: https://www.legislation.gov.uk/ukpga/2010/15/introduction.

30. **HM Government**. Health and Social Care Act 2008. 2008. Available from: https://www.legislation.gov.uk/ukpga/2008/14/introduction

31. **National Development Team for Inclusion**. Reasonably adjusted? Mental health services and support for people with autism and people with learning disabilities. 2012. Available from: https://www.ndti.org.uk/assets/files/Reasonably-adjusted_2020-12-30-150637.pdf

32. **Mencap**. Treat me well. 2022. Available from: https://www.mencap.org.uk/get-involved/campaign-mencap/treat-me-well

33. **NHS Digital**. Measures from the Adult Social Care Outcomes Framework, England – 2020–21. 2022. Available from: https://digital.nhs.uk/data-and-information/publications/statistical/adult-social-care-outcomes-framework-ascof/england-2020-21

34. **National Development Team for Inclusion**. Supported living – making the move. Developing supported living options for people with learning disabilities. 2010. Available from: https://www.ndti.org.uk/assets/files/Supported_Living-Making_the_Move2C_May_2010.pdf

35. **Burge P, Ouellette-Kuntz H, Lysaght R.** Public views on employment of people with intellectual disabilities. Journal of Vocational Rehabilitation 2007;**26**(1):29–37.

36. **Brindle D.** Remploy factories shut up shop—the end of an era for disabled workers. The Guardian 20 Oct 2013. Available from: https://www.theguardian.com/society/2013/oct/30/remploy-factories-close-disabled-workers#comment-28428969

37. **NHS Digital**. Measures from the Adult Social Care Outcomes Framework England, 2017–18. 2018. Available from: https://files.digital.nhs.uk/51/9D4229/meas-from-asc-of-17-18-report-v2.pdf

38. **Scottish Commission for People with Learning Disabilities**. Learning Disability Statistics Scotland, 2018 provisional statistics. 2018. Available from: https://www.scld.org.uk/wp-content/uploads/2019/12/Learning-Disability-Statistics-Scotland-2018.pdf

39. **National Health Service**. The NHS Long Term Plan. 2019. Available from: https://www.longtermplan.nhs.uk/wp-content/uploads/2019/08/nhs-long-term-plan-version-1.2.pdf

40. **Nind M, Coverdale A, Croydon A.** Learning from each other in the context of personalisation and self-build social care. Disability & Society 2021;**36**(10):1553–73.

41. **Moore T, Carey L.** Friendship formation in adults with learning disabilities: peer-mediated approaches to social skills development. British Journal of Learning Disabilities 2005;**33**(1):23–6.

42. **Alexandra P, Angela H, Ali A.** Loneliness in people with intellectual and developmental disorders across the lifespan: a systematic review of prevalence and interventions. Journal of Applied Research in Intellectual Disabilities 2018;**31**(5):643–58.

43. **Marlow E, Walker N.** Does supported living work for people with severe intellectual disabilities? Advances in Mental Health and Intellectual Disabilities 2015;**9**(6):338–51.

44. **Treanor DP.** Social inclusion: culture and disability. In: Intellectual Disability and Social Policies of Inclusion. Singapore: Palgrave Macmillan; 2020: 129–50.

45. **Hill A.** Winterbourne View care home staff jailed for abusing residents. The Guardian 26 Oct 2012. Available from: https://www.theguardian.com/society/2012/oct/26/winterbourne-view-care-staff-jailed

46. **Department of Health**. Transforming care: a national response to Winterbourne View Hospital. Department of Health Review: final report. 2012. Available from: https://assets.publishing.service.gov.uk/government/uploads/system/uploads/attachment_data/file/213215/final-report.pdf

47. **Department of Health**. DH Winterbourne view review. Concordat: programme of action. 2012. Available from: https://assets.publishing.service.gov.uk/government/uploads/system/uploads/attachment_data/file/213217/Concordat.pdf

48. **Odiyoor M, Tromans SJ, Alexander RT, Akbari S, Bell G, Bering S**, et al. The role of specialist inpatient rehabilitation services for people with intellectual disability, autism and mental health, behavioural or forensic needs. Advances in Mental Health and Intellectual Disabilities 2019;**13**(5):204–15.

49. **Department of Health**. Mental Health Act 1983: code of practice. 2015. Available from: https://assets.publishing.service.gov.uk/government/uploads/system/uploads/attachment_data/file/435512/MHA_Code_of_Practice.PDF

50. **Hollins S, Lodge K, Lomax P.** The case for removing intellectual disability and autism from the Mental Health Act. British Journal of Psychiatry 2019;**215**(5):633–5.

51. **Department of Health & Social Care**. Reforming the Mental Health Act. London: Stationery Office; 2021. Available from: https://assets.publishing.service.gov.uk/government/uploads/system/uploads/attachment_data/file/951398/mental-health-act-white-paper-web-accessible.pdf

52. **Tromans S, Biswas A.** Potential unintended consequences of removal of intellectual disability and autism from the Mental Health Act. British Journal of Psychiatry 2021;**218**(3):173.

53. **McCarthy J, Duff M.** Services for adults with intellectual disability in Aotearoa New Zealand. BJPsych International 2019;**16**(3):71–3.

54. **Branford D, Gerrard D, Saleem N, Shaw C, Webster A.** Stopping over-medication of people with intellectual disability, autism or both (STOMP) in England part 1—history and background of STOMP. Advances in Mental Health and Intellectual Disabilities 2019;**13**(1):31–40.

55. **Sheehan R, Hassiotis A, Walters K, Osborn D, Strydom A, Horsfall L.** Mental illness, challenging behaviour, and psychotropic drug prescribing in people with intellectual disability: UK population based cohort study. BMJ 2015;**351**:h4326.

56. **Public Health England.** Prescribing of psychotropic drugs to people with learning disabilities and or autism by general practitioners in England. 2015. Available from: https://www.gov.uk/government/publications/psychotropic-drugs-and-people-with-learning-disabilities-or-autism/psychotropic-drugs-and-people-with-learning-disabilities-or-autism-executive-summary

57. **National Health Service.** Stopping over medication of people with a learning disability, autism or both (STOMP). n.d. Availablefrom: https://www.england.nhs.uk/learning-disabilities/improving-health/stomp/

58. **Health and Social Care Information Centre.** National dementia & antipsychotic prescribing audit 2012. 2012. Available from: https://digital.nhs.uk/data-and-information/publications/statistical/national-dementia-and-antipsychotic-prescribing-audit/national-dementia-and-antipsychotic-prescribing-audit-national-summary-report

59. **Glover G, Williams R, Branford D, Avery R, Chauhan U, Hoghton M**, et al. Prescribing of psychotropic drugs to people with learning disabilities and/or autism by general practitioners in England. Public Health England; 2015. Available from: http://clok.uclan.ac.uk/17970/

60. **Gov.UK.** Psychotropic drugs and people with learning disabilities or autism: executive summary. 2019. Available from: https://www.gov.uk/government/publications/psychotropic-drugs-and-people-with-learning-disabilities-or-autism/psychotropic-drugs-and-people-with-learning-disabilities-or-autism-executive-summary

61. **Heslop P, Blair PS, Fleming P, Hoghton M, Marriott A, Russ L.** The Confidential Inquiry into premature deaths of people with intellectual disabilities in the UK: a population-based study. Lancet 2014;**383**(9920):889–95.

62. **Mencap.** Treat me right! Better healthcare for people with a learning disability. 2004. Available from: https://www.mencap.org.uk/sites/default/files/2016-08/treat_me_right.pdf

63. **Mencap.** Death by indifference. 2007. Available from: https://www.mencap.org.uk/sites/default/files/2016-06/DBIreport.pdf

64. **Michael J.** Healthcare for all: report of the independent inquiry into access to healthcare for people with learning disabilities. 2008. Available from: https://webarchive.nationalarchives.gov.uk/ukgwa/20130105064250mp_/http://www.dh.gov.uk/prod_consum_dh/groups/dh_digitalassets/@dh/@en/documents/digitalasset/dh_106126.pdf

65. **Heslop P, Blair PS, Fleming P, Hoghton M, Marriott A, Russ L.** The Confidential Inquiry into premature deaths of people with intellectual disabilities in the UK: a population-based study. Lancet 2014;**383**(9920):889–95.

66. **Gov.UK.** Mental Capacity Act 2005. 2005. Available from: https://www.legislation.gov.uk/ukpga/2005/9/contents

67. **National Health Service.** Learning from lives and deaths—people with a learning disability and autistic people (LeDeR) policy 2021. 2021. Available from: https://www.england.nhs.uk/wp-content/uploads/2021/03/B0428-LeDeR-policy-2021.pdf

68. **National Health Service.** About LeDeR. n.d. Available from: https://leder.nhs.uk/about

69. **NHS Improvement.** The learning disability improvement standards for NHS trusts. 2018. Available from: https://www.england.nhs.uk/wp-content/uploads/2020/08/v1.17_Improvement_Standards_added_note.pdf

Chapter 18

Intellectual disability services in European countries

Ken Courtenay, Romanie Dekker-Couchman, and Rajnish Attavar

Introduction

The population of Europe is 747 million people across 46 countries with a diverse range of people, languages, and cultures (1). Historically, ethnic groups in Europe included Slav, Germanic, and Franco people spanning the continent. It has a long history in social and political terms that spawned the industrial revolution and great changes and upheavals in social systems across the continent over the centuries. Present-day Europe comprises the 46 countries affiliated to the Council of Europe (2).

An estimated 100 million Europeans, 10% of the population, were registered as having a disability of some form by the European Disability Forum in 2007 (3). Further, it is estimated that over 4.2 million people have intellectual disability (ID), costing approximately €43.3 billion annually in support services (4).

There are significant differences in the quality and organisation of services for people with ID across European countries. Such diverse political and social systems lead inevitably to a range of models to support people with ID. For this reason, international declarations and policies such as the United Nations Convention on the Rights of Persons with Disabilities (UN CRPD) are important in raising awareness of standards in models of care and support in societies and political systems (5). The movement to support people to move out of long-stay institutions (deinstitutionalisation) is an example of how changes in attitudes and policies can effect positive social change for people with ID. Deinstitutionalisation has taken place at various rates across European countries where early adopters of international policies have led the way on models of care for more integration in communities. Such social progress demonstrates the interplay between political action and culture, where one influences the other and can lead to greater social change. This chapter describes and explores systems supporting people with ID in European societies and how they vary between countries. The attitudes of people towards ID and the contributions of social policies to changing attitudes and practice are also discussed.

Political changes

A reflection on historical events and their impacts on European societies is important to understand the context in which people with ID have lived over the centuries. Political and social changes have had direct and sometimes dramatic effects on the lives of people that have not always been positive or supportive.

With industrialisation in the eighteenth and nineteenth centuries came shifts in social networks and supports with people moving to urban areas to work in factories (6). The breakdown of traditional social supports in communities led to the creation of institutional care in asylums and workhouses in nineteenth-century societies where people with ID, even from childhood, were housed and often at great distances from their communities of origin, living in large shared dormitories where they spent their lives (7). In Austria, psychiatric institutions homed long-term, and often lifelong, admission units for people with ID that were described as highly restrictive environments (8). Over time, many innovations in institutional care were undertaken with the right intentions of supporting people with ID, including utilitarian models of state-led interventions such as in former Soviet bloc countries (9).

Second World War

During the Second World War (1939–1945) under the Nazi regime, many people with disabilities were murdered under the 'T4 Action' regime. In Austria, a special concentration camp was set up in Schloß Hartheim where people with disabilities, most of them people with ID, were killed. In total, 275,000 children and adults with disabilities were murdered in special death and experimentation camps in Nazi Germany (8). The impact of such genocide in Europe has affected how people with disabilities and their families view authority and society in general.

European Union

With the formation of the European Union (EU) and its predecessors, more progressive policies in human rights, rights to family life, employment, and voting have led to more positive impacts in the lives of people with ID and attitudes towards them as full citizens (10,11). In 1993, the UN published 'Standard Rules on the Equalization of Opportunities for Persons with Disabilities' following which disability rights in Europe received more attention. The EU disability strategy emphasizes the importance of 'a society open and accessible to all' and the identification and removal of barriers (12).

Within the EU, disability is considered a human rights issue and as a matter of law (13). In 2007, the UN CRPD was adopted at the European Disability Forum and signed by the EU member states (14). The UN CRPD focuses on the principles of non-discrimination, participation and inclusion in society, equal opportunities, and accessibility. In member countries and those that aspire to join the EU, such standards can influence the care that people with ID receive (14,15).

States of the former Soviet Union

In the former socialist states of the Soviet Union there is a long history of treatment of people with disabilities. The concept of 'defectology' originated in 1912 as a science that allowed the categorization of those considered to be educable and those not (16). The non-educable were deemed incapable of contributing to the economy and were often housed in institutions rather than remaining in their communities. Under defectology, a medical model of special needs was adopted where medical language was used to categorize people with disabilities.

The advent of political changes in 1989 raised the curtain on systems of care in the former Soviet bloc countries. Certain strides have taken place in the Baltic and Central European nations where access to the EU has accelerated changes in social attitudes and care with advances towards deinstitutionalization (15). The same is less evident in non-EU countries of the former Soviet Union where the legacy of such practices and attitudes are present with significant stigma among the general population towards people with disabilities (17).

In post-communist countries the need to develop mental health services is great and there is evidence of investment in mental health services occurring (18,19). Changes have also taken place in some countries by providing more legal supports to people with ID, as in Latvia (20) and Lithuania (21); however, reforms may be well intentioned but need to be improved further (22). The approach to supporting people in the community has been described as paternalistic with limited resources made available to deliver effective supports (23). There has been pressure from the EU and international disability rights organizations to change to more inclusive systems in living and education in member countries but the slow progress may be related to negative public opinion, lack of political will, and general inadequate financing of care services (14).

European countries do not exist within a homogeneous system and there are clear disparities in the care that people with ID receive across the continent and even between member countries of the EU (24). The issue of equality in care was highlighted where promoting policy development in effecting change is essential (25). While people in some countries enjoy good standards in care services, others do not, such as in Bulgaria, where rights and opportunities are limited (26). A related issue is how people with ID perceive themselves and their perceptions could be related to culture. A study on the role of stigma in the UK, Germany, and Austria reported that in the latter two, people with ID were less likely to take pride in their ID (27).

Moving from institutional care

Many Western and Northern European countries have worked towards total deinstitutionalisation and inclusion of people with ID in general society. From the 1960s onwards, deinstitutionalisation was underway in countries in Europe in response to political and ideological opposition to institutions, but by 2007 up to 1.2 million people across 25 countries remained in residential care (28,29). Initially, countries focused on reforming and improving institutions with reductions in their size and the closure of dormitory living. In Norway, the mean size of homes in the community reduced from 60 to 25 residents from 1970 to 1989 (30). In Sweden and Norway, the large residential institutions for people with ID have been completely closed. In countries such as Belgium, the Netherlands, Germany, Spain, Greece, Italy, and Portugal, there is still a varying pattern of institutional care, even though the number of people in large residential institutions has been decreasing (31).

The background to such changes was the changing attitudes among families about where their family members should live. Concern among families for their children growing up in institutions has led to not admitting them to hospitals. In Norway in 1963, 35% of the residents were under the age of 16; by 1989 that proportion fell to 3% (30). In Scandinavia, parental associations had advocated closing institutions while others opposed it. In Norway, support among families for resettlement rose from 17% to 73% after closures with similar rates in Sweden (30). In general, institutions were replaced by family living environments and day services. Special education settings changed from being 24-hour residential schools to schools with normal school days.

In the 1990s, policies moved from improving institutions to full deinstitutionalisation that were sometimes triggered by scandals in institutions, and frustration at the slow pace of discharges in previous decades. The aim of full deinstitutionalisation was to provide 'living conditions in keeping with what one expects for all citizens' (30).

Health and social care systems developed their own approaches to the process of closing the institutions. In Spain, deinstitutionalisation was organised by local governments where Andalusia and Asturias opted for the complete closure of psychiatric hospitals, while the Basque Country and Catalonia re-modelled and included these institutions in their strategies (8). Despite this, the proportionate rate of discharges over time for people with ID was low, where 24% of inpatients of all psychiatric beds were people with ID (8). Greece achieved a 35% reduction in institutional beds and admissions were for shorter periods.

In a comparison of 'countries with an advanced stage of deinstitutionalisa-tion' and 'countries with an early stage of deinstitutionalisation' revealed that for those in the advanced stage, the average number of people per home was 2.99 (standard deviation (SD) 1.54) in unstaffed services. For those in the early stages the number was 3.58 (SD 1.85) in unstaffed homes. In advanced systems, the average number of places per home in staffed residences was 12.38 (SD 14.62) compared with 42.66 (SD 27.42) in early systems (24).

The benefits of moving from institutions to living in the community are greatest for those moving out of institutions with enhanced quality of life and improved skills (32,33). There have been improvements in levels of functioning and access to community services that have not been universal in all European countries, leading to disparity between countries in the care that people receive (24). This is most obvious when comparing Eastern European with Western European states. Hungary, Poland, Romania, Czechia, and in Central and Eastern Europe generally, large institutional settings remain the main place of living for people with ID (24). Support from EU funding has facilitated the move from institutional settings to community living (34).

Despite policies across Europe aimed at people with ID living their lives in the community, some of these expectations were not realized and this has been described as 'the revolution that disappeared' (30). The expectations that people with ID would be included in regular employment, to have normal social net-works, and to be socially integrated, have only succeeded to a limited extent. It has been postulated that since the 1990s another process has developed that is referred to as 're-institutionalisation' where new models of accommodation group more people together in individual apartments. In Norway, for example, the mean size of groups grew from 3.8 in 1994 to 8.1 in 2010 where 40% lived in a group home with seven people or more which could be a worrying trend (30). The common themes and trends going forward include further deinstitutional-isation in many countries of Europe especially in the Eastern Europe supported by the EU. The trend is not uniform across all European countries where many Central and Eastern European countries have been slow or have failed to imple-ment reforms in community living (17).

Inclusion of people with intellectual disability in Europe

There has been a general aim across Europe for people with ID to be included in life in the community, to have jobs and paid employment, and have opportunities and live life as other people without disabilities. Countries are at different stages regarding inclusion of people with disabilities.

The Commission of the EU issued a Council Resolution in 1996,— 'Collectivity of the member states for the goals of achieving equal opportunity and non-discrimination'—with the focus on people with ID to be included in normal working life to stop discrimination and achieve inclusion. Such policies are based on human rights with integration of people with disabilities as a fundamental right for citizens of the EU (35).

In the former Soviet Union countries, people with disabilities usually worked in segregated workplaces and would generally receive small state benefits. Countries are increasingly promoting employment for all citizens, including people with disabilities, but reforms have proven difficult to put into practice partly because of high rates of unemployment generally. In Macedonia, there have been efforts for workplace integration, but most disabled people who are employed work in protected or 'sheltered' enterprises that receive subsidies for hiring a large percentage of disabled workers. There is also significant stigma and negative perceptions among employers regarding hiring people with disabilities. In Bulgaria, most people with disabilities continue to be employed in segregated work cooperatives similar to the historic cartels for the disabled in the Soviet Union (14). Such contrasts between European societies in the models of support for people with ID appear to align with more progressive attitudes in the less authoritarian systems compared with authoritarian ones. Post-communism comparisons appear to support this perspective where in spite of regime changes, cultures of care persist and are slow to change without external pressure to support internal activities for change (15).

Education for people and children with intellectual disability in Europe

Education for children and people with disabilities is organised differently across European countries. In some countries, legislation is focused on including people with disabilities in general education, while in others most people with disabilities are in separate, specialist educational systems (36).

In countries in Eastern Europe, there is generally a pattern of segregated education for people with disabilities, despite policies and legislation aimed

Table 18.1 Adherence to inclusive education

Country	Inclusive education (%)	Segregated education (%)
Spain	83	17
Germany	17	83
Norway	84	16
Portugal	85	15
Latvia	20	80
Belgium	9	91

Source data from Taub D, Foster M. Inclusion and intellectual disabilities: a cross cultural review of descriptions. International Electronic Journal of Elementary Education 2020;12(3):275–81.

at inclusion in general education (14). The EU and international disability rights organisations have encouraged countries to implement more inclusive education for children with disabilities; however, progress has been slow (14) (Table 18.1). Explanations for the rate of progress include negative public opinion, a lack of political will, institutional inertia, and a lack of resources and finances. In Bulgaria, legislation on education reform through the Public Education Reform Act of 2003 is in place to facilitate deinstitutionalization and support to children with special needs to access mainstream education but implementation has been slow to progress.

In Macedonia, a government report stated that only 20% of children with special needs received any form of education, despite laws stating that all people with disabilities should receive an education. As in other Eastern European countries, many children with disabilities are educated separately from mainstream schools. There are special schools as well as 'satellite' classes within regular schools. The situation is worse for children of minorities in some countries, such as Roma children educated in special schools, where they are assumed to have ID (14).

The impact of inclusive education depends on the attitudes of educators and legislators towards students with ID. Legislation and policy support inclusive education, but funding is required to realise ambitions (37). A survey of the general public on attitudes to inclusive education conducted in 2007 reported that 85% of people generally disapprove of inclusive education for children with disabilities (14). In Bosnia, positive attitudes towards inclusive education were reported in more than 50% of respondents, but they did not feel prepared to support students (38). This is an improvement in attitudes over time as compared with previous attitudinal survey in Bulgaria in 1996 (39). Internal structural change is key to changing attitudes towards inclusive education among educators and policymakers (40).

Healthcare for people with intellectual disability in Europe

The life expectancy of people with ID has increased significantly during the past few decades, but they continue to experience a greater number of co-occurring physical health conditions than the general population (41,42). Rates of obesity are high in people with ID in Europe, predisposing them to developing comorbid disorders, while participation in health screening and vaccination programmes is low (25,43). For countries at the early stages of deinstitutionalisation, the prevalence of respiratory, cardiovascular, and gastroenterological disorders is high (24).

People with ID are more likely to experience mental health problems, but there are few specialists in mental health dedicated to supporting people with ID in most European countries (44). Services are developing in Germany and the Netherlands with the development of inpatient care and community provision (45–47).

The POMONA study across 14 European countries, reported that people living in staffed residences consumed a higher proportion of services and used more medication than people living in unstaffed homes (24,48). This may be related to a higher level of need among residents of staffed accommodations. They are also likely to be treated by professionals with little knowledge of or experience in the health needs of people with ID. Interestingly, living in staffed residences increased the uptake of health promotion programmes such as vaccinations and health screening (49).

Public health policies in European countries do not always give attention to the health needs of people with ID that perpetuates their poor health outcomes (50). Data are required in national healthcare systems on the health needs of people with ID to make progress in reducing health inequalities. It is feasible to construct meaningful data collection systems across healthcare systems on the health needs of people with ID (51).

Training in intellectual disability in Europe

Across Europe, people with ID access mainstream healthcare in secondary and primary care services. There are significant gaps in training and education of health and support care staff on the needs of people with ID, where care for people is not part of the core training curricula. Such gaps result in negative attitudes towards people with ID (52). In Czechia, many surveyed doctors were in favour of advocating for termination of the pregnancies of women with ID (53). Similarly, in Greece, social care support staff perceive that people with ID have few skills in independent living and require greater education (54). Surveys of healthcare students reveal the attitudes towards people with ID and the positive impact of training (55). Overall, there is a general lack of education and training about people with ID in healthcare training systems in Europe.

In contrast to many countries, the Netherlands has developed the role of the ID physician since 2000, where doctors specialise in the healthcare of people with ID (56). The training programme is a 3-year postgraduate programme 'Artsen voor Verstandelijk Gehandicapten' ('Doctors for the Mentally Handicapped'), focusing on the health needs of people with ID in community and hospital care. Similar roles exist in Germany known as 'Geistig Behinderten Arzt' ('Mentally Handicapped Doctor') or 'Arzt für Mensen mit geistiger oder mehrfacher Behinderung' ('Doctor for People with Mental or Multiple Disabilities'), supported by the Federal Association of Physicians for People with Intellectual and Multiple Handicaps (45).

Professional training in the mental healthcare of people with ID is limited in European countries. A survey of psychiatric training programmes in Europe found that ID was mandatory in only five countries. This compared sharply with training in psychotherapy (18), community psychiatry (19), and old-age psychiatry (14). The mental health needs of people with ID are not a key feature of training curricula in Europe (4).

Conclusion

It is clear from an examination of the literature on the life experiences of people with ID in Europe the extent to which culture and political ideology and systems interplay to shape the experiences of people. Mass movements, such as those that occurred with the industrial revolution, and political changes through the twentieth century have had far-reaching consequences for people with ID who are least likely to have the power to exert control over the impacts of external changes in their lives. Changes in social attitudes are likely to lead to policy changes and behaviour to empower and support the inclusion of people with ID. Such changes require leadership that has been most evident among the families and carers of people with ID.

While it is clear what impact political changes have had on societal attitudes and behaviour, it is not always apparent what the role of religious belief and practice has had on the lives of people with ID. Indeed, many of the formal institutions in some European countries were provided by religious orders with the support of churches that may not have had incentives to deviate from the institutional model, similar to state-sponsored care systems in the absence of religious observance. In more progressive social systems, religious groups are at the forefront of innovation in services for people with ID that can reflect the culture of a society and how it perceives and values its citizens who have ID.

Globalisation and the sharing of information on lifestyles for people with ID should facilitate the exchange of views and innovations in service developments along with adopting a human rights approach to supporting people with ID as full citizens. Great political frameworks can enable change to take place even in societies that do not appear to be motivated to support people with ID and, therefore, it is essential that countries perceived to be leaders in social change support their neighbours to enhance the lives of their citizens.

References

1. **Statista.** Estimated population of Europe. 2021. Available from: https://www.statista.com/statistics/1106711/population-of-europe/

2. **Council of Europe.** 46 member states. 2023. Available from: https://www.coe.int/en/web/portal/46-members-states

3. **European Disability Forum.** Homepage. 2007. Available from: https://www.edf-feph.org/

4. **Salvador-Carulla L, Martínez-Leal R, Heyler C, Alvarez-Galvez J, Veenstra MY, García-Ibáñez J,** et al. Training on intellectual disability in health sciences: the European perspective. International Journal of Developmental Disabilities 2015;**61**(1):20–31.

5. **McSherry B.** The United Nations Convention on the rights of persons with disabilities. Journal of Law and Medicine 2008;**16**(1):17–20.

6. **Åkerman S.** Internal migration, industrialisation and urbanisation (1895–1930): a summary of the Västmanland study. Scandinavian Economic History Review 1975 Jul 1;**23**(2):149–58.

7. **van Drenth A.** The 'truth' about idiocy: revisiting files of children in the Dutch 'School for Idiots' in the nineteenth century. History of Education 2016;**45**(4):477–91.

8. **Holt G, Costello H, Bouras N, Diareme S, Hillery J, Moss S,** et al. BIOMED-MEROPE* project: service provision for adults with intellectual disability: a European comparison. Journal of Intellectual Disability Research 2000;**44**(6):685–96.

9. **Kalinnikova L, Trygged S.** A retrospective on care and denial of children with disabilities in Russia. Scandinavian Journal of Disability Research 2014;**16**(3):229–48.

10. **Priestley M.** In search of European disability policy: between national and global. Alter 2007;**1**(1):61–74.

11. **O'Mahony C, Quinlivan S.** The EU disability strategy and the future of EU disability policy. In: Research Handbook on EU Disability Law 2020 Nov 17. Edward Elgar Publishing.

12. **Priestley M.** We're all Europeans now! The social model of disability and European social policy. In: **Barnes C, Mercer G,** editors. The Social Model of Disability: Europe and the Majority World. Leeds: The Disability Press; 2005: 17–31.

13. **Commission of the European Communities.** Communication from the Commission to the European Parliament and the Council. A Strong European Neighbourhood

Policy. 2007. Available from: https://eur-lex.europa.eu/LexUriServ/LexUriServ.do?uri=
COM:2007:0774:FIN:EN:PDF

14. **Phillips SD.** EU disability policy and implications of EU accession for disability rights
in education and employment in Bulgaria, Romania, Croatia, and the Former Yugoslav
Republic of Macedonia. Journal of Disability Policy Studies 2012;**22**(4):208–19.

15. **Mladenov T, Petri G.** Critique of deinstitutionalisation in post-socialist Central and
Eastern Europe. Disability & Society 2020;**35**(8):1203–26.

16. **Grigorenko EL.** Russian 'Defectology' anticipating perestroika in the field. Journal of
Learning Disabilities 1998;**31**(2):193–207.

17. **Turnpenny A, Petri G, Finn A, Beadle-Brown J, Nyman M.** Mapping and
understanding exclusion: institutional, coercive and community-based services and
practices across Europe. Mental Health Europe; 2017. Available from: https://mhe-sme.
org/wp-content/uploads/2018/01/Mapping-and-Understanding-Exclusion-in-Eur
ope.pdf

18. **Jenkins R, Klein J, Parker C.** Mental health in post-communist countries. BMJ
2005;**331**(7510):173–4.

19. **Krupchanka D, Winkler P.** State of mental healthcare systems in Eastern Europe: do we
really understand what is going on? BJPsych international 2016;**13**(4):96–9.

20. **Kulačkovska J.** The legal situation of people with disabilities in Latvia. Society,
Integration, Education. Proceedings of the International Scientific Conference
2018;**3**:107–116.

21. **Raudeliunaite R, Gudžinskienė V.** The development of independent living skills
in young adults with intellectual disability in sheltered housing accommodation.
Society, Integration, Education. Proceedings of the International Scientific Conference
2017;**3**:265–76.

22. **Mazecaite-Vaitilaviciene L, Owens J.** Children with disabilities at risk of poor oral
health in the Republic of Lithuania: a retrospective descriptive service evaluation.
World Medical & Health Policy 2018;**10**(3):246–58.

23. **Wapiennik E.** Comparative policy brief: status of intellectual disabilities in the Republic
of Poland. Journal of Policy and Practice in Intellectual Disabilities 2008;**5**(2):137–41.

24. **Martínez-Leal R, Salvador-Carulla L, Linehan C, Walsh P, Weber G, Van Hove G,**
et al. The impact of living arrangements and deinstitutionalisation in the health status of
persons with intellectual disability in Europe. Journal of Intellectual Disability Research
2011;**55**(9):858–72.

25. **Meijer MM, Carpenter S, Scholte FA.** European manifesto on basic standards of health
care for people with intellectual disabilities. Journal of Policy and Practice in Intellectual
Disabilities 2004;**1**(1):10–15.

26. **Kukova S.** Fundamental rights situation of persons with mental health problems and
persons with intellectual disabilities: desk report Bulgaria. Commissioned by the
European Union Agency for Fundamental Rights. Bulgarian Helsinki Committee; 2011.
Available from: www.bghelsinki.org/media/uploads/special/bg_fra_mh.pdf

27. **Zeilinger EL, Stiehl KA, Bagnall H, Scior K.** Intellectual disability literacy and its
connection to stigma: a multinational comparison study in three European countries.
PloS One 2020;**15**(10):e0239936.

28. **Novella EJ.** Mental health care in the aftermath of deinstitutionalization: a retrospective
and prospective view. Health Care Analysis 2010;**18**(3):222–38.

29. **Mansell J, Knapp M, Beadle-Brown J, Beecham J.** Deinstitutionalisation and Community Living–Outcomes and Costs: Report of a European Study. Volume 2: Main Report. Canterbury: Tizard Centre, University of Kent; 2007.

30. **Tøssebro J.** Scandinavian disability policy: from deinstitutionalisation to non-discrimination and beyond. Alter 2016;**10**(2):111–23.

31. **Beadle-Brown J, Mansell J, Kozma A.** Deinstitutionalization in intellectual disabilities. Current Opinion in Psychiatry 2007;**20**(5):437–42.

32. **Tideman M, Tøssebro J.** A comparison of living conditions for intellectually disabled people in Norway and Sweden: present situation and changes following the national reforms in the 1990s. Scandinavian Journal of Disability Research 2002;**4**(1):23–42.

33. **Bredewold F, Hermus M, Trappenburg M.** 'Living in the community' the pros and cons: a systematic literature review of the impact of deinstitutionalisation on people with intellectual and psychiatric disabilities. Journal of Social Work 2020;**20**(1):83–116.

34. **Parker C, Bulic Cojocari I.** European structural and investment funds and people with disabilities in the European Union. European Parliament, Directorate-General for Internal Policies; 2016. Available from: https://www.europarl.europa.eu/RegData/etu des/STUD/2016/571386/IPOL_STU(2016)571386_EN.pdf

35. **Walsh PN.** Old World—new territory: European perspectives on intellectual disability. Journal of Intellectual Disability Research 1997;**41**(2):112–19.

36. **Buchner T, Shevlin M, Donovan MA, Gercke M, Goll H, Šiška J,** et al. Same progress for all? Inclusive education, the United Nations Convention on the Rights of Persons with Disabilities and students with intellectual disability in European countries. Journal of Policy and Practice in Intellectual Disabilities 2021;**18**(1):7–22.

37. **Ruškus J.** Right to inclusive education for children with disabilities at stake in Lithuania. Special Education 2020;**1**(41):10–52.

38. **Memisevic H, Hodzic S.** Teachers' attitudes towards inclusion of students with intellectual disability in Bosnia and Herzegovina. International Journal of Inclusive Education 2011;**15**(7):699–710.

39. **Cholakova M, Georgieva D.** The present situation and the future development of special education in Bulgaria. Paper presented at the Annual World Congress of the International Association for the Scientific Study of Intellectual Disabilities (10th), Helsinki, Finland, 8–13 July 1996.

40. **Stepaniuk I.** Inclusive education in Eastern European countries: a current state and future directions. International Journal of Inclusive Education 2019;**23**(3):328–52.

41. **Emerson E, Hatton C.** Health Inequalities and People with Intellectual Disabilities. Cambridge: Cambridge University Press; 2014.

42. **Kinnear D, Morrison J, Allan L, Henderson A, Smiley E, Cooper SA.** Prevalence of physical conditions and multimorbidity in a cohort of adults with intellectual disabilities with and without Down syndrome: cross-sectional study. BMJ Open 2018;**8**(2):e018292.

43. **Sadowsky M, McConkey R, Shellard A.** Obesity in youth and adults with intellectual disability in Europe and Eurasia. Journal of Applied Research in Intellectual Disabilities 2020;**33**(2):321–6.

44. **Cooper SA, Smiley E, Morrison J, Williamson A, Allan L.** Mental ill-health in adults with intellectual disabilities: prevalence and associated factors. British Journal of Psychiatry 2007;**190**(1):27–35.

45. **Elstner S, Theil MM.** The health and social care of people with disabilities in Germany. Advances in Mental Health and Intellectual Disabilities 2018;**12**(3/4):99–104.

46. **Wieland J, ten Doesschate M.** Awareness and accessibility of the Dutch mental health care system for people with borderline intellectual functioning or mild intellectual disabilities. Advances in Mental Health and Intellectual Disabilities 2018;**12**(3/4):114–20.

47. **Bakken TL, Evensen OO, Bjørgen TG, Nilsen IT, Bang N, Pedersen U,** et al. Mental health services for adolescents and adults with intellectual disabilities in Norway: a descriptive study. Advances in Mental Health and Intellectual Disabilities 2018;**12**(3/4):121–34.

48. **Haveman M, Perry J, Salvador-Carulla L, Walsh PN, Kerr M, Van Schrojenstein Lantman-de Valk H,** et al. Ageing and health status in adults with intellectual disabilities: results of the European POMONA II study. Journal of Intellectual and Developmental Disability 2011;**36**(1):49–60.

49. **Wahlström L, Bergström H, Marttila A.** Promoting health of people with intellectual disabilities: views of professionals working in group homes. Journal of Intellectual Disabilities 2014;**18**(2):113–28.

50. **Linehan C, Walsh PN, Van Schrojenstein Lantman-de Valk HM, Kerr MP, Dawson F, Pomona-1 Group.** Are people with intellectual disabilities represented in European public health surveys? Journal of Applied Research in Intellectual Disabilities 2009;**22**(5):409–20.

51. **van Bakel M, Einarsson I, Arnaud C, Craig S, Michelsen SI, Pildava S,** et al. Monitoring the prevalence of severe intellectual disability in children across Europe: feasibility of a common database. Developmental Medicine & Child Neurology 2014;**56**(4):361–9.

52. **Kritsotakis G, Galanis P, Papastefanakis E, Meidani F, Philalithis AE, Kalokairinou A,** et al. Attitudes towards people with physical or intellectual disabilities among nursing, social work and medical students. Journal of Clinical Nursing 2017;**26**(23–24):4951–63.

53. **Strnadová I, Bernoldová J, Adamčíková Z, Klusáček J.** Medical personnel's knowledge, attitudes, and experiences with regard to mothers with intellectual disability in the Czech Republic. Journal of Intellectual & Developmental Disability 2019;**44**(1):81–91.

54. **Kartasidou L, Dimitriadou I, Pavlidou E, Varsamis P.** Independent living and interpersonal relations of individuals with intellectual disability: the perspective of support staff in Greece. International Journal of Learner Diversity and Identities 2013;**19**(1):59–73.

55. **Packer TL, Iwasiw C, Theben J, Sheveleva P, Metrofanova N.** Attitudes to disability of Russian occupational therapy and nursing students. International Journal of Rehabilitation Research 2000;**23**(1):39–47.

56. **Evenhuis HM, Penning C.** Eight years of specialist training of Dutch intellectual disability physicians: results of scientific research education. Journal of Policy and Practice in Intellectual Disabilities 2009;**6**(4):276–81.

Chapter 19

Intellectual disability services in Africa

Aisha M. Bakhiet, Mo Eyeoyibo, and Mohamed O. El Tahir

Introduction

Health systems in Africa show wide variation between countries, with many challenges in service provision with constant changes as countries are developing. The poverty, wars, conflicts, and political reforms have had significant impacts on health planning and service development. People with intellectual disability (ID) are often catered for within broader disability services. Thus, they have no specified resources to meet their needs. This leaves people with ID remaining a major disadvantaged group within African societies.

Eighty per cent of the estimated 140 million out-of-school children worldwide, the majority of whom are girls and/or children with disabilities, live in Africa (1). Most disabilities in Africa can be traced to poverty, malnutrition, and restricted access to basic services (1). The large-scale exclusion of children with disabilities from education services is concerning; one in every 100 children with a disability are denied access to education services (1). This can be attributed to complex factors, mainly the limited appreciation of the right to education of children with disabilities, particularly when market forces govern public expenditure, and the instrumental view of education is prevailing (2).

Prevalence rates of ID vary widely across the world, depending on many factors. According to the World Health Organization (WHO), the true prevalence of ID is close to 3%; however, there are no research reports from African countries (3). Based on this 3% prevalence estimate and a total African population of 1.2 billion people, this would equate to approximately 36 million people with ID in Africa.

Current trends and perspectives on education of children with disabilities require a proper law and policies for schooling of children with disabilities. A preliminary investigation by the African Child Policy Forum revealed that most African countries lack a proper law and policy strategy for the schooling of children with ID (2). They are not in compliance with international and regional human rights instruments.

In this chapter, we will explore healthcare provision and service models in different countries in Africa, taking into consideration the available literature and information. We attempt to answer questions on the availability of support for people with ID, national programmes and funding, as well as reflecting on system-wide strengths and weaknesses. Information is summarized to reflect on the African continent population, due to similarities across countries.

Policy

There is a dearth of information on the policies and practices to support individuals with ID in Africa. Available policies emphasize the need to include people with disability in education, but tend to place less emphasis on access to health facilities (4).

The United Nations (UN) has proposed measures to ensure the rights of people with ID to access health services (5,6). There is an expectation for countries to conduct a review or scope all legislations and policies that concern people with ID, and through this process identify gaps or areas for development. This way, foundations are set for a comprehensive policy framework to support access to healthcare.

The UN Convention on the Rights of Persons with Disabilities (CRPD) (5) aims to change attitudes and approaches to people with ID. Instead of being viewed as objects of charity, people with ID can be capable of claiming their rights if offered the correct support. They can take part in making decisions for their lives, as well as being active members of society.

South Sudan is one of the few countries yet to endorse the UN CRPD, and has no legislation or policies relating to the rights of people with disabilities, despite references in the constitution to the special needs of people with disabilities.

South Sudan has a 'National Disability and Inclusion' policy and an 'Inclusive Education' policy that are yet to be implemented due to a lack of political will and government funding (2,6). However, there are a number of organizations involved in raising awareness around the needs of people with ID, promoting their rights and advocating for greater socioeconomic and political empowerment. Most awareness campaigns are through the country's main radio outlet in Juba, using arts and sports to challenge stereotyping of people with disabilities.

In contrast, the government of Sudan had signed up to the UN CRPD and established a Ministry for Social Planning with an Office for Disability. The Ministry of Social Planning in collaboration with the Ministry of Education are responsible for formulating activities for people with disabilities, and have responsibility for organizing forums on disability for participants from the government and the private sector.

In Nigeria, the Lagos state disability bill was passed into law in 2010 (7). This was the first law in the country relating to discrimination against people with disability. Eight years later, following pressures from many disability groups, the country passed into law the first Disability Act (8). The essence of the Act is to promote awareness about disability and ensure access to social amenities, including transport, education, employment, and participation in politics. More importantly, the Act stipulates unfettered access to adequate healthcare and without discrimination.

There is provision within the Act in Nigeria for individuals with disability to be identified and certified as such when they contact healthcare services. This registration could be temporary, to allow for immediate support to access health facilities, and once disability is firmly confirmed, a permanent certificate can be issued. The Act mentioned that 'a person with mental disability' is entitled to free medical and health services in all public institutions and that there should be access to 'special communication' such as sign language, augmentative, and alternative communication when required.

There is a provision within the Nigerian Act for the establishment of a national commission for people with disabilities with a governing council (8). The governing council is expected to include a person with disability and a wide range of representation, including from health and education, and representation from the national human rights commission and the office of national planning. The commission is required to take measures to reduce stigma, promote access to public facilities, ensure public offices recognize the needs of people with disability, and prosecute anybody or any organization that contravenes the provisions of the Act. Penalties are stated in the act, especially for corporate bodies, and may include 6-month prison sentences for individuals' violations.

Many agencies welcome the Disability Act, as it demonstrates the government intention to remove barriers that hinder access to services, but they remain sceptical about its application across all sectors, including health. Again, the lack of political will and poor funding of health and education have made implementation of the act across the country a challenge.

South Africa's mental health strategy ranks mental health burden as third, after HIV and other infectious diseases (9). The country's provision of care and rehabilitation services for mental healthcare remain under the responsibility of the Department of Health. Vocational-related service needs for people with mild and moderate ID is under the responsibility of the Department of Education for the young population, and under the Department of Labour for adults. There is recognition of inequity between provinces in the distribution of the mental health services and resources.

Healthcare in Africa

Healthcare systems and provisions among African countries have similarities, as all are classed within the low- and middle-income countries. The population demographics and resources for healthcare are affected significantly by social determinants such as poverty, poor education and work environments, and conflicts and wars. However, health service provision for people with ID may vary depending on many factors. We discuss here the healthcare in four countries as examples of currently existing health systems.

Healthcare system

The health system in South Africa includes three concurrent health systems, the National Health, Provincial Health, and District Health systems. The National Department of Health coordinates the public and private healthcare provisions at national, provincial, district and local levels. The healthcare system, described as fragmented and poorly organized, has two tiers:

1. A poorly financed and human resource-poor public sector; with a lack of personnel training and specialized curriculum for children with IDs.
2. A well-resourced and fast developing private sector.

ID in South Africa was estimated to have a prevalence of 35.6 per 1000 children (10). This prevalence rate seems high relative to most estimates from other populations (3), suggesting that local factors may have contributed, especially socioeconomic factors (10). The impact of environmental and societal factors on the health of people with ID is well recognized in Africa. Attempts to address disparities between health of people with ID and the general population is an imperative goal for health services (10).

The health system in South Africa underwent major reforms with the adoption of the Mental Health Act 2002 (11), emphasizing the human rights of patients and the development of the National Mental Health Strategy and Action Plan 2013–2020 (11) in line with the WHO Mental Health Action Plan (11). The scope of the strategy included ID, as the Department of Health is responsible to provide developmentally appropriate services for those with severe and profound ID.

Sudan has been torn by civil wars. The war and its related effects have led to millions of deaths and people have been displaced, with additional strain on limited health and educational resources. Many research areas in Sudan have not been investigated, including those relating to disability.

There is no official prevalence estimate of ID in Sudan; according to the 2008 census (14,15) there were 1,463,034 people with disabilities (4.8% of the total population). The highest rates of disability were among the category of 5–14 years of age (14.9%). However, there were no specific figures for ID as a specific subgroup of people with disability. However, ID is observed to be increasing in prevalence, mainly because of poverty, consanguinity, and iodine deficiency in Western Sudan, as well as poor medical care. Furthermore, families are becoming more aware about the availability of help, via efforts to raise public awareness through the media, including radio and television programmes (15).

The Sudanese community is culturally diverse, with a very close social fabric and strong religious beliefs (15). Stigma against disabled people and mental illnesses is still a great obstacle for accessing services. Sudanese patients prefer seeking traditional healing, as this is more culturally accepted than going to see a psychiatrist. However, in some Sudanese communities a disabled child is perceived as a holy gift to the family (15). This can also expose them to exploitation, as they can be used as a source of money, when people come to them seeking blessings or healing of their ill patients. This can discourage families from seeking healthcare or education for disabled children, as they get used to their disability as a source of income for the family (15).

The global review on stigma and awareness raising in low- and middle-income countries by Scior et al. (2015) reported that in Africa children and adults with ID experience high levels of stigma, and are denied many rights and freedoms enjoyed by people without ID (16).

In Nigeria, there are about 25 million people with disability according to the WHO (17). This estimate may be inaccurate, as there is no epidemiological study to support it. There is a dearth of information on policies and practices to support individuals with ID in Nigeria. The term disability is often used broadly to represent impairments, activity limitations, and participation restrictions, and includes individuals with physical disabilities, as well as those with ID. Available policies emphasize the need to include people with disability in education, but places less emphasis on access to health facilities.

Long years of conflict and its impact on poverty and services have left many South Sudanese people with different types of disabilities. However, there are no official statistics in relation to disability prevalence. People with disabilities accounted for 5.1% of the population (2), though this was believed to be an underestimate, due to both issues with how disability was defined and the stigma towards disability that prevented people from identifying themselves as disabled. There have been no ID prevalence studies conducted for the Sudanese population. However, the 2008 census and a 2011 disability assessment reported a range of impairments, including intellectual impairments and mental illness (10–17% overall prevalence; 1.6% intellectual impairments; 8.3% mental illness); these figures give an estimate of the magnitude of support needs (18). According to the 2016 household survey by the Food Security and Livelihood Cluster in South Sudan, 15% of households have at least one disabled family member (16).

Due to war in South Sudan, poverty, and poor access to services, people with disabilities have become more marginalized and excluded, as they face numerous attitudinal, environmental, and institutional barriers, as well as a lack of concerted efforts to include them in mainstream society. Lack of data on disability in South Sudan has made lobbying for rights of people with disabilities and access to services difficult. There are numerous evidence gaps in relation to the experiences of people with disabilities in South Sudan. Very little research has looked at disability in South Sudan and the available evidence base is extremely limited, being focused mostly on Juba rather than the rest of the country.

Care provisions for people with intellectual disability

In South Africa, the service provision at provincial and district levels led by health and social service departments are based on the financial responsibilities. As an example, the Western Cape policy framework indicates that the care needs of children and adults with severe and profound ID are provided by the Department of Health through 24-hour care provision, while children and adults with moderate and low ID needs are provided for by the Department of Social Development through protective workshops and special care centres.

The provision of care and rehabilitation services for mental healthcare remain under the responsibility of the Department of Health (12), while vocationally related service needs of people with mild and moderate ID are kept under the responsibility of the Department of Education at a younger age and the Department of Labour as adults (12).

Community service needs and housing provision in some provinces are under the Department of Social Development. For people with ID and co-occurring mental disorders, their treatment and care needs are the responsibility of the Department of Health. However, the challenges remain in the collaborative approaches needed between different governmental departments and the delivery of such responsibility.

In Sudan, health expenditure represents 1.6% of the country's budget (18). The expenditure on disability and mental health is unknown. Health services for people with ID in Sudan present a challenge to families and healthcare providers alike. Scarcity of specialized healthcare services for people with ID exposes these children and their families to a difficult journey, adding to their pain of caring after a disabled child. Paediatricians are the main gatekeepers for service provision. There is only one psychiatrist with specialist training in ID, based in Khartoum, the nation's capital.

The first unit of ID psychiatry was established in 2010, looking after children with ID in Taha Baashar Psychiatric Teaching Hospital (Fig. 19.1). It provides care for children with IDs and their families within an adult psychiatry service. This not an ideal set-up, but still preferable to the absence of an ID psychiatry service. The service has a lack of trained psychologists with experience in ID psychiatry, as well as scarcity of social support. There are significant barriers to diagnosis of ID in Sudan, with no clear referral pathway and a lack of a proper multidisciplinary network. These services are mainly clustered in the capital Khartoum, leaving other parts of the country with no specialized services for people with ID (15).

South Sudanese people with disabilities face a struggle to access and pay for healthcare, and are also vulnerable to malnutrition; thus, the struggle for those with ID is magnified. Evidence has shown that people with disabilities in South Sudan are hit hardest by recent crises (2). People with disabilities have restricted access to humanitarian services, like food distributions, education, and healthcare. A lack of mobility devices and challenging and unfamiliar environments in displacement sites make it hard for people with disabilities to access aid services (19).

According to Light for the World, 250,000 people with disabilities live in displacement camps in South Sudan (19). Some organizations are providing services to people with disabilities in internal displacement people sites,

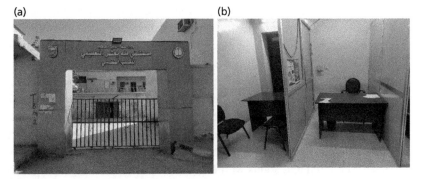

(a)　　　　　　　　　　　　(b)

Fig. 19.1 Taha Baashar Psychiatric Teaching Hospital, Sudan. (a) Hospital entrance. (b) Clinical area.

including community-based rehabilitation, focusing on education, health, social inclusion, empowerment, and livelihoods (20,21).

Several disabled people's organizations exist in South Sudan; they are involved in rights advocacy, raising awareness, and socioeconomic and political empowerment (1,22). Most awareness-raising campaigns on disability rights are concentrated in the capital Juba. Radio programmes running since 2010 have helped raise awareness of disability in Juba. Organizations have helped people with disabilities using arts and sports to challenge stereotypes in society about people with disabilities (1).

Education

A lack of educational facilities is not the sole reason for the limited access to education for children with disabilities. Household deprivation and the attitudes of parents and the wider community towards people with ID can go as far as causing parents to hide children from public view, or to think they are uneducable—playing an equally important role in limiting access to education (1). A recent study carried out by the African Child Policy Forum on the situation of children with disabilities in Ethiopia showed that many children are not going to school because their parents cannot afford transportation and related costs (23). A UNESCO review showed that provision of early childhood education was deplorably low or non-existent in half the countries covered (1). The review also revealed that most existing services were urban based, and focused only on children with overt physical or sensory impairments.

There are several challenges facing the provision of specialized care for Sudanese children with ID. The government and decision-makers do not prioritize services for the disabled, perhaps in part because of a lack of epidemiological data pertaining to people with ID. After effective lobbying by disabled people's organizations, the government decided that all children with disabilities would be entitled to free education from 2002. There are various special institutions catering to people with disabilities; education in these institutions has been supported by public efforts and voluntary organizations. In 2013, the Ministry of Education offered free education for children with disabilities (18). In reality, this has not been applied yet, as many schools lack the minimum resources to meet the needs of this marginalized sector of community. There are some individual efforts to provide services for people with disabilities, especially those with ID. Most of the specialized schools for children with ID are owned and run by parents of disabled children. These centres offer a lifespan service for children and adults with ID. However, they are not purpose built and provide care for different ages under the same roof, including sharing toilets and other facilities. This unsuitable environment exposes people with ID to risks of different types of abuse. These specialized schools for children with ID are not governed by any official supervisory body to monitor them, and there are no protocols or guidelines to guide practice of these centres (15). Most of these centres are privately run and not sponsored by the government; they are too expensive for poor families to afford. Interestingly, there is only one project providing a hybrid service, led by an individualistic initiative in collaboration with the government. This special centre is promoted as a charitable service providing an early intervention service for disabled children across Sudan. However, these kinds of services are still only available in the capital Khartoum, and are not accessible to a wide sector of those who need it, because of logistic reasons like limitation of places and poor transport. Furthermore, the staff are poorly paid and receive no official training. What training that does exist is inconsistent, and does not follow evidence-based practice.

In South Sudan, children with disabilities have very limited access to any educational opportunities, especially outside Juba, if they are girls, or if they have intellectual, psychosocial, and multiple impairments. Barriers to education for children with disabilities include the school's location and accessibility, negative attitudes, and lack of teacher experience. Efforts are being made by the government and other parties to foster inclusive education.

Social determinants of health in Africa

Most African countries have sizeable proportions of their respective populations living in poverty, which significantly affects mental health. Although social determinants of mental health such as education, employment, environment, relationships, and support can be different between countries in Africa, they still have a significant impact on the mental health and well-being of the African population at large, and more specifically on people with ID.

Stigma against disability and mental illness is another hindrance for families to seek advice and help from specialists. ID is perceived differently in different cultures but in most parts of Africa, people with ID are alienated because ID is perceived to be caused by evil eye or black magic (15). In most African nations, traditional healers are more acceptable than medical professionals, this enhances the stigma even further. Stereotyping of people with ID is another hurdle on the way of recognizing their needs, as they are frequently perceived as untrainable and educable.

Furthermore, there are limited educational opportunities for people with ID in Africa, as their needs are not perceived as a priority by different governments across the continent. Additionally, war and conflict often lead to displacement and interruption of continuity of support.

Additional challenges facing people with intellectual disability in Africa

The dearth of evidence about the prevalence of ID and magnitude of support needs remains a key obstacle to identifying the needs of such a vulnerable group. For example, many research areas in Sudan have not been investigated—disability is one of these areas. Although the limited literature available indicates that the Sudanese have negative attitudes towards disabled people, there is still a shallow evidence base pertaining to how people with disabilities are perceived in Sudan (2).

A major obstacle across African countries facing the care for people with ID is the development and vocational training opportunities and career pathways. This challenging situation leaves many families struggling to deal with their disabled youngsters after leaving school. Furthermore, integrating people with ID into the education system, in collaboration with the Department of Health, to promote ongoing rehabilitation and re-entry to education and learning following a period of illness is needed.

This situation is mirrored in South Africa, where mental health services have been marked by discriminatory divisions established in the apartheid era, when access to healthcare facilities for Black people in the Western Cape was severely compromised (24).

People living in certain parts often travel long distances to access basic mental health services in institutions and significant language barriers has been identified. Provision of services should be in a language that is well understood by patients and their caregivers, as this forms the basis for establishing a common ground between carers and clinicians to agree interventions and care planning. Inaccessibility to formal ID health services may contribute to parents seeking alternative healthcare systems to receive support related to their children's ID. Caregivers may seek help from traditional healers in isolation, or dually accessing both Western formal health systems and traditional healers.

South African families of children with ID sometimes react with negative feelings such as relating to bewitchment and fear of the ancestors. As a result, some families would take their children with ID to traditional healers seeking a 'cure' and performing rituals for the ancestors. This suggested using traditional healers and other alternative forms of care are utilized by parents and caregivers of children with ID and should be explored as alternative models of care.

Parents and primary caregivers of children with ID living in poor, marginalized settings in South Africa experience living with their children in contexts of poverty, indicating a need for support for both carers and children in low-resourced environments. They also experience isolation and stigma in their communities, and parents and caregivers use both biomedical and sociocultural terms to describe their children's ID.

Provision of educational and vocational support to children and adults with ID through non-profit organizations has been an alternative approach that developed in many countries to bridge service gaps. However, access to these organizations may be limited to urban areas, where volunteers are available. Alternative private care provisions may only be affordable to a minority of the population. Funding to support access to such provisions is not usually available, and hence the reliance on families' own resources with limited support from local society.

Care and responsibility for Sudanese disabled people is shared between the Ministry of Social Planning, Ministry of Education, and Ministry of Health (18). The division of responsibility adds to the challenge of funding allocation and execution of assigned programmes.

Key strengths and weaknesses of intellectual disability care in Africa

- People with ID in many African countries seem to live in similar environmental and social situations, with major issues pertaining to healthcare provision. The healthcare systems are developing with differing rates, with limited information available about the needs of the most vulnerable groups.
- The conflicts and wars, together with poverty and poor education, significantly affect access to health services in many African countries. However, the closed communities are often supportive to their members and sharing the difficulties may help in coping with atrocities and can be supportive to people with ID.
- Most people with ID live at home with their families, and receive support from extended families and communities in the absence of institutional care.
- Most government expenditures on health and social care in African countries are very low; hence there are very limited resources allocated to support people with ID and their families and carers.
- Governments that signed up to the UN CRPD made efforts to adopt legislations, policies, and service planning strategies to comply with the convention. However, protection of these rights needs more lobbying, advocacy, and support to implement such plans.
- Health systems in Africa remain fragile, leaving people with ID highly vulnerable, and further development requires improvements in ID recognition, resource allocation, and professional training.

- A lack of epidemiological data about the prevalence and characteristics of ID within African countries stands as a barrier to identifying the needs of this important sector of the community. Decision-makers, such as the governments and human right organizations, need to have more reliable figures available to support budgeting for service provision.

References

1. **African Child Policy Forum.** Educating Children with Disabilities in Africa: Towards a Policy of Inclusion. Addis Ababa, Ethiopia: African Child Policy Forum; 2011.

2. **Rohwerder B.** Disability in South Sudan. K4D Helpdesk Report. Brighton: Institute of Development Studies; 2018.

3. **Maulik P, Mascarenhas M, Mathers C, Dua T, Saxena S.** Prevalence of intellectual disability: a meta-analysis of population-based studies. Research in Developmental Disabilities 2011;**32**(2):419–36.

4. **World Health Organization.** WHO Global Disability Action Plan 2014–2021: Better Health for All People with Disability. Geneva: World Health Organization; 2015.

5. **Kanter AS.** The United Nations Convention on the Rights of Persons with Disabilities and its implications for the rights of elderly people under international law. Georgia State University Law Review 2009;**25**(3). Available from: https://readingroom.law.gsu.edu/gsulr/vol25/iss3/4/

6. **Virendrakumar B, Jolley E, Badu E, Schmidt E.** Disability inclusive elections in Africa: a systematic review of published and unpublished literature. Disability & Society 2018;**33**(4):509–38.

7. **Lagos State House of Assembly.** Lagos State Special People's Law. Lagos, Nigeria: Lagos State House of Assembly; 2010.

8. **Federal Government of Nigeria.** Discrimination Against Persons with Disability (Prohibition) Act. Abuja, Nigeria: Federal Government of Nigeria; 2018.

9. **Pretoria University Law Press (PULP).** African Disability Rights Yearbook. Pretoria, South Africa: Pretoria University Law Press; 2013.

10. **Conmy A.** South African health care system analysis. Public Health Review 2018;**1**(1):1–8. Available from: https://pubs.lib.umn.edu/index.php/phr/article/view/1568

11. **South African Non-Communicable Diseases Alliance.** National mental health policy framework & strategic plan 2013–2020. 2013. Available from: https://www.sancda.org.za/knowledge-base/national-mental-health-policy-framework-and-strategic-plan-2013-2020

12. **Katuu S.** Healthcare systems: typologies, framework models, and South Africa's health sector. International Journal of Health Governance 2018;**23**(2):134–48.

13. **Lord JE, Ashley Stein M.** Prospects and practices for CRPD implementation in Africa. 21 Oct 2014. Available from: https://upjournals.up.ac.za/index.php/adry/article/view/400

14. **Christianson AL, Zwane ME, Manga P, Rosen E, Venter A, Downs D,** et al. Children with intellectual disability in rural South Africa: prevalence and associated disability. Journal of Intellectual Disabilities 2002;**46**(2):179–86.

15. **Bakhiet AM.** Challenges of practicing learning disability psychiatry in Sudan. Sudanese Journal of Paediatrics 2015;**15**(1):96.

16. **Scior K, Hamid A, Hastings R, Werner S, Belton C, Laniyan A,** et al. Intellectual Disabilities: Raising Awareness and Combating Stigma—A Global Review. Executive Summary and Recommendations. London: University College London; 2015. Available from: https://www.ucl.ac.uk/ciddr/publications

17. **Institute of Development Studies.** What is the current situation for persons with disabilities in Nigeria? 2020. Available from: https://opendocs.ids.ac.uk/opendocs/han dle/20.500.12413/15561

18. **ILO InFocus Programme on Skills, Knowledge and Employability in the framework of a project funded by Development Cooperation Ireland (DCI).** Employment of People with Disabilities: The Impact of Legislation (East Africa): Sudan Country Profile. Geneva: International Labour Office; 2004.

19. **Amnesty International.** Our Hearts Have Gone Dark: The Mental Health Impact of South Sudan's Conflict. Amnesty International; 2016. Available from: https://www.amne sty.org/en/documents/afr65/3203/2016/en/

29. **Anyang M.** Presentation by the Education Secretary of South Sudan Association of the Visually Impaired. 2016. Available from: https://worldinstituteondisabilityblog.files. wordpress.com/2016/11/mauots-presentation.pdf

21. **Ayazi T, Lien L, Eide AH, Jenkins R, Albino RA, Hauff E.** Disability associated with exposure to traumatic events: results from a cross-sectional community survey in South Sudan. BMC Public Health 2013;**13**(1):469.

22. **African Child Policy Forum.** Children with Disabilities in Ethiopia: The Hidden Reality. Addis Ababa, Ethiopia: African Child Policy Forum; 2011.

23. **Nyere L.** Understanding disability in Sudan. 2011. Available from: https://mspace.lib. umanitoba.ca/bitstream/handle/1993/5223/Nyerere_Leon.pdf?sequence

24. **Cummins P.** Access to health care in the Western Cape. Lancet 2002;**360**(Suppl):s49–50.

Chapter 20

Intellectual disability services in the Middle East (with a focus on Iran)

Javad Alaghband-Rad, Mahtab Motamed, and Mohammed Al-Uzri

Introduction

It has not been long since a relatively modern system of care with limited re-sources for people with intellectual disability (ID) was put in place in Iran. The reasons behind the underdeveloped status of such services are manifold, ranging from stigma and prejudiced attitudes towards this population to inad-equate commissioning and funding of already established services. These have inevitably led to the complex health and social care needs of people with ID being overlooked. Traditionally, like many other societies with a preponderance of extended families, care and support of those with ID has been considered a task carried out by the remaining family members. However, like many other countries, civil society and non-governmental organizations (NGOs) in Iran have taken the first steps to address the multifaceted needs of this population by raising awareness, providing person-centred training, and advocating on behalf of people with ID and their carers/families to influence further service develop-ment by the local authorities.

Intellectual disability in Iran

Historical perspective, legal frameworks, and national initiatives

Interestingly, a German priest, in his role as a missionary, established the first education centre for the blind in Iran in 1920 (1). This was then followed by the setting up of other institutions for different populations with disabilities, including those with ID. In 1959, a law was passed by the Iranian Parliament granting some vocational and rehabilitation rights to people 'whose prospects of securing and retaining sustainable employment are substantially reduced as a result of physical and mental impairment'. This law was also included in the new constitution under a section called 'Social welfare' (2). The Iranian constitution states that those with disabilities should benefit from Iran's social security system. This legislation which originated in 1959 was the first that granted some vocational rehabilitation rights to people with physical disabilities and mental impairments (3).

In 1968 another law was passed to establish an organization called the 'Rehabilitation Organization' under a newly established Ministry of Labour and Social Affairs (4). The bulk of activities at that organization, initially, was to rehabilitate physically disabled people. Very little had been planned or organized to do the same for people with ID. However, over time, people with ID were also included in various programmes. With the establishment of the Special Education Organization in 1991 under the Ministry of Education, it was hoped that various efforts in educating children with ID would get more recognition and become more organized. However, there have been no formal processes or mechanisms to coordinate various medical, rehabilitative, and educational programmes for this population and these are currently delivered by three separate state ministries, namely the Ministry of Health, Ministry of Welfare, and Ministry of Education (5).

In 2003, the 'Comprehensive Law on Protection of the Rights of Persons with Disabilities' was passed which puts Iran among 50 other nations with a comprehensive and progressive legal safeguard for people with a disability. The Disability Protection Act (6), a progressive legislation in its nature, contains 16 articles providing legal protection for disabled people in multiple areas, including one which ensures that employment and reintegration rights of this population are taken seriously and as a high priority. For instance, organizations receiving state funding are mandated to offer employment opportunities to people with disabilities so that at least 3% of their workforce are from this population (and 10% from veterans) (7).

Iran's Parliament modified the United Nations Convention on the Rights of Persons with Disabilities (UN CRPD) for domestic purposes on 23 October 2009, using the word 'reservations' in their ratification that: 'with regard to Article 46, the Islamic Republic of Iran declares that it does not consider itself bound by any provisions of the Convention, which may be incompatible with its applicable rules'. This has of course the potential to change the Convention's legal impact on the rights of people with ID.

In Iran, mental disability (including ID and autism) is one of the four disability categories formally recognized by the State Welfare Organization (SWO)

(7). The other categories are hearing, visual, and physical disabilities. As high-lighted above, Iran has a progressive legal framework for safeguarding the rights of people with disabilities; however, much of these remain underutilized in real life due to the lack of commissioned resources allocated to improve service provision for these populations (8). The SWO offers services through three different means: social support, prevention, and rehabilitation. However, due to the lack of resources and support, they fall short to meet the complex needs of people with physical disability and ID. To some extent, NGOs and the civil society have been active in closing the gap in service provision. Despite all their commendable efforts, an acceptable minimum standard of service delivery has not been achieved for this population so far.

Epidemiology, facts, and figures

Iran is a vast country with a population of about 82 million. Data on the health and social care status of people with disabilities in Iran are usually collected in two ways: (1) via the statistics of population and housing censuses, conducted every 5 years; and (2) through the statistics available on people with disabilities who have been registered with the SWO.

Since not everyone with a disability is registered with the SWO, the welfare statistics do not include all people with disabilities in the country. As a result, both aforementioned data sources can have significant errors.

Furthermore, there is no official data on the prevalence of ID in Iran based on different age groups, sex, or geographical distribution (e.g., urban vs rural areas). According to the census results in 2011, the prevalence of disability was around 13/1000 of the population (9) with ID as the most prevalent type of disability with a rate of 0.419% of the general population. This gives a total of about 400,000 individuals with ID in the country (10). In general, the prevalence of ID was found to be higher among men (5.3/1000) than women (3.5/1000). This, as mentioned by the authors, unusually low rate would perhaps reflect methodological issues and should not be considered a basis for comparison with other countries. The reported prevalence was also highest in the adolescent and younger age groups.

The prevalence of autism in Iran is perhaps close to its global prevalence (11). Considering the lifetime prevalence of approximately 1% for autism, there are close to 820,000 individuals with autism in Iran who need help and support in different medical, psychological, and social domains.

There is generally no national programme for screening for ID or autism in children. However, developmental milestones and delays are recorded in primary healthcare records and all children are neuropsychologically assessed prior to initiating school. Once someone is diagnosed as autistic, he or she is registered with the SWO and would receive a monthly allowance, which is small as a result of devaluation of the national currency due to financial sanctions imposed on the country. Furthermore, autism has been included among categories of 'Special Diseases' (as of 2021) that automatically make them eligible to receive a wide range of benefits and medical services. These benefits are offered by an NGO operating at the national level, the Charity Foundation for Special Diseases (https://cffsd.org/).

Current service models

Training of professionals

There are formal training sessions on autism in different formats for medical students, interns, residents, and the fellows of child and adolescent psychiatry, delivered in all medical schools and residency programmes throughout the country. All students and trainees therefore have opportunities to train on how to assess, diagnose, and manage the health needs of autistic children and adolescents both on the wards and in outpatient settings. Furthermore, there is one academic training site for autistic adults at Roozbeh Hospital in Tehran (12). With regard to the field of ID psychiatry, however, there is no formal training at any level including for psychiatric residents and fellows who are responsible for the clinical care of this population.

Services available for people with intellectual disability

Currently, there is no stand-alone psychiatry service for people with ID in Iran. There are two national governmental organizations for people with ID: the State Welfare Organization of Iran (https://www.behzisti.ir; affiliated with the Ministry of Cooperatives, Labour, and Social Welfare) and the Special Education Organization (http://csdeo.ir; affiliated with the Ministry of Education).

The Special Education Organization is responsible for the education and training of the 'educable students' with ID. There are also private services registered with and regulated by the above-named state organizations complementing the above-mentioned services as there are huge amounts of unmet educational needs for those with ID, though the exact numbers and types of services they offer are not well documented or reported.

Residential rehabilitation centres across the country
There are currently about 388 rehabilitation centres (Fig. 20.1) with 23,827 beds offering 24-hour support/7 days of the week to 14,273 people with ID. Out of these, 54 centres are dedicated for individuals under the age of 14 years (13,14). There are four temporary housing facilities for autistic people which

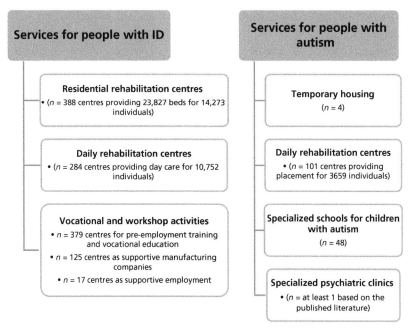

Fig. 20.1 Services available for people with ID and autism in Iran.

offer placement for 55 individuals. People with severe disability that cannot be supported within the family environment or those without a caregiver are accepted in these centres.

These centres are often privately run and therefore the families and carers need to pay a fee to access them. According to Article 7 of the Law on the Protection of Persons with Disabilities, the government must provide funding and carers' allowances to families who have a relative with a disability. The government should also provide grants to centres for service provision to people with ID. Not all the NGOs can apply for this grant as it is only available to those centres which are registered as charity organizations.

Services provided in these centres include outpatient and emergency medical and psychological appointments and 24-hour nursing and nursing assistance input. There are also inputs from other multidisciplinary agencies, including rehabilitation and occupational therapy services, social and pre-employment skills training, art therapy, speech and language therapy, and physiotherapy.

While there is no fixed psychiatry input assigned to these centres, if there is a need, patients can be referred to access specialized psychiatric clinics. The main service providers in these centres, as a minimum, have a high school diploma and have been trained as carers.

The centres act as bridges or half-way houses for helping people with ID to return to the community by equipping them with life skills following a period of rehabilitation work. In this regard, two other types of services are provided to these people. One is provided by the mobile care teams for people who are temporary residents at the centres and have the opportunity to go back to the family home. The other provides services for those with profound and multiple ID at home.

In general, caregivers affiliated to the centres aim to proactively manage the families' and carers' difficulties so that people with ID can be discharged back home as soon as possible. Given that the centres benefit from social workers' input, they can also offer advice on financial matters or even provide financial assistance if indicated.

Daily rehabilitation centres

About 284 centres (with capacity for 10,752 individuals) (Fig. 20.1) provide daily rehabilitation services for people with ID under the age of 14 years (13,14). There are also about 101 day centres with capacity for 3659 autistic individuals. Eighteen centres provide services for people with a wide range of disabilities, including both physical disabilities and ID. Every family can register their child in these centres by paying tuition. However, as part of their inclusion criteria, these centres only accept children who have the ability to go through their formal educational curricula.

Vocational and workshop activities

There are approximately 379 centres (Fig. 20.1) for pre-employment training and vocational education, 125 supportive manufacturing companies, and 17 centres for supportive employment for people with ID (14).

Services for autistic people

There are few national reports with estimated prevalence of autism in children. This ranges from 6.26 per 10,000 (11) to 1.9% (15).

Specialized healthcare services for autistic children with or without intellectual disability

Although general practitioners, paediatric neurologists, paediatricians, and psychiatrists are all involved in diagnosis and management of autistic children, most of the services are delivered by the child and adolescent psychiatrists. There are approximately 80 child and adolescent psychiatrists in Iran who work in private and public sectors, which gives a ratio of approximately one child and adolescent psychiatrist per 300,000 children (16). Psychologists and social workers are part of the multidisciplinary team, who collaborate with psychiatrists to provide a holistic management plan to those with autism and ID.

Currently there are 48 public schools which provide specialized educational input for approximately 2800 autistic students. There are also several private schools for this group. However, these facilities are not equally distributed in the country; for example, 14 out of 31 counties in Iran lack any kind of specialized schools for autistic students (17).

In the last two decades there has been an increase in the number of NGOs for autistic people that have taken significant steps in improving the quality of life of this population and their families. An example would be the recent activities of the Charity Foundation for Special Diseases (https://khaspress.ir).

The most influential and well-known among these NGOs is the Iran Autism Association, which is a non-governmental, non-profit, educational, supportive, and rehabilitation organization established in 2013. There are approximately 6500 individuals registered with the association, 3500 of who are residing in Tehran (18). Some of the educational activities of the association include organizing autism-related conferences, seminars, and workshops. Sport activities, art classes, play therapy and behaviour therapy, social gatherings, and vocational education are offered to autistic individuals in the rehabilitation section of the association. The support section provides advocacy services for individuals and their carers/families. The association provides some limited financial assistance to families and individuals and has also been lobbying for useful legislations and regulations for autistic people. The association has made significant contributions to amend the relevant laws and legislations, including the reform of the regulations for the complete exemption of autistic people from military service obligation (2020) and for including autism in the list of 'specific diseases' to secure appropriate benefits or social grants/funds for autistic people and their carers/families (2019).

Services specialized for autistic adults with or without intellectual disability
Many autistic children lose their access to the health and social care facilities when they graduate into adulthood. There is no established transition programme to hand over their care to the adult services. There is also no reliable data available on the prevalence of autism among the adult population in Iran. No specialized autism or ID services for the adult population are available in Iran, except for the Roozbeh Hospital's Adult Autism Clinic, which is affiliated to the Tehran University of Medical Sciences. The Roozbeh Adult Autism Clinic was established in 2019 and is the first and only specialized academic clinic nationwide. A general adult psychiatrist, a child and adolescent psychiatrist, together with three psychologists and a social worker are assigned to the clinic to work collaboratively with the families and carers aiming to address complex needs of autistic adults (12).

Intellectual disability services in other countries of the Middle East

The picture varies across Arab countries in the Middle East when it comes to prevalence and services for people with ID. There is a clear link between sociopolitical stability of a country and services provided in general, but this link is stronger when it comes to services for this vulnerable population. Countries in the Middle East vary from relatively stable and well-resourced ones like Saudi Arabia and Gulf states to countries where resources were once abundant but have been depleted with decades of wars and conflicts. There are yet other countries that have been consistently limited in resources, which make it hard to provide services to vulnerable people in the first place. An example would be Jordan, which is a relatively stable country, but has had to deal with large numbers of refugees as consequences of war and conflict in neighbouring countries. This could be compared with Lebanon, where limited resources have been compounded by decades of wars and internal conflict. It is not possible to cover all Middle East countries in this chapter, but the above-mentioned countries will be covered as examples of different categories of countries in the region according to resources and stability.

One of the main challenges in this region is the lack of accurate data on the prevalence of ID, as most countries include these people under the wider definition of 'disability'. However, some countries provide detailed numbers for the different types of disability. For example, accurate figures are not available for Saudi Arabia (19) but the General Authority for Statistics reports that 7.1% (1,445,723) of the population (approximately 21 million) have a disability. It is not clear how many of these individuals meet the definition of ID, but they report 19,428 with Down syndrome and 53,282 with autism. As one of the more settled countries in the Middle East, Saudi Arabia has more services for people with disabilities and legislations that protect their rights compared to many of their neighbouring countries (20). The government provides most services to people with ID, complemented by community and family support.

Iraq, a country which experienced decades of wars, international sanctions, and internal conflict, produces regular reports on service utilization by different groups of patients. The term 'mental retardation' (F70–79, International Classification of Diseases, 10th Revision) was included in the Ministry of Health, National Adviser Office for Mental Health report for the year 2021 (personal correspondence). The report describes 10,125 patients with 'mental retardations' accessing the service as outpatients and 123 as inpatients. A total of 3758 'autistic persons' were accessing services as outpatients during 2021. These figures are unlikely to be accurate in reflecting the prevalence of ID and autism in Iraq but demonstrate the limited access to and large gap in services in a country with a population of over 30 million. The federal ministry of health has nine centres for child mental health (not including the Kurdistan Regional Government) that provide health services for all children with autism and ID, which is inadequate. In addition, the Ministry of Social Affairs has centres for people with 'special needs' to address their social care needs, but it is unclear how many people with ID are provided for. However, more private centres and NGOs were established post 2003 for people with ID, in recognition of the gap between needs and services provided. The families remain the main source of care for people with ID and autism. Of note is that these families established the only service-users' families' association for psychoeducation in the country.

For Lebanon, another country in the Middle East with decades of wars and conflicts, it is also difficult to get precise figures on the prevalence of ID. This is largely due to reports and literature including both mental and physical disabilities in their figures. Additionally, it is hard to have accurate figures with continued changes in demographics either, with waves of refugees from neighbouring countries, and internally displaced people due to civil war and conflicts. According to the K4D report, between 10% and 15% of the population has some kind of disability (physical and/or mental) (21). The report identifies a systemic lack of provision for rights, resources, and services and blames 'inaction by state', which exacerbates stigma and discrimination against people with disability in the country. The absence of accurate figures for those with ID makes it hard to say with confidence who is providing care and support for this population group. However, it is safe to say that families, private sector, and NGOs supported by international donors are taking a bigger role in the provision of care and support for people with ID, with the state preoccupied with political instability and conflict. Regarding the prevalence of autism, evidence from a national survey of 818 children (age 16–48 months) in all regions indicate a conservative estimate of up to 513 per 10,000 (5.13%), which is higher when compared to other Arab-speaking countries in the region (22).

Jordan is a relatively stable country in the Middle East but with limited resources, where prevalence of people with disability reported to be 13% within a total population of around 4 million when UNICEF supported Jordan with a technical assistance and disability module in 2015 according to The K4D report on disability in Jordan (23). This percentage was confirmed in 2017 which is significantly different to other reports that varies from 1.8 to 2.7 using census data. However, it is less clear what proportion of this disability is ID. There has been an influx of refugees after the Iraq invasion in 2003 and following the start of the civil war in Syria in 2011. International support is crucial to delivering the needs of people with ID in such a country with limited resources. The UN and other international donors are major sources of support in Jordan. Stigma and discrimination are significant barriers for people with ID in Jordan to live independently and fulfil their potential, much like for other countries in the region. Of note, is that attitudes towards people with sensory and physical disabilities is improving by society but not towards people with ID. The UNHCR Health Working Group—Jordan report (24) highlights the difficulties with obtaining reliable data when it comes to the refugee population. However, it is estimated that up to 30% of Syrian refugees, which form 90% of total refugee number of 750,000, are suffering some kind of disability. People with intellectual impairment, which does not necessarily equate to ID, were estimated to represent up to 13.4% of the total refugee population with disability, based on a 2014 survey. The prevalence of ID was reported to be between 7 and 12% among mental health conditions in one of the large refugee camps (Azraq) as reported by Health Working Group—Jordan in 2022. Services are limited and legislations to protect the rights of people with disability are often inadequate or not implemented. However, Jordan produced number of legislations such as "the Law of Disabled people care (1993), Law on the rights of persons with disabilities (2007) and Law on the rights of persons with disabilities (2017). Jordan has a national disability strategy, a specific disability law, articles on disability included in the constitution, focal points for disability in line ministries, direct involvement of persons with disabilities in government mechanisms, indicating its position as a regional leader for disability rights" (23). International agencies work with the government and local NGOs, as well as community and national leaders, including the royal family, to raise awareness of disability issues and improve services for them.

Conclusion

While Iran is fairly advanced in terms of having legislations and reviewing these pertaining to the care of people with ID and autism to safeguard their rights and entitlements, there are generally significant deficits in resource allocation at various levels. There are also barriers to make concerted efforts to provide this population with comprehensive packages of care. The distribution of services also seems to be limited to larger cities. Civil society and NGOs try to bridge this gap; however, the complex needs of this vulnerable group are greater than what these agencies can meet at this time. Provision of adequate services for adults with ID, including establishment of specialist healthcare services, vocational training, and supported employment opportunities, is of high priority. The historical barriers of stigma and cultural ignorance remain today and are equally challenging to tackle. There is also a lack of robust epidemiological data on the mental and physical health comorbidities in this population group in Iran and on the stigma, prejudices, barriers, and challenges that they and their families/carers face to access services.

To our knowledge, there are no data on the mortality and the causes of death in this population in Iran. This includes the lack of data on the impact of the COVID-19 pandemic on the ID population in Iran. One could, however, make inferences from recently published literature (25,26) on the same topics in high-income countries to generalize the findings to low- and middle-income countries including Iran to draw conclusions on the estimates of the statistical figures. Given the general lack of appropriately allocated resources and absence of dedicated and adequately commissioned specialist multiagency and multidisciplinary social and healthcare services, it can be deduced that health inequalities and gaps in service provision/delivery and premature mortality should be higher in Iran when these statistical figures are compared to those which have been published for the high-income countries.

As recommended by Tyrer et al. (25), population-level approaches such as specially tailored health promotion strategies, prevention programmes, and staff training across health and social care settings should be commissioned centrally to address health inequality and premature mortality for this vulnerable group of people. The generic services should also make reasonable adjustments for people with ID to make sure that services are easily accessible for them (25,26). These interventions, however, need to be backed up by legislations and centrally approved policies and initiatives that are guaranteed to be implemented in daily practice by allocation of enough resources and meaningful commissioning if low- and middle-income countries similar to Iran aspire to develop person-centred services in support of their ID population and those with autism.

The rest of the Middle East also generally faces similar problems with legislation, resource allocation, and lack of reliable data on people with ID.

Acknowledgement

The authors wish to thank Dr Maryam Abbasinejad for her tremendous help with piecing together the available data and formal reports published for people with ID in Iran.

References

1. **Salehpour Y, Adibsereshki N.** Disability and Iranian Culture. Tehran: University of Social Welfare and Rehabilitation Sciences; 2001.

2. **International Labor Organization.** R99 Vocational Rehabilitation (Disabled) Recommendation, 1955. n.d. Available from: https://www.ilo.org/dyn/normlex/en/f?p= NORMLEXPUB:12100:0::NO::P12100_INSTRUMENT_ID:312437

3. Iranian Constitution 1979; amended in 1989.

4. **Noori M.** History of rehabilitation in Iran. Handicap Cultural Center; 2019. Available from: http://www.handicapcenter.com/2018/12/31/19865

5. **Moore A, Kornblet S.** Advancing the Rights of Persons with Disabilities: A US–Iran Dialogue on Law, Policy, and Advocacy. Washington, DC: Henry L. Stimson Center; 2011.

6. **Islamic Republic of Iran.** Comprehensive Law on Protection of the Rights of Persons with Disabilities. Official Gazette, 1383-2-16, (2003-05-06) No. 17264. 2003. Available from: http://www.rooznamehrasmi.ir/

7. **Alaedini P.** Training and Employment of People with Disabilities: Iran 2003. Bangkok: International Labour Office; 2004.

8. **Bahreini R.** Understanding disability as a human rights issue. In: Gozaar: A Forum on Human Rights and Democracy in Iran. 2007. Message posted to: http://www.gozaar.org/english/articles-en/Understanding-Disability-as-a-Human-Rights-Issue html

9. **Statistical Centre of Iran.** Iran Statistical Yearbook. Tehran: Statistical Centre of Iran; 2015.

10. **Soltani S, Khosravi B, Salehiniya H.** Prevalence of ID in Iran: toward a new conceptual framework in data collection. Journal of Research in Medical Sciences 2015;**20**(7):715–16.

11. **Samadi SA, Mahmoodizadeh A, McConkey R.** A national study of the prevalence of autism among five-year-old children in Iran. Autism 2012;**16**(1):5–14.

12. **Alaghband-Rad J, Jamaloo S, Motamed M.** Roozbeh adult autism spectrum disorder clinic: lessons learned from first 34 cases. International Journal of Developmental Disabilities 2020;**68**(5):766–72.

13. **State Welfare Organization of Iran.** Clinical criteria and guidelines for people with autism and ID. 2018. Available from: https://www.behzisti.ir/

14. Data obtained through verbal communication with Dr Maryam Abbasinejad, Senior officer, Department for Mental Health and Substance Abuse, Deputy for Health, Ministry of Health and Medical Education, Islamic Republic of Iran and Farideh BaghAlishahi, Director, office.

15. **Ghanizadeh A.** A preliminary study on screening prevalence of pervasive developmental disorder in schoolchildren in Iran. Journal of Autism and Developmental Disorders 2008;**38**(4):759–63.

16. **Sharifi V, Amin-Esmaeili M, Hajebi A, Motevalian A, Radgoodarzi R, Hefazi M,** et al. Twelve-month prevalence and correlates of psychiatric disorders in Iran: the Iranian Mental Health Survey, 2011. Archives of Iranian Medicine 2015;**18**(2):76–84.

17. **Islamic Republic News Agency.** No Title [Internet]. Available from: www.irna.ir/news/83740885

18. **State Welfare Organization of Iran.** No Title [Internet]. Available from: https://behzisti.ir/xhG8

19. **Alrowili NO.** ID in Saudi Arabia between reality and ambition. Global Journal of Intellectual & Developmental Disabilities 2017;**2**(5):153–4.

20. **GOV.SA**. Rights of People with Disabilities. n.d. Available from: https://www.my.gov.sa/wps/portal/snp/careaboutyou/RightsOfPeopleWithDisabilities

21. **Combaz E.** Situation of persons with disabilities in Lebanon. K4D; 2018. Available from: https://assets.publishing.service.gov.uk/media/5b584da340f0b633af812655/Disability_in_Lebanon.pdf

22. **Richa S, Khoury R, Rouhayem J, Chammay R, Kazour F, Khalil RB**, et al. Estimating the prevalence of autism spectrum disorder in Lebanon. L'Encephale 2020;**46**(6):414–19.

23. **Thompson S.** The current situation of persons with disabilities in Jordan. K4D; 2018. Available from: https://assets.publishing.service.gov.uk/media/5bb22804ed915d258 ed26e2c/Persons_with_disabilities_in_Jordan.pdf

24. The UNHCR Health Working Group—Jordan Working Group: Health Working Group-Jordan (unhcr.org)

25. **Tyrer F, Kiani R, Rutherford MJ.** Mortality, predictors and causes among people with ID: a systematic narrative review supplemented by machine learning. Journal of Intellectual & Developmental Disability 2021;**46**(2):102–14.

26. **Tyrer F, Morriss R, Kiani R, Gangadharan SK, Rutherford MJ.** Mortality disparities and deprivation among people with ID in England: 2000–2019. Journal of Epidemiology and Community Health 2022;**76**(2):168–74.

Chapter 21

Intellectual disability services in the Indian subcontinent

Ayomipo J. Amiola, Asif Zia,
Chandanie G. Hewage, Varghese Punnoose,
Satheesh Kumar Gangadharan, and
Regi T. Alexander

Introduction

The Indian subcontinent includes the countries of Bangladesh, Bhutan, India, Maldives, Nepal, Pakistan, and Sri Lanka. The terms Indian subcontinent and South Asia are often used interchangeably to denote the region (1). Although there are variations in economic status and political situations in the different countries included within this chapter, the region shares a common cultural background which influences the perception of its inhabitants to life, including disability. In addition, all the countries included belong to the category of low- and middle-income (LAMI) countries. Many LAMI countries face several challenges in relation to intellectual disability (ID).

The concept of ID was recognized in ancient Indian literature (2). As in most LAMI countries, their care rests with the family. True to its collectivistic moorings, the cultural ethos of communities in the Indian subcontinent generally encourages the family to give compassionate care. A strong emphasis is placed on family values and giving support to women before, during, and after birth. Breastfeeding is encouraged, and children are brought up in a joint family system where they are supported by their mothers or extended family. All of this comes at the cost of significant burden for the caretakers in the family, especially the parents (3,4).

Limited financial resources, lack of access to healthcare, emergence of behavioural problems, social stigma, worry about the future care of children as the parents become older, and concerns about possible sexual abuse and so on contribute to parental distress and burnout. There is a view that urbanization and Westernization of the society has eroded the support systems which existed within the extended family and has necessitated a shift from care within the family to more formal care systems in the community. However, this rosy picture may not be entirely reflective of the reality and discrimination against differently abled children that has been described (5). Though the gap between the needs of the individuals with ID and their families and the existing services are very wide, there have been several changes in a positive direction for the last five or six decades (2).

Epidemiology

The prevalence of people with an ID is almost double in developing countries compared to high-income countries (6). Prevalence estimates of ID in India have wide variance. Prevalence has clustered around 1–4 per 1000 population in studies which included only severe forms whereas those which included all degrees of severity showed figures around 10–30 per 1000 population. Adjusting for methodological differences in the available studies, it has been estimated that the prevalence of ID including all grades of severity in the general population is around 2.5%, with excess prevalence in males, rural areas, and low-income groups. If this is translated to absolute figures, there are 40 million people requiring care (7). These figures correspond to the entire population of countries like Canada.

Pakistan has one of the highest reported rates of childhood ID in the world. Prevalence estimates vary from 19.1 per 1000 for serious ID to 65 per 1000 for mild ID (8).

According to the Society for the Welfare of the Intellectually Disabled, Bangladesh (SWID Bangladesh) annual report 2017, there are 116,771 people with ID in Bangladesh (9). There is very limited information on the prevalence of ID in Nepal with only one reference in the literature to a survey of ID conducted in 1989 showing a prevalence rate of 4.9% (10). There are some pointers to significant regional variations within Nepal with prevalence as high as 10% in the northern mountainous region with significantly lower prevalence in other parts (11).

The prevalence of ID in Sri Lanka is not accurately assessed. Based on the findings of the World Health Survey, prevalence of disability was considered to be 12.9%. This includes all types of disabilities. Out of this, 25.12% was considered 'mental disability', which may encompass intellectual or psychosocial impairment. Nevertheless, the Department of Census and Statistics of Sri Lanka, in a survey in 2001, estimated 1.6% of the Sri Lankan population had ID (12).

Cultural issues

Culturally, communities in the Indian subcontinent share many features of LAMI countries regarding ID. The close-knit kinship systems have always cared for their members with ID and families generally take care of their needy relatives with compassion, because of a sense of duty (2). However, there is a low level of awareness about the nature, causes, and interventions in ID. Superstitions, myths, and misconceptions abound. In an agrarian environment with little or no mechanization, people with mild ID could assume valued roles. That did not preclude the possibility of rampant discrimination against the differently abled. A study among children in rural Indian communities described several unwelcome attitudes and beliefs. These included denial of disability, denial of property rights, social boycott, use of physical restraints, suppression of any expressions of sexuality particularly of women, and a perceived reduction in the marital prospects of family members. Difficulties in the management of challenging behaviours and stigma led to the ostracizing of entire families. Inhuman treatment like being chained to 'keep them safe' and 'out of danger' was reported (5).

The delay in early detection and seeking of professional help of ID in the Indian subcontinent can have cultural determinants. More visible disabilities like visual, hearing, or motor disorders are easily identified, and help is sought. Since the concept of ID is a somewhat alien entity in the local culture, parents may neglect seeking intervention until their child develops behavioural problems (13). Stigma associated with ID may also prevent parents from seeking help. The parents who experience shame for having a child with ID may prevent the child from going out and being exposed to peer interaction and play time. The superstitious beliefs about the aetiology and expectations of magical cure and the resigned attitude of therapeutic nihilism can also be impediments in seeking help. Within the more urbanized and middle-class populations, there is an emphasis on education and many people with mild ID encounter services only when they struggle with academic work.

The rapid transition within societies in the Indian subcontinent, driven by urbanization, Westernization, market economics, and globalization, is making it more individualistic. The support of the extended family or joint family is slowly disappearing. A child with ID is expected be looked after almost exclusively by the mother at the cost of her career and personal life. This can lead to caretaker distress, burnout, and even create a fertile ground for child abuse (14).

Patka and colleagues in their study among 262 community members and 190 disability service providers in Pakistan found more positive attitudes in staff serving people with ID, females, Christians, Hindus, Sunnis, and people with greater education (15).

As most of the services for people with ID are limited to childhood, issues of caring for adults and the conflicts about issues of sexuality and marriage continue to remain as sociocultural dilemmas. Clinicians (and borne out by research evidence) are often faced with questions like 'Who will care for my intellectually disabled son after we die or become incapable of supporting him?', 'Our 20-year-old daughter with ID is showing sexual interests which are embarrassing. Can we think of an arranged marriage for her?', 'I can't keep an eye over my teenage daughter always as I must go for my work as a maid. She does not have the skill to keep herself safe from sexual exploitation. Is it possible to sterilize her by an operation?' These are issues that services for people with ID in the Indian subcontinent grapple with regularly (16–18).

Legislation and health policies

India

In the last seven decades, lots of progress has been made in terms of legislations and inclusive health policies for people with ID. With the enactment of the Mental Health Act in 1987 and the Persons with Disability Act, 1996, 'mental retardation' which was initially part of the Indian Lunacy Act, 1912, along with 'insanity', was seen as distinct from mental illness (19). The Persons with Disabilities Act, 1996 (further revised in 2016 as the Rights of Persons with Disabilities Act (RPWD Act), 2016) emphasized equality of opportunity and non-discrimination, together with the range of services that needed to be developed, such as prevention, early intervention, education, training, and social benefits.

The setting up of the National Institute for the Mentally Handicapped (now known as the National Institute for the Empowerment of Persons with Intellectual Disabilities (NIEPID)) in 1984 was a milestone for people with ID (20); the National Trust Act, 1999 for people with 'mental retardation', cerebral palsy, autism, and multiple disabilities specifically addressed those with ID. This Act was intended to empower people who could not speak for themselves, as well as their families. It was envisaged that it would permit greater participation of parents' associations and non-governmental organizations (NGOs) in service development (2). It also provides for establishment of the National Trust for the welfare of people with ID and their families. This Act provides for health insurance, establishment of training centres, and residential care centres funded by the trust and run by parent associations. The issue of guardianship for adults with ID is also covered in this Act.

The RPWD Act, 2016 emphasizes the rights perspective of people with disabilities and signifies a major shift from the welfare perspective of its predecessor law enacted in 1995. This Act makes equal opportunities, protection from discrimination, and dignified living of people with disabilities legally binding. Unique Identity Cards issued to the disabled citizens make them eligible for pension, free travel, and health insurance. It has created a system of implementing and monitoring the benefits and rights through the office of the Disability Commissioner with enhanced powers in every state. A separate track in the legal system for the disabled has been established. In short, the RPWD Act, 2016 has become a landmark legislation which has improved the services provided to people with disability, especially those with ID as it ensures inclusive education from age 6 to 16 years and 4% reservation of jobs in government services.

As highlighted previously, social security benefits for people with ID include disability pensions, family pensions to be carried over from parent/guardian, travel concessions, income tax exemption for guardians, scholarships, health insurance, and customs duty exemption for import of assistive devices. The Social Security Mission under the Ministry of Social Justice and Empowerment is effectively monitoring these services in states. Local self-governments (three-tier panchayat systems with village, block, and district levels) and municipalities have schemes to ensure that these benefits reach all the deserving individuals in a hassle-free manner.

Pakistan

At the time of independence in 1947, there were no special education schools for children with ID in Pakistan. The history of working with this population started in the 1950s at an individual level. The success of individual efforts motivated and encouraged the private sector to get involved in this noble task. The first government initiative for the education of special children can be traced back to the report of National Commission on Education, 1959, which recommended vocational education for children and adults with ID. The movement spread all over the country but slowly. The period 1980–1990 is considered a boom time in the history of prevention, treatment, education, and rehabilitation for children with disabilities and now Pakistan is moving towards inclusive education and social inclusion through employment opportunities for children with ID (21).

Bangladesh

The Bangladeshi government adopted the National Disability Policy in 1995 and in 2001 the Disabled Welfare Act (Protibandhi Kallayan Act-2001) was passed by the parliament. The National Co-ordination Committee for the Disabled, Bangladesh Disability Trust, and Committee for Inclusive Education were formed by the government to promote development of people with ID along with people with other forms of disabilities. In addition, Bangladesh maintains working relationship with international organizations related to the care of the ID population (22).

Bhutan

Bhutan started its journey of modernization only in the 1960s but has made some significant changes in its approach to inclusive education (23). Bhutan's Gross National Happiness, a constitutional aim, includes people with disability. Bhutan signed the United Nations Convention on the Rights of Persons with Disabilities in 2010 and set the standards for inclusive education in 2016. In 2018, Bhutan set the 10-year roadmap for inclusive and special education. A national policy for people with disabilities was introduced in 2019 followed by a multisectoral action plan to operationalize the policy in 2020.

Nepal

The Protection and Welfare of the Disabled Persons Act 1982 was replaced with the Disability Rights Act of 2017 with a significant change in emphasis from a welfare-based approach to a rights-based approach to disability. The act focuses on measures to address rights to health, education, and livelihood of people with disabilities. The National Childhood Disability Management Strategy (2008) outlines the measures for detecting, supporting, and preventing childhood disabilities (24). The constitution emphasizes the rights of people with disabilities and criminalizes any infringement of rights. The key challenge, however, is in the identification of people with disabilities including those with ID, provision of infrastructure, and support for enacting the national policies.

Sri Lanka

In Sri Lanka, a 'National Council for Coordinating the Work of Disability Organizations', appointed by the Minister of Social Services, was established in 1989. The Act for the Protection of the Rights of Persons with Disabilities came into effect on 24 October 1996 by proclamation in the Gazette of the Democratic Socialist Republic of Sri Lanka (25).

The Act had five major provisions: firstly, the establishment of a National Council for Persons with Disabilities which is concerned with all matters concerning the promotion, advancement, and protection of the rights of people with disabilities in Sri Lanka. Secondly, the establishment of a 'National Secretariat for Persons with Disabilities'; thirdly, establishment of a 'National Fund for Persons with Disabilities' which deals with all the financial transactions of the Council, both receiving funds voted by the parliament for the use of the Council donations, aid, and grants, and paying out all such finances required for expenditure by the Council. Fourthly, registration of NGOs working in the disability field are required, under the Act, to prevent the exploitation of individuals who have disabilities and disabilities itself; and finally, protection of individual rights in terms of discrimination in employment and educational aspects and access to public places (26).

Service models

Service models describe what relevant services there are and how they are provided to a special group of people having a defined condition throughout the period of illness (if a lifelong condition through the lifespan of such a person). The key areas in the concept of service models include health promotion and prevention, early detection and intervention, integration, community care, and encouragement of self-management.

In the Indian subcontinent, there are many prevention and promotion programmes that concern ID. These services for people with ID are provided based on the internationally accepted key concepts. It is multisectoral in nature and the key partners include community and hospital-based healthcare teams, education services, vocational training, rehabilitation, social services, labour department, transport services, housing, international collaborators, philanthropists, parent groups, private sector, and NGOs. We discuss below, the service models for clinical services, community-based services, special education, role of NGOs, role of families, social care, and training.

Clinical services

India

Perhaps the earliest model of care in India is hospital-based services provided in the departments of paediatrics or psychiatry. Child guidance clinics in teaching hospitals and multispecialty hospitals are functioning in almost all medical college hospitals, the primary aim of which is to incorporate basic training for psychiatrists and paediatricians during their postgraduate training. These centres unfortunately do not function all the time and often lack the ideal multidisciplinary team to render the services needed for children with ID under one umbrella team. Babies born in public health facilities and at home (domestic deliveries) will be screened at 6 weeks after birth, preschool children in rural areas and urban slums will be screened at 6 years, and children in government and government-aided schools will be screened from class 1 to class 12 (until 18 years) under this scheme.

Screening is done by trained health workers using special tools developed for the purpose. Children who are picked up by the screening team are directed to District (Regional) Early Intervention Centres (DEIC) attached to district hospitals or designated government medical colleges. These children undergo comprehensive evaluation and management by medical professionals and allied professionals such as a nutritionist, audiologist cum speech therapist, optometrist, special educator and clinical psychologist. Children who are beneficiaries of DEICs are given a unique identification number through which mother and child tracking can be facilitated. DEICs can have MoU with 13 tertiary centres geographically distributed across the nation for training and referral of people requiring advanced interventions.

Nepal

Nepal has a focus on a community-based rehabilitation model. The key focus within this model is for the local communities to integrate and provide support for people with disabilities including those with ID in all aspects of life. The role of professionals and professional organizations is to facilitate and support. NGOs play a key role in the provision of support. Some of the NGOs provide sheltered workshops allowing some limited skills development and employment opportunities for people with ID. However, there is very limited provision for the rural population with the NGO support mostly limited to main towns (10). Like in other LAMI countries, the family is the main source of support for adults with ID (27). Access to healthcare is variable, based on rural–urban variations as well as the family's attitude to ID. Improving awareness, access to support, as well as employment opportunities for people with ID are the key challenges that Nepal is facing in this context.

Bhutan

Bhutan supports the integration of children with disability into mainstream schools, but the actual implementation of this approach is not successful with many of the schools segregating children with disability from other students and some children with disability are supported in schools or organizations admitting only those with disabilities. There are no special facilities for supporting the health needs of people with ID and they access mainstream healthcare provisions with support from their families. Access to healthcare is determined by the location as well as awareness of families, as in other countries in the region.

Sri Lanka

Paediatric teams at community levels and small hospitals, neonatal services including intensive care units, specialized paediatric services, and child psychiatry/guidance clinics in major hospitals in Sri Lanka are involved in early detection and management of ID. Specialist teams including audiology, speech and language therapy, physiotherapy, occupational therapy, clinical, and educational psychology teams work together with paediatric teams in early detection and intervention activities.

Community-based interventions

India

Programmes were introduced by the Government of India with the aims of reducing maternal and child mortality, ensuring universal vaccinations as per the national immunization schedule, and providing adequate nutrition in childhood. These programmes, supported by an extensive network of field staff and trained health workers, have access even to the most rural and underprivileged areas of this vast country. These services are integrated with the general healthcare system through the primary health centres. The efficacy of this system varies from state to state, but the trend of growth of these services are in a positive direction. The focus on reproductive health, nutrition, and chance of getting access to the modern medical system early in life is believed to have resulted in primary prevention and early detection of developmental disorders, especially ID, though good-quality data are not available.

The National Rural Health Mission (NRHM) was set up in 2005. The aim of this mission is to ensure simultaneous action on a wide range of determinants of health such as safe drinking water, nutrition, sanitation, education, and social and gender justice. Community health workers from the same community called Accredited Social Health Activists (ASHAs), trained in early identification of various diseases, make house-to-house visits and identify the health needs of the individual. The effective links between the community and the public health system provided by ASHAs are expected to clear the pathways for early intervention in ID. A scheme named Rashtriya Bal Swasthya Karyakram for child health screening and early intervention was launched in 2013 under the NRHM to screen specifically for developmental disorders, disabilities, and birth defects. The mammoth initiative spread across 718 revenue districts of India is expected to cover 270 million children between 0 and 18 years and offers to provide free treatment of problems detected; hopefully this will help in the early identification of and multidisciplinary interventions for ID in India.

Sri Lanka

In Sri Lanka, promotion, prevention, early detection, early intervention, and rehabilitation are part of the national health plan. These include vaccination of all children for rubella in childhood, preconception care for young couples, prenatal care for pregnant mothers, professional care for childbirth, neonatal screening for hypothyroidism and deafness, regular monitoring of growth and development parameters of babies during early childhood at community level, nutrition supplementation when indicated, screening at various ages, referral for assessments, and specialized care for children having such needs. Primary care health teams functioning at grassroot level in the community play a large role in these activities and there is regular monitoring of these programmes with in-service training, improvement of infrastructure, and human resources. Community health teams conduct regular screening of school-aged children in school medical inspections, and this contributes significantly to the detection of children who need interventions.

Special education

India

Community-based early childhood development programmes of the health sector work in collaboration with education and social services. Special education services also play a large role in early identification of children with ID and planning appropriate educational interventions in normal stream or in special education units. The social services department plays a major role in arranging vocational training and arranging suitable employment opportunities. Concerning mainstreaming, the launching of a national programme called Sarva Siksha Abhiyan (SSA) in India for children between 6 and 14 years of age has boosted the inclusion of children with ID into mainstream schools (27). The zero-rejection policy in this programme asserts the right of children with ID to receive state-supported educational services without restrictions or discrimination. Though challenges like attitudinal problems, adaptation of school pedagogy, and lack of trained human resources exist, this scheme has covered around 90% of children with special needs.

Role of non-governmental organizations

India

In India between the 1950s and 1980, several NGOs established special schools, initially in cities and later in smaller towns. These schools aimed to provide individualized education of basic academic skills, training in basic self-support skills, and occupational skills, though highly trained professionals were not adequately available. Provision of mid-day meals and day care were huge respites provided by these institutions for parents with a low income. Various state governments are giving partial financial support to these institutions in the form of annual grants. In addition, driven by the philosophy of reaching the unreached, these NGOs established strong community links and later obtained governmental support. Using grassroot-level workers who survey the geographical area they cover, the NGOs help individuals with ID to access services and social security benefits, and transfer skills to families for home-based training and enrolment in school, thus assisting community activities and reducing social exclusion.

Bangladesh

Before 1977, people in Bangladesh were unaware of the concept of ID, hence those with ID were often treated as 'mad' with little or no access to educational or vocational services. In 1977, SWID Bangladesh was established by parents and professionals to provide services to children with ID, and develop human resources and social awareness, including advocacy to establish the rights of people with ID. Currently, more than 1000 people with ID have been rehabilitated by SWID Bangladesh. Another NGO, the Bangladesh Protibondhi Foundation, provides services to children with ID (22).

Role of family-based interventions and parent associations

India

The close-knit kinship systems have always cared for their members with ID. Institutionalization, unlike in the West, has never been a major movement in the Indian subcontinent and families largely take care of their needy relatives. In the 1980s and 1990s, professionals working with people with ID started exploring the possibility of involving families in management. They were successful in training parents to use behaviour modification techniques and in teaching self-help skills. The approach has now found widespread application, albeit with wide variations in goals and approaches (28), affirming the strength of parent–professional partnerships (2). Parent self-help groups which were formed in the 1980s soon gathered momentum and spread all over India. More than 250 parental associations across the nation have come together under an umbrella organization called PARIVAR (meaning extended family). This National Confederation of Parental Organizations is playing an increasing role in advocacy, policy planning, and legislation. Self-advocacy training of people with ID is an innovative programme by this Confederation.

Social care

Sri Lanka

In Sri Lanka, the social services department plays a major role in arranging vocational training and suitable employment opportunities; also, when needed, social benefits, housing, respite, and/or long-term accommodation are arranged for the disabled and their carers. A disability allowance and payment of parental pension to those with ID help these people to become independent. There are many services run by local and international NGOs, various religious groups, philanthropists, and parent groups who contribute significantly to providing special education, training life skills, vocational training, care homes, and long-term residential care as required.

Training

India

NIEPID (formerly the National Institute for the Mentally Handicapped) was established by the Government of India in 1984 at Secunderabad with a primary aim of building human resource potential at all levels. Apart from this primary goal, NIEPID is active in promoting community awareness, research, publishing educational materials and a directory of services all over India. Premier institutes such as the National Institute of Mental Health and Neuroscience (NIMHANS), Bengaluru, the Christian Medical College, Vellore, and the Postgraduate Institute of Medical Education Research, Chandigarh, are contributing to the development of human resources and quality of services in ID.

Bangladesh

The Bangladesh Government (separate from the University of Dhaka) runs the National Centre for Special Education where educational facilities for people with ID and the 'Teachers' Training Program on Special Education' are available (22).

Nepal

The Association for the Welfare of the Mentally Retarded is the key umbrella organization in Nepal providing leadership for improving the education and training of people with ID. A national special education programme facilitated the introduction of 'resource classes' within mainstream schools where children with disabilities including ID could be accommodated. However, only a small proportion of mainstream schools have this provision. While children with mild ID and some with moderate ID could be supported in these facilities, children with severe or profound ID will not be able to access this. There are limited number of special schools and counselling centre. Vocational programmes for people with ID and community-based employment opportunities are extremely limited and centred mostly around the bigger cities like Kathmandu.

Key strengths and weaknesses

Care given in the community by families is a major strength of the service model in this part of the world. Individuals with ID become part of the community which ensures normalization and integration into the larger society. Nevertheless, family members can experience high levels of stress, caregiver burden, and burnout (2,29). Also, stigma and myths concerning the cause of ID are still widely prevalent making it difficult to access services and ensure the inclusion of those with ID. Overprotection of children with ID by family members and other forms of paternalistic care likely based on social, cultural, or religious factors can hamper their independence and autonomy.

Current health indicators prove that Sri Lanka has a very comprehensive and widespread primary healthcare system which can promote preventing, detecting, and intervening early for children with ID. Paediatric and neonatal services provide a high level of care and this contributes significantly to care. The establishment of child psychiatry as a subspeciality in psychiatry and compulsory training of all general adult psychiatrists in child psychiatry has contributed significantly to the care of individuals with ID. Training special education teachers and establishment of a special education service and units in education department provide equal opportunities and fulfil the right of individuals with ID to receive education. Human resources of the social services department have increased significantly over last decade with improvement of services and care available to those with ID.

Clinical services for ID in India include clinical evaluation, physical and psychological testing, parent counselling, treatment of comorbid physical and mental disorders, and genetic counselling. Mental hospitals, general hospital psychiatric units, paediatric clinics and child guidance clinics, and ID clinics provide mental health services and there are referral centres that provide good-quality care; they also undertake some professional training and research. Unfortunately, these services are often inadequate and unevenly distributed.

Development of culture- and language-appropriate assessment methods to identify ID and training healthcare workers to use them is a priority in this region. Also, provision of easily accessible genetic counselling services would be helpful in preventing ID due to genetic causes.

References

1. **Wikipedia contributors**. Indian subcontinent. Wikipedia, The Free Encyclopedia; 2022. Available from: https://en.wikipedia.org/wiki/Indian_subcontinent

2. **Girimaji SC**. Intellectual disability in India: the evolving patterns of care. International Psychiatry 2011;**8**(2):29–31.

3. **Seshadri M, Verma VK, Verma SK, Pershad D**. Impact of a mentally handicapped child on the family. Indian Journal of Clinical Psychology 1983;**10**(2):473–8.

4. **Sethi S, Bhargava SC, Dhiman V**. Study of level of stress and burden in the caregivers of children with mental retardation. Eastern Journal of Medicine 2007;**12**(1–2):21–4.

5. **Janardhana N, Muralidhar D, Naidu D M, Raghevendra G**. Discrimination against differently abled children among rural communities in India: need for action. Journal of Natural Science, Biology, and Medicine 2015; **6**:7–11.

6. **Maulik PK, Mascarenhas MN, Mathers CD, Dua T, Saxena S**. Prevalence of intellectual disability: a meta-analysis of population-based studies. Research in Developmental Disabilities 2011;**32**(2):419–36.

7. **Gururaj G, Varghese M, Benegal VN, Rao GN, Pathak K, Singh LK, Misra R**. National Mental Health Survey of India, 2015–16: Summary. Bengaluru: National Institute of Mental Health and Neurosciences; 2016: 1–48.

8. **Mirza I, Tareen A, Davidson LL, Rahman A**. Community management of intellectual disabilities in Pakistan: a mixed methods study. Journal of Intellectual Disability Research 2009;**53**(6):559–70.

9. **Islam K, Uddin MS, Islam MS, Siddiqui SA, Hussain MS, Millat MS**. Profile for people with intellectual disabilities in the Dhaka and Pabna regions of Bangladesh. Journal of Disability Studies 2022;**8**(1):1–6.

10. **Crishna B, Prajapati SB**. Comparative policy brief: status of intellectual disabilities in Nepal. Journal of Policy and Practice in Intellectual Disabilities 2008;**5**(2):133–6.

11. **Ali A**. Mental Retardation in Nepal. Kathmandu, Nepal: Association for the Welfare of Mentally Retarded/Maryknoll Fathers. 1991.

12. **Department of Census and Statistics**. Information on disabled persons, census of population and housing 2001, Colombo c2016. Available from: http://www.statistics. gov.lk/page.asp?page= Population %20and%20Housing

13. **Ginige P, Wijesinghe WH, Tennakoon SU**. An epidemiological study of clinic attendees at the first specialised clinic for individuals with intellectual disability in Sri Lanka. Sri Lanka Journal of Psychiatry 2016;**7**(2):8–11.

14. **Majumdar M, Pereira YD, Fernandes J**. Stress and anxiety in parents of mentally retarded children. Indian Journal of Psychiatry 2005;**47**(3):144–7.

15. **Patka M, Keys CB, Henry DB, McDonald KE**. Attitudes of Pakistani community members and staff toward people with intellectual disability. American Journal on Intellectual and Developmental Disabilities 2013;**118**(1):32–43.

16. **Chandra P, Kar N**. Sexual education in intellectually disabled persons: an exploratory study on challenges and resources. Indian Journal of Social Psychiatry 2014;**30**(3–4):A22.

17. **Soniya AM**. Notions of sexuality: an analysis of the interplays of gender and care among adults with intellectual disabilities in Kerala. Journal of Gender Studies 2022;**31**(3):1–11.

18. **Chavan BS, Ahmad W, Arun P, Mehta S, Nazli, Ratnam V**, et al. Sexuality among adolescents and young adults with intellectual disability: knowledge, attitude, and practices. Journal of Psychosexual Health 2021;**3**(2):140–5.

19. **Murthy RS, Divya B, Nischitha S.** Vision for total care of persons with developmental disabilities. Indian Journal of Social Psychiatry 2021;**37**(4):346.

20. **National Institute for the Empowerment of Persons with Intellectual Disabilities (formerly National Institute for the Mentally Handicapped).** Homepage. n.d. Available from: https://www.niepid.nic.in/index.php

21. **Bano H, Anjum N.** Therapeutic, educational and employment services for children with intellectual disability in Pakistan. New Horizons 2013;**7**(1):51.

22. **Mamun JI.** State of the Persons with Intellectual Disability in Bangladesh.

23. **Dukpa D, Kamenopoulou L.** The conceptualisation of inclusion and disability in Bhutan. In: **Kamenopoulou L**, editor. Inclusive Education and Disability in the Global South. Cham: Palgrave Macmillan; 2018: 53–79.

24. **Adhikari KP.** Realising the rights of persons with disability in Nepal: policy addresses from the health, education and livelihoods perspectives. Nepalese Journal of Development and Rural Studies 2019;**16**:23–34.

25. **The Gazette of the Democratic Socialist Republic of Sri Lanka.** Bill for the Protection of the Rights of Persons with Disabilities (Supplement Part II of 09th August 1996). Sri Lanka: Department of Government Printing; 1996.

26. **Mendis P.** Act for the Protection of the Rights of Persons with Disabilities in Sri Lanka. Asia and Pacific Journal on Disability 1997;**1**(1):6–9.

27. **Das A, Kattumuri R.** Children with disabilities in private inclusive schools in Mumbai: experiences and challenges. Electronic Journal for Inclusive Education 2011;**2**(8):7.

28. **Russell PS, John JK, Lakshmanan JL.** Family intervention for intellectually disabled children: randomised controlled trial. British Journal of Psychiatry 1999;**174**(3):254–8.

29. **Girimaji SC, Srinath S, Seshadri S, Krishna DS.** Family interview for stress and coping in mental retardation (FISC-MR): a tool to study stress and coping in families of children with mental retardation. Indian Journal of Psychiatry 1999;**41**(4):341.

Chapter 22

Intellectual disability services in Australia and New Zealand

Dhara N. Perera and Soman Elangovan

Introduction

In 2018, 4.4 million Australians were documented as having a disability (compared to 4.3 million in 2015), defined by restrictions in ability to perform and participate in everyday activities lasting for up to or at least 6 months. Of these, 1.9 million people with disability were aged 65 years and over (increased from 1.8 million in 2015) (1). Based on 2012 data 668,100 Australians (2.9%) suffered from an intellectual disability (ID) which was a 2.6% increase from 2009 (2).

In 2012, 4% of children aged 0–14 years were identified as having an ID, with children making up the largest proportion of the population with ID. Boys aged 0–14 were twice as likely to have an ID than girls in the same age group (2). Among Aboriginal people and Torres Strait Islander people, in 2015, 23.9% of the 523,200 Aboriginal people and Torres Strait Islander people living in households were reported to be living with a disability (Figs. 22.1 and 22.2). This has remained largely unchanged since 2012 (23.4%). In 2015, the disability rate among non-Indigenous people was 17.5%. Disability prevalence rates for Aboriginal and Torres Strait Islander males and females were similar (3).

Many of these individuals (57%) suffer from a psychiatric disorder (4). Compared with the general population, people with ID experience poorer health, suffer more from common mental disorders, and have higher mortality (5–9).

In Australia, the healthcare system is funded by the Commonwealth and State Governments. A minority of the population is serviced by private specialists and hospital services. These are largely inaccessible to a majority of those with ID having complex needs (10). Furthermore, there are very few consultants, clinicians, or services at a tertiary level that can support those with ID with mental illnesses in the public sector. Although public mental health services are responsible for servicing all mental health conditions, there are no specific inpatient facilities for people with ID. As such, admissions occur to general

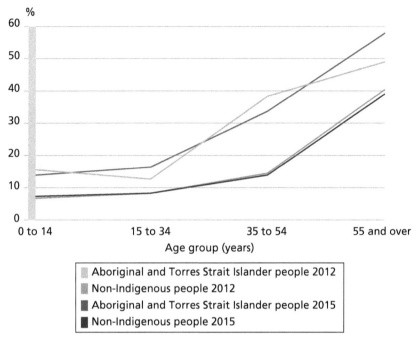

Fig. 22.1 Disability rates among Aboriginal and Torres Strait Islander people and non-Indigenous people.
Source: ABS Survey of Disability, Ageing and Carers: Summary of Findings—2012 and 2015.

mental health facilities where they receive care from staff with limited skills or no experience in working with people with ID (10).

Definitions

ID is a word used to when someone has 'a significantly reduced ability to understand new or complex information and to learn and apply new skills (impaired intelligence)'. This results in a reduced ability to cope independently (impaired social functioning), and begins before adulthood, with a lasting effect on development. Disability is acknowledged as being influenced by not only a person's health conditions or impairments but also environmental factors that could affect their participation in the community.

Similarly, the American Association on Intellectual and Developmental disabilities, formerly known as American Association of Mental Retardation, defines ID as being characterized by significant impairment in both intellectual functioning and in adaptive behaviour affecting everyday social and practical skills in a person under 22 years of age (11).

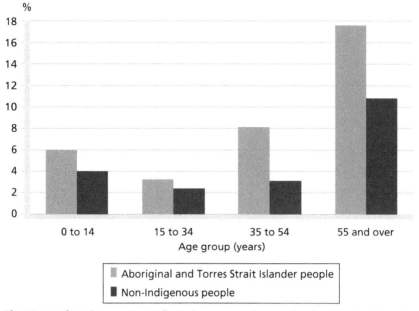

Fig. 22.2 Profound or severe core limitation among Aboriginal and Torres Strait Islander people and non-Indigenous people.
Source: ABS Survey of Disability, Ageing and Carers: Summary of Findings—2015.

In comparison, the Survey of Disability, Ageing and Carers conducted by the Australian Bureau of Statistics (12) defined ID as being characterized by having difficulty learning or understanding things; and or having one or more intellectual impairments. In contrast, a profound disability was defined as occasional or regular need for personal assistance or supervision in domains of self-care, mobility, or communication (4).

Disability services in Australia

There is limited availability and quality of data regarding adults with ID in Australia. It has been demonstrated by Dintino et al. that disability rates are higher in rural and remote areas of Australia (13). Reasons for this include wide variations in operational definitions, measurements, survey approaches, data sources, and geographic locations. There is also considerable variation in the underlying concepts, definitions, and classifications of ID adopted in Australia (14).

Sixty-one per cent of this population experience profound limitation in their activities of daily living and are heavily reliant on the disability support services

(4). In recognition of this demand, the Australian Government introduced the National Disability Insurance Scheme (NDIS) (15–17). The NDIS was legislated in 2013 but only became fully operational in 2020 (18,19). Therefore, the NDIS is currently the primary disability support service in Australia, which underpins the tenets of the United Nations Convention on the Rights of Persons with Disabilities following significant reforms in this sector.

National Disability Insurance Scheme

Background

The purpose of the NDIS is to support those with a significant and permanent disability, who struggle to perform everyday tasks or participate in activities (17,20). The NDIS supports individuals with psychosocial disability and extends support to their families and carers (15,19,21). While the NDIS is the primary organization providing disability support, other support services are also available (15).

This initiative was introduced in July 2013 as a trial and rolled out in July 2016 to sites across Australia, in recognition of the significant deficits in the existing disability services that did not meet the needs of people with disabilities. The NDIS serves to help disabled individuals who are consenting to access services, by linkage with appropriate agencies. This scheme does not provide clients with an allowance, nor does it replace the Disability Support Pension. As such, a client may receive a Disability Support Pension but not be eligible for NDIS or vice versa. The NDIS is expected to serve approximately 460,000 participants (15,16,18,19).

NDIS hierarchy

See Fig. 22.3.

Access and eligibility criteria

Accessing support via the NDIS can be a lengthy and complicated process, and in view of this a website has been created (Reimagine) to facilitate those with mental health conditions to navigate the NDIS (16).

The NDIS is an area-based service with differences in the application process between State and Territory governments. To access services, participants need to be between 7 and 65 years of age, require support to perform everyday tasks, be a citizen or permanent resident of Australia, or hold a Protected Special Category Visa. Children under the age of 7 can access support under the Early Childhood Early Intervention approach which also falls under the NDIS. Those over 65 years of age can gain support via My Aged Care services.

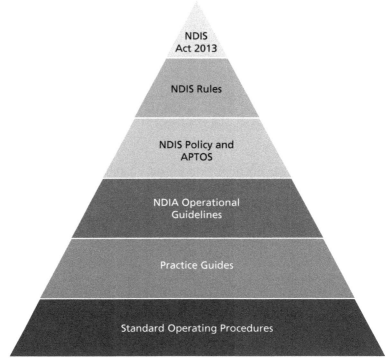

Fig. 22.3 NDIS hierarchy.
Source: www.anao.gov.au/work/performance-audit/decision-making-controls-ndis-particip ant-plans

If eligible to apply, individuals then need to contact their local area coordinator office to check if the NDIS is available in their area. Based on the availability of services locally, an application form for NDIS—an Access Request Form— needs to be submitted by the participant, along with evidence to support that their diagnosis or condition is permanent. This can be provided by their general practitioner, mental health service (psychiatrist), or local area coordinator. In particular, the evidence provided needs to confirm the presence of an enduring severe disability with significant impairment in various psychosocial domains. For example, these domains broadly consist of mobility, communication, social interaction, learning, self-care, and self-management. Depending on the area(s) of disability, the details of those difficulties need to be highlighted under each domain including previous treatments tried for same. Notably, psychiatrists play a key role in providing supporting evidence as part of the assessment process for NDIS, particularly in public mental health services where a greater level of disability secondary to chronic severe mental illness is likely to be observed. The applications for NDIS occur via the National Disability Insurance Agency (NDIA) which is the local agency that processes individual applications. Interestingly, according to the NDIS criteria, a specific diagnosis (including that of an ID) is not required given that the focus is on functional disability and its impact on day-to-day living (16). Once an application is submitted to the local NDIA, they will determine whether an individual is eligible based on the eligibility criteria and provide a response in 21 days (Fig. 22.4).

As part of the assessment there are various tools that can be used including the Health of Nation Outcome Survey (HoNOS), Life Skills Profile (LSP-16 item), and WHO Assessment Schedule.

When an individual is deemed eligible for NDIS support, they are assigned a care coordinator and invited to participate in a planning meeting to create an individualized care plan based on their identified goals and needs. This

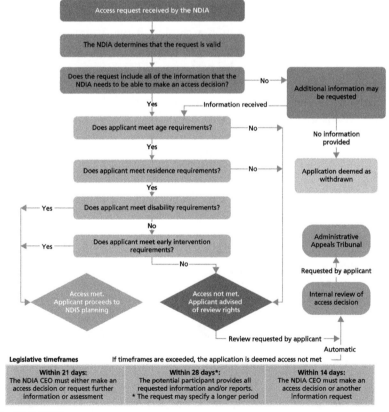

Fig. 22.4 NDIS access.

Source: www.anao.gov.au/work/performance-audit/decision-making-controls-sustainability-ndis

allows each individual a better choice and control over the support they receive. Accordingly, they will be linked in with the relevant support agencies which are funded via NDIS. This allows for support workers assigned to assist the individual with actioning their goals and to offer practical and psychological support as required. After 12 months of initiating the plan, it is reviewed to make any changes based on client needs. The organizations and case workers involved in care provision are via NDIS-funded support agencies (14–16,18).

NDIS for NDIA system
See Fig. 22.5.

School disability support services

Children and young adults with ID experience significant challenges in education, in the context of their disability. Options for these individuals include attending 'special' schools or mainstream schools with 'special' classes that address their specific educational needs. Students with ID experienced significant difficulties with learning, problems with socializing or fitting in, as well as difficulties with communication according to the Australian Institute of Health and Welfare (4). In Australia, children with special needs at school are supported by government-funded programmes. For example, in Victoria it is called the Programme for Students with Disabilities (PSD) (22).

Learning difficulties and fitting in at school were the predominant impairments experienced by 66% and 41%, respectively, among children and young adults. Therefore, a Disability Support Person, special tuition, and a special assessment procedure were introduced (4).

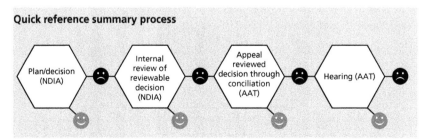

Fig. 22.5 NDIA planning process which involves going through an Administrative Appeal Process.
Source: https://www.disabilityloop.org.au/resources/reviews_appeals_flow_chart.html

Disability services for over 65-year-olds

For people over 65 years of age or Aboriginal people aged over 50, an assessment is required to access Commonwealth Government-funded services for older people. These assessments determine an aged person's eligibility to access services. There are two levels of assessment. The Regional Assessment Services (RAS) performs basic Home Support Assessments via the Commonwealth Home Support Programme (CHSP) (23). If a higher level of care is required, the Aged Care Assessment Services are required to conduct comprehensive assessments. This allows for people to be assessed for eligibility to access higher-level services, including Commonwealth-funded residential aged care, residential respite care, Transition Care Programme, Short Term Restorative Care Programme, Home Care Packages, as well as the CHSP (23).

State-based variations in application and service delivery

In all the states the NDIS works with qualified partner organizations to facilitate care provision to individuals with a disability or developmental delay. The partner organizations enable service delivery through local area care coordination to individuals aged between 7 and 64 years (15).

Victoria

According to the data from the Publication of Disability Support Services 2003–2004, Victoria was reported to have the highest proportion of service users, accounting for 68,238 out of a total 187,806 (36%) (4,21,24). Recent data from Victoria from March 2021 indicated that 122,772 people were receiving NDIS support (25).

From a diagnostic and management perspective, the Victorian Dual Disability Services (VDDS) offer support for people with ID (26). VDDS is a service offered by St Vincent's Hospital and Melbourne Health. VDDS provides assessment and consultation services to staff and consumers of Victorian Area Mental Health Services. The service promotes access to those with a dual disability, for example, people with an ID as well as other comorbidities such as autism spectrum and borderline personality disorders. VDDS serves as a consultation–liaison service by facilitating partnerships and offering collaborative treatment planning (26).

To access services in Victoria, the Victorian Partners in the Community can assist to identify local partner offices in the local government area. The services are wide ranging and include personal care services (24) such as assistance with transportation to appointments, facilitating outings and participation in activities, household cleaning services, occupational therapy, behavioural assessments (to implement behaviour management care plans), physiotherapy, speech therapy, sourcing housing, podiatry services, and psychology services. Other roles played by NDIS case workers may include supervision of medication and liaison with mental healthcare providers as well as carer support.

New South Wales

Data from the Australian Institute of Health Welfare, from March 2021, revealed 144,204 people were receiving support in New South Wales.

In New South Wales, the Council for Intellectual Disability is a not-for-profit organization that serves to support people with ID, their families, and carers through advocacy (27). Furthermore, the New South Wales Agency for Clinical Innovation Intellectual Disability Health Network has created a website with resources entitled 'The Essentials' (28). Following consultation with local and specialty health districts, the Agency for Clinical Innovation serves to improve and enhance service delivery to those with an ID with a view to addressing service delivery at organizational and local levels (28). It also provides resources on issues that matter to people with ID such as NDIS, education, jobs, transport, and linkage with justice advocacy services. It focuses on inclusion services which include 'Easy Read' to facilitate understanding by those with low literacy levels, as well as making information available in different languages. Additionally, it supports people with ID navigate the justice system via linkage with Justice Advocacy Service through the Intellectual Disability Rights Service (29).

Australian Capital Territory

In 2014, Wurth and Brandon highlighted the significant deficit in services for people with an ID in the Australian Capital Territory (30). Since the introduction of NDIS, in the Australian Capital Territory, the Integrated Service Response Programme (ISRP) (31) in conjunction with NDIA, is now able to serve this population. Currently 8503 people benefit from NDIS according to data from March 2021 (32). ISRP serves as a short-term source of support for people with complex needs including provision of funding for people with disabilities to purchase emergency support and services through non-government agencies. Additionally, for children under 16 with significant disability requirements who are unable to live at home due to their disability, funding for accommodation is provided by ISRP. ISRP works with NDIA and liaises with key stakeholders to coordinate services. However, they do not provide ongoing long-term case management, specialist care, or supported accommodation (32). As such, there are gaps or deficits in long-term service provision for those with ID requiring access to those services. These gaps become more evident at the time of reviewing of individual plans.

Western Australia

In Western Australia, Developmental Disability Western Australia supports those with developmental disability, ID, and autism spectrum disorder (33). It serves to offer NDIS independent support coordination which includes making sense of the NDIS application process or plan, family peer support to connect families experiencing challenging behaviour, and individual advocacy. Developmental Disability Western Australia services people of all ages who have a developmental disability and have complex needs.

South Australia

In South Australia, disability services were provided by the Department of Human Services (DHS) before NDIS was established (34). At present, the DHS provides disability support to those with a NDIS plan, or to existing clients via Accommodation Services and Northgate Aged Care, Equipment Programme and Independent Living Centre, and the Continence Resource Centre. Furthermore, a Disability Access and Inclusion Plan 2020–2024 was created to improve accessibility and inclusiveness of these services (34). Other services unique to South Australia, provided via DHS, include a mobile-friendly database to improve access to parking spaces for those with a disability. Furthermore, DHS in South Australia is also in the process of creating a new inclusive app that will display existing and future services and facilities for people with a disability.

Tasmania

Service provision in Tasmania is based on division into metropolitan and regional local area coordinators and regional early childhood partners. Based on the regional division, South East and North West Tasmania are serviced by Mission Australia, and North and South West Tasmania are serviced by Baptcare. Support coordination for NDIS participants is provided by a registered NDIS provider, Human Resources Plus, through which individuals with disabilities are supported to maximize their NDIS benefits, supported to build capacity to self-manage, encouraged to explore vocational opportunities, celebrate milestones, and apply for community and government grants to improve community participation (35). Another service provider for NDIS participants is OnTrack who provide support with getting into housing, joining fun community groups, and gaining access to employment (36).

Queensland

In Queensland, the services are provided by Queensland Health, Mental Health Services, and Disability Support Queensland which is an online community resource for people with disabilities, families, friends, and carers. However, the NDIS provides maximum support for intellectually disabled clients. The Queensland Centre for Intellectual and Developmental Disability, as part of the University of Queensland, provides additional services in relation to assessment and treatment and other support services (37). Non-governmental organizations and the private sector service providers also play a major role in providing support to NDIS stakeholders. The Disability Information and Awareness Line (DIAL) is a free, state-wide information, resource and referral service maintained and operated by Disability Services Queensland (38). Information available through DIAL addresses all disabilities and includes information about services for people with a disability for anyone wanting to know about supports and services for people with a disability in Queensland.

Alternative options

If individuals with reduced psychosocial functioning, such as those with ID, are unable to access psychosocial support via the NDIS, or deemed ineligible for NDIS, they can access services via government-funded Primary Health Networks. A 4-year funding initiative was made by the Australian Government which commenced in January 2019 (19). The support services are the National Psychosocial Support Measure, Psychosocial Transition Support, and Continuity of Supports programmes. All these services have certain criteria such as applicability based on access to previously available services. Fundamentally, these services include one-on-one support at times of increased need, and group activities that build capacity and life skills. These services aim to promote social connectedness and well-being (39).

Special populations

Based on data from the Australian Bureau Statistics 2015 (12), rural and remote areas are reported to have a greater rate of disability with 23.1% reporting a disability compared to 16.4% in major cities (40). There is a lack of access to allied health services in rural and remote areas, where the introduction of NDIS had failed to adequately deliver (40). In New South Wales, there are significant challenges faced by rural and remote clinicians in providing care to people with a disability as there appears to be inconsistent and inadequate funding via NDIS. Additionally, there are complexities around accessing NDIS services via local area coordinators. There is a lack of data pertaining to Aboriginal people and Torres Strait Islander people in terms of accessibility to disability services. A strong criticism of the NDIS is that the inadequate support for existing service providers in these areas is likely to adversely affect the recruitment and retention of new therapists to work in these regions. Additionally, there is a risk of physical and emotional exhaustion of existing therapists (40).

Barriers to accessing services

There are several barriers to accessing services and in providing effective care. These include the complicated application process for the NDIS, the challenges of navigating the websites, gathering evidence, and, at times, lengthy waiting periods for processing of applications to occur. The challenges associated with accessing services form the primary barrier relating to the inclusion and exclusion criteria mentioned above. There is no uniform system across different states either. Additionally, the referral processes are multipronged, with clients being referred for NDIS via their general practitioner or psychiatrist through the public or private sector (41).

Currently, there is no formal training required for NDIS support workers and how this may impact care provision for this vulnerable population also needs due consideration. This lack of training is also reflected in the current Royal Australian and New Zealand College of Psychiatrists training programme which does not offer specialist training in ID. Thus, there is a lack of subspecialist psychiatrists trained in this field to support people with ID (42).

In summary, the Australian disability system is provided by the NDIS which is a complex system to navigate to gain access to services. Gaining access requires multiple layers which can be challenging for people with disability and for their carers. The process remains difficult to understand even for healthcare professionals.

New Zealand or Aotearoa (in Maori)

Overview

In a population of 5 million, in 2017, there were 96,800 people with ID (2% of the population) (43). Five per cent of children aged 0–14, 3% of adults aged 15–44 years, and 1% of people aged 45 years and over suffered from an ID (44). It was noted that a higher proportion of males lived with ID. Notably, Māori and Pacific people had higher rates of disability after adjusting for differences in ethnic population groups. Furthermore, the ethnicity of the person with ID is a factor which may influence their experience of health services, as is seen in the wider population of New Zealand (44). Seventy-four per cent of the population identify as being of European descent and 14.9% of Maori descent, who are the Indigenous people of New Zealand. The other groups are comprised of 11.8% Asian and 7.4% Pacific ethnic origin. The percentage of ID in the various ethnic groups is unknown. People with ID were more likely to live in the most socioeconomically deprived areas of New Zealand, had poorer health, were 2.5 times more likely to have health problems, and had a lower life expectancy (43–46). In New Zealand, males with an ID had a lower life expectancy of 59.7 years compared to 78.4 years in all males. The life expectancy in females with an ID was 59.5 years compared to 82.4 years in all females.

Services available in New Zealand

Services for people with ID are provided via the Ministry of Health disability support services (45,46). In addition to disability support services, screening tools that assess a person's physical health status and health documentation indicating a person's conditions are made available to facilitate tailored care provision.

For example, Intellectual Disability Empowerment in Action (IDEA) Services (46), has developed its own health assessment tool, based on the Cardiff Health Assessment, developed in the UK. IDEA Services strongly encourage annual health screening which facilitates early detection of health issues in these individuals who may not be able to report these conditions themselves. This screening tool includes syndrome-specific screening as well as completion of a health checklist with the person with an ID along with their family or support worker (46).

Another screening tool is the Comprehensive Health Assessment Programme (CHAP) (46) which has enabled improved, thorough assessments for those with ID to establish their physical health status based on investigations they have undergone. This helps to gain insight into their day-to-day difficulties, facilitating tailored care for these people (46).

Additionally, a support document called the Health Passport containing essential disability support information was created in response to concerns expressed by families about the lack of understanding of health professionals of client difficulties (46). This document serves to inform health professionals of a person's wishes during consultations. Unique to this record is that it is owned by the patient and is always kept with them. This initiative is led by New Zealand's Health and Disability Commissioner and is based on a similar passport developed in the UK, modified to suit the New Zealand standards and practices. The Health Passport is now established at Waitemata and Waikato. Furthermore, it is also being implemented in hospitals throughout New Zealand, including Northland, Auckland, Whanganui, and South Canterbury (46).

Another initiative of the Ministry of Health is 'Explore', which is a service that provides specialist behaviour support for people with disabilities of all ages

(46), their families/whānau, and their support networks. They provide in-home care by working with people with an ID in their homes until their services are no longer required (46). Explore facilitates provision of holistic care to the person and their support network through a multidisciplinary team which includes services such as speech and language therapists, specialist nurses, occupational therapists, behaviour support specialists, and psychologists. This team offers support with health issues that commonly affect those with ID such as swallowing and feeding problems, and epilepsy. Additionally, there is a focus on supporting healthy nutrition, increased activity, and participation at home and in the community. Following referral and completion of a core assessment, an individual plan is developed based on all identified concerns and agreed goals. A lead specialist worker is assigned to each client to help coordinate the support provided in a minimally intrusive manner. The Explore specialist workers ensure ongoing support, monitoring, and review of the goals in the individual plan in collaboration with the client, their family and whānau, and their support team.

Through the core assessment, certain patterns and causes of behaviour are identified to better support clients by tailoring services to the individual needs. A specialist nurse serves to provide key liaison between people with ID, their families, support workers, and the hospital's nurses, clinicians, and other staff. This would include assessing the needs of people in hospital with ID and liaising with the staff about treatment plans for them. Sharing this knowledge with hospital staff, including nurses, clinicians, and registrars, helps to provide better care to this special population along with their health passport which allows the essential information about their care to be recorded or identified. It also becomes part of their documentation in hospital that a specific care plan is in place for them. The nurse specialist also assists with preparation for surgery and home visits, as well as ensuring that clear communication is maintained. There are several training programmes that are also facilitated including 'Voice Thru Your Hands' which teaches clinicians who treat patients with ID.

Additionally, a programme known as 'The Healthy Athletes' serves to monitor the health of Special Olympics participants through a series of screenings, called Fit Feet (podiatry check), Healthy Hearing (audiology checks), MedFest (sports physical exam), Opening Eyes (vision), FUNfitness (physical therapy), Health Promotion (better health and well-being), and Special Smiles (dentistry). The support workers who carry out these screenings are volunteer nurses, doctors, and dieticians, and this programme provides them with an opportunity to develop their skills in providing care for people with ID. Prior to the events they receive a 3-hour educational training session (46).

Concluding remarks

ID has been noted to be higher in Maori and Pacific populations as compared to the non-Indigenous people in New Zealand with the disability services being primarily governed by the Ministry of Health and Health and Disability Commissioner. These services seem to be quite comprehensive, recognizing the importance of tailoring services to cater for the individual needs through use of screening tools, Health Passports, and support workers through various support organizations. It takes into consideration information essential for the person with ID, their family, and healthcare professionals.

Services for people with intellectual disability in Australia and New Zealand services: views of the authors

Having reviewed the services available in Australia and New Zealand, there are notable differences as well as similarities. While both provide myriad services, designed to cater to the needs of individuals with ID and their carers, the pathway to gaining access to services in Australia appears to be quite complicated and difficult to navigate. Comparatively, the services made available in New Zealand are seemingly more streamlined and easier to access without the requirement of complex application processes. Improving access to services is important to enhance the well-being of these generally underserved people who require additional support to be able to participate in the community and be able to contribute to society. It may be useful to consider revising the Australian disability services to streamline services across the states and implement a uniform system to facilitate navigating this complex and multilayered disability support service to make it more accessible and thus meaningful. Furthermore, providing skills training for those working in disability services is important in terms of improving understanding of manifestations of ID for support workers to provide effective care. Healthcare professionals would also benefit from having training and education in the field of ID, which should be included as part of the Royal Australian and New Zealand College of Psychiatrists training programme for psychiatrists. This would allow for ID specialists to be able to provide meaningful specialist care for this population.

References

1. **Australian Bureau of Statistics**. Disability, Ageing and Carers, Australia: Summary of Findings. Canberra: Australian Bureau of Statistics, Australia; 2018. Available from: https://www.abs.gov.au/statistics/health/disability/disability-ageing-and-carers-australia-summary-findings/latest-release#key-statistics
2. **Australian Bureau of Statistics**. Intellectual Disability, Australia, 2012. Catalogue no. 4433.0.55.003. Australian Bureau of Statistics; 2012. Available from: https://www.abs.gov.au/ausstats/abs@.nsf/Lookup/4433.0.55.003main+features102012

3. **Australian Bureau of Statistics**. Disability, Ageing and Carers, Australia: Summary of Findings. Catalogue no. 4430.0. Australian Bureau of Statistics; 2015. Available from: https://www.abs.gov.au/AUSSTATS/abs@.nsf/Lookup/4430.0Main+Feature s802015?

4. **Australian Institute of Health and Welfare**. Disability in Australia: Intellectual Disability. Cat. no. AUS 110. Canberra: **Australian Institute of Health and Welfare**; 2008.

5. **Bittles AH, Petterson, BA Sullivan, SG, Hussain R, Glasson EJ, Montgomery PD.** The influence of intellectual disability on life expectancy. Journal of Gerontology: Series A, Biological Sciences and Medical Sciences 2002;**57A**(7):M470–2.

6. **Einfeld SL, Ellis LA, Emerson E.** Comorbidity of intellectual disability and mental disorder in children and adolescents: a systematic review. Journal of Intellectual & Developmental Disability 2011;**36**(2):137–43.

7. **Smiley E, Cooper SA, Finlayson J, Jackson A, Allan L, Mantry D,** et al. Incidence and predictors of mental ill-health in adults with intellectual disabilities: prospective study. British Journal of Psychiatry 2007;**191**:313–19.

8. **Trollor, JN.** It's time to address the mental health needs of people with intellectual disability. Australasian Psychiatry 2018;**26**(6):575–7.

9. **Davies K, Eagelson C, Weise J, Cvejic RC, Trollor JN.** Clinical capacity of Australian and New Zealand psychiatrists who work with people with intellectual and developmental disabilities. Australasian Psychiatry 2019;**27**(5):506–12.

10. **Evans, E, Howlett, S, Kremser T, Simpson J, Kayess R, Trollor J,** et al. Service development for intellectual disability mental health: a human rights approach. Journal of Intellectual Disability Research 2012;**56**(11):1098–109.

11. American Association on Intellectual and Developmental Disabilities (AAIDD). Homepage. n.d. Available from: https://www.aaidd.org/intellectual-disability

12. **Australian Bureau of Statistics**. Disability, Ageing and Carers, Australia: Summary of Findings. Canberra: Australian Bureau of Statistics; 2015.

13. **Dintino R, Wakely L, Wolfgang R, Wakely KM, Little A.** Powerless facing the wave of change: the lived experience of providing services in rural areas under the National Disability Insurance Scheme. Rural and Remote Health 2019;**19**:5337.

14. **Australian Health Ministers Advisory Council.** Evaluation of the National Mental Health Strategy, Final Report. Canberra: Health Services Division, Commonwealth Department of Health and Aged Care; 1997.

15. **National Disability Insurance Scheme.** Government announces improved NDIS mental health support. 2018. Available from: https://www.ndis.gov.au/news/400-gov ernment-announces-improved-ndis-mental-health-support

16. **National Disability Insurance Agency.** Accessing the NDIS: A guide for mental health professionals. 2017. Available from: https://www.ndis.gov.au/media/121/download

17. **Williams TM, Smith GP.** Can the National Disability Insurance Scheme work for mental health? Australian & New Zealand Journal of Psychiatry 2014;**48**(5):391–4.

18. **Buckmaster L, Clark S.** The National Disability Insurance Scheme: a chronology. Research paper series, 2018–19. Parliament of Australia; 2018. Available from: https:// parlinfo.aph.gov.au/parlInfo/download/library/prspub/6083264/upload_binary/6083 264.pdf

19. **Royal Australian College of Psychiatrists**. Section of Psychiatry of Intellectual and Developmental Disabilities. n.d. Available from: https://www.ranzcp.org/membership/faculties-sections-and-networks/intellectual-developmental-disabilities

20. **Troller J.** Making mental health services accessible to people with an intellectual disability. Australian & New Zealand Journal of Psychiatry 2014;**48**(5):395–8.

21. **Hayes L, Brophy L, Harvey C, Tellez JJ, Herrman H, Killackey E.** Enabling choice, recovery and participation: evidence-based early intervention support for psychosocial disability in the National Disability Insurance Scheme. Australasian Psychiatry 2018;**26**(6):578–85.

22. **Department of Education**. Program for Students with Disabilities (PSD) supports. Victoria State Government; n.d. Available from: https://www.education.vic.gov.au/school/teachers/learningneeds/Pages/psdhandbook.aspx

23. **Commonwealth Home Support Programme** (CHSP). My Aged Care assessment services. n.d. Available from: https://www.health.vic.gov.au/ageing-and-aged-care/my-aged-care-assessment-services

24. **Australian Institute of Health and Welfare**. Disability support services 2003–04. National data on services provided under the Commonwealth State/Territory Disability Agreement. 2005. Available from: https://www.aihw.gov.au/reports/disability-services/disability-support-services-2003-04/contents/table-of-contents

25. **National Disability Insurance Scheme.** Disability services and support Victoria. n.d. Available from: https://www.vic.gov.au/ndis-disability-services-and-support-victoria

26. **Victorian Dual Disability Service.** St. Vincent's Hospital. n.d. Available from: https://www.svhm.org.au/our-services/departments-and-services/v/victorian-dual-disability-service

27. **Council for Intellectual Disability**. Homepage. n.d. Available from: https://cid.org.au

28. **New South Wales Agency for Clinical Innovation.** The essentials. n.d. Available from: https://aci.health.nsw.gov.au/networks/intellectual-disability

29. **New South Wales Justice Advocacy Service**. Homepage. n.d. Available from: https://idrs.org.au/jas/

30. **Wurth P, Brandon S-A.** The ACT mental health service for people with intellectual disability, 10 years on. Australasian Psychiatry 2014;**22**(1):52–5.

31. **Integrated service response program**. ACT community services. n.d. Available from: https://www.communityservices.act.gov.au/disability_act/integrated-service-response-program

32. **National Disability Insurance Scheme.** Australian Capital Territory. n.d. Available from: https://www.ndis.gov.au/understanding/ndis-each-state/australian-capital-territory

33. **Developmental Disability Western Australia** (DDWA). Homepage. n.d. Available from: https://ddwa.org.au/

34. **Department of Human Services**. Homepage. n.d. Available from: https://dhs.sa.gov.au/services/disability

35. **HR+**. Homepage. n.d. Available from: https://ds.hrplustas.com.au/about-hr-plus

36. **OnTrack Tasmania**. Homepage. n.d. Available from: https://ontracktasmania.com.au

37. The Queensland Centre for Intellectual and Developmental Disability (QCIDD). Homepage. n.d. Available from: https://qcidd.centre.uq.edu.au

38. **Disability Information and Awareness Line (DIAL).** A free, state-wide information, resource and referral service maintained and operated by Disability Services Queensland. n.d. Available from: http://www.disability.qld.gov.au/dial.cfm

39. **Australian Department of Health.** Psychosocial support for people with severe mental illness. 2019. Available from: https://www.health.gov.au/internet/main/publishing.nsf/Content/psychosocial-support-mental-illness

40. **Keane S, Lincoln M, Rolfe M, Smith T.** Retention of the rural allied health workforce in New South Wales: a comparison of public and private practitioners. BMC Health Services Research 2013;**13**(1):32.

41. **Doherty AJ, Atherton H, Boland, P, Hastings R, Hives L, Hood K,** et al. Barriers and facilitators to primary health care for people with intellectual disabilities and/or autism: an integrative review. BJGP Open 2020;**4**(3):1–10.

42. **Hill H.** Is it time to include people with intellectual disabilities in Royal Australian and New Zealand College of Psychiatrists' treatment guidelines? Australasian Psychiatry 2019;**27**(5):519–21.

43. **In Your Community.** Valuing All and leaving no one behind. 2017. Available from: https://ihc.org.nz/sites/default/files/documents/Valuing%20All%20Leave%20no%20one%20behind%20-%20Report.pdf

44. **McCarthy J, Duff M.** Services for adults with intellectual disability in Aotearoa New Zealand. BJPsych International 2019;**16**(3):71–3.

45. **Ministry of Health.** Health Indicators for New Zealanders with Intellectual Disability. Wellington: Ministry of Health; 2011. Available from: https://www.health.govt.nz/publication/health-indicators-new-zealanders-intellectual-disability

46. **Ministry of Health.** Providing Health Services for People with Intellectual Disability: Case Studies of Programmes and Tools Used in New Zealand. Wellington: Ministry of Health. 2013. Available from: https://www.health.govt.nz/publication/providing-health-services-people-intellectual-disability-new-zealand-literature-review-and-case

47. **Ministry of Health.** Innovative Methods of Providing Health Services for People with Intellectual Disability: A Review of the Literature. Wellington: Ministry of Health. 2013. Available from: https://www.health.govt.nz/publication/providing-health-services-people-intellectual-disability-new-zealand-literature-review-and-case

Index

For the benefit of digital users, indexed terms that span two pages (e.g., 52–53) may, on occasion, appear on only one of those pages.

Tables and boxes are indicated by *t* and *b* following the page number